DIALOGUES WITH
FORGOTTEN VOICES

DIALOGUES WITH FORGOTTEN VOICES

*Relational Perspectives on
Child Abuse Trauma and
Treatment of Dissociative Disorders*

HARVEY L. SCHWARTZ, PH.D.

BASIC
BOOKS

A Member of the Perseus Books Group

Published by Basic Books,
A Member of the Perseus Books Group

Library of Congress Cataloging-in-Publication Data
Schwartz, Harvey L., 1955–
   Dialogues with forgotten voices : relational perspectives on child abuse trauma and
treatment of dissociative disorders / Harvey L. Schwartz.
      p.   cm.
   Includes bibliographical references and index.
   ISBN 0-465-09573-9
   1. Adult child abuse victims—Rehabilitation.   2. Adult child abuse victims—Mental
health.   3. Sexual abuse victims—Mental health. 4. Dissociative disorders—Treatment.
I. Title.

RC569.5.C55 S395   2000
616.85'82239—dc21

                                                                                    00-058557

00 01 02 03 / 10 9 8 7 6 5 4 3 2 1

I gratefully dedicate this book to my patients and to my colleagues:

to my patients, who have courageously sought wholeness and
healing against great odds, and who have been
my most challenging and important teachers;

to my colleagues treating trauma and dissociation,
who have continued to find ways of reaching profoundly
violated human beings in a time of increasing
professional and cultural adversity.

It is often said that in today's modern and postmodern world, the forces of darkness are upon us. But I think not; in the Dark and the Deep there are truths that can always heal. It is not the forces of darkness but of shallowness that everywhere threaten the true, and the good, and the beautiful, and that ironically announce themselves as deep and profound. It is an exuberant and fearless shallowness that everywhere is the modern danger, the modern threat, and that everywhere nonetheless calls to us as Savior. We might have lost the Light and the Height; but more frightening, we have lost the Mystery and the Deep, the Emptiness and the Abyss, and lost it in a world dedicated to surfaces and shadows, exteriors and shells, whose prophets lovingly exhort us to dive into the shallow end of the pool head first.

—Ken Wilber

Contents

PART III
SURVIVAL, TRANSFORMATION, AND TRANSCENDENCE

Acknowledgments

All books are written within the context of a community of discourse, and this one is no exception.

My reflections on clinical work have been continuously nourished and revitalized by my interactions with my patients, who never cease to surprise me, change me, and inspire me.

My ideas about trauma, dissociative experience, and clinical process have also evolved through dialogues with colleagues and consultees over the years in a variety of settings. Witnessing the perseverance, dedication, and courage of many of my colleagues who continue to offer state-of-the-art treatment to severely traumatized patients in the era of managed care, the "false memory" backlash, the remedicalization of psychiatry and psychology, and a waning cultural investment in healing and reparation processes has been a truly moving experience. This book evolved through many of our individual and group consultation sessions and is in large part dedicated to supporting and recognizing your efforts.

There are many who have read chapters or sections of this book or who have offered ideas or constructive critiques or who have offered support and encouragement of one kind or another. Along these lines I would like to thank:

Suzan Harvey, Jay Rosenblatt, Cal Gough, Mary Ciofalo, Melissa Farley, Bobbie Schear, Suzanne Chassay, Leah Lazar, Joan Hertzberg, Susan Sands, Catharine MacKinnon, Sherry Brown, Robert Wilk, Marleen Norman, Patti McWilliams, June Madsen-Clausen, Karen Peoples, Randall Alifano, Martha Monetti, Jordana Schwartz, Marcia Rosenberg, Bobby Weinstock, Jim Reed, Elizabeth Pelzner, Rita Cristman, Roy Bonney, Nora Chen, Min Chen, Alicia Rause, Anne Uemura, Linda Burge, and special thanks to Lew Aron and Jeffrey Moulton-Benevedes for their extensive reading of, and valuable feedback on, an earlier version of this book. I would also especially like to thank

Cal Gough for his intensive editorial work, sound advice, and the enormous time and energy he devoted to bringing several earlier versions of this book into fruition. My heartfelt appreciation to Jay Rosenblatt and Suzan Harvey who kept believing in my creative abilities, helping me find my own voice when I could not do this for myself, and who have continued to offer love, friendship, and grounding.

My own thinking and professional and intellectual development have been inspired and influenced by the work and the writing of psychoanalysts, traumatologists, dissociation theorists, and other teachers:

Lew Aron, Jessica Benjamin, Christopher Bollas, John Briere, Philip Bromberg, Elias Canetti, Pema Chodron, Noam Chomsky, Christine Courtois, Jody Davies, Lloyd DeMause, Andrea Dworkin, Darlene Ehrenberg, Michael Eigen, Frantz Fanon, Sandor Ferenczi, Mary G. Frawley-O'Dea, Emmanuel Ghent, Emma Goldman, Judith Herman, bell hooks, Carl Jung, Richard Kluft , R. D. Laing, Lawrence Langer, C. S. Lewis, Robert Jay Lifton, Deborah Lipstadt, Catharine MacKinnon, Karen Maroda, Alice Miller, Stephen Mitchell, Adam Phillips, Frank Putnam, Wilhelm Reich, Colin Ross, Anna Salter, Gershom Sholem, Malidoma Some, Charles Spezzano, Rudolf Steiner, Robert Stolorow, Harry S. Sullivan, Bessel Van der Kolk, Cornel West, Elie Wiesel, D. W. Winnicott, and Howard Zinn.

Finally, I want to acknowledge my appreciation to my editor, Cindy Hyden, at Basic Books for her immediate and forthright response to my work, for her extensive editorial assistance, great sense of humor, and her unwavering belief in a new, unknown, relatively unaffiliated author. More than any other contributor, Cindy's gifts with words, concepts, and rhythms brought this book into fruition in the best of possible forms. My gratitude also to Basic Books—and its editorial staff, including Joan Miller, Jessica Callaway, Felicity Tucker, and Norman MacAfee—for their willingness to take on this difficult, controversial, and often misunderstood clinical subject area and their willingness to take a chance on a new and unknown writer.

Introduction

This breach of a child's body does count. It does register. The boundary of the body itself is broken by force and intimidation, a chaotic but choreographed violence. The child is used intentionally and reduced to less than human by the predator's intelligence as well as his behavior. The commitment of the child molester is absolute, and both his insistence and his victory communicate to the child his experience of her—a breachable, breakable thing any stranger can wipe his dick on. When it is family, of course, the invasion is more terrible, more intimate, escape more unlikely.

—Andrea Dworkin

Child abuse is our most powerful and successful ritual, according to psychohistorian Lloyd DeMause (1998). Some of the most egregious crimes against humanity involve the sexual abuse, abandonment, and torture of children in isolated families or in organized perpetrator groups. The fractured psyches and easily misrecognized voices and behaviors of many of the world's traumatized individuals are still not being heard or completely understood. And, while society debates, the belief systems of child-abuse perpetrators continue to pervade the minds of victims decades after the abuse has ended. As a result, far too many people live in the trap of a marginalizing psychological system of horror and terror characterized by unforgiveness, self-hatred, and dislocated accountability and responsibility. Because of their confusing symptoms and behaviors, many severely traumatized individuals are thwarted (or limited) for reasons they cannot understand when they seek to elicit help from various mental health, social services, and medical professionals, and these people remain ambivalently treated within a culture that benefits from their marginalization—primarily through a peculiar combination of fear, fascination, and incredulity.

Humility and open-mindedness are essentials in our collaborative under-standing of the impact and spiraling consequences of chronic childhood trauma, including its persistent denial and frequently camouflaged effects. Successful treatment of individuals who are severely dissociative trauma survivors requires a compassionate witness sufficiently informed about the forms and transformations of trauma—and his/her own responses to them—to navigate the perils endemic to the traumatic transference/countertransference matrix so that mutuality, self-respect, and compassion may replace the tyranny of isolation and self-hatred. The severely dissociative patient's re-ownership of his/her mind, body, and spirit by means of a regenerated and reclaimed voice is the only hope. Without a therapist who is both willing to struggle with the internalized perpetrator ideologies and malignant attachments, and able to engender in the patient a deeply felt level of valuation and validity, there can be no revelation or reparation.

Contemporary relational movements within psychoanalysis have begun to respond to the clinical and sociopolitical challenges involved in recognizing and treating severely traumatized children and adults; the inclusion of feminist perspectives and the maturing response to trauma and dissociative phenomena have led to refined psychoanalytic conceptualizations of the self under siege. The integration has yielded new and creative visions of the essential reciprocities that make for mutative therapeutic interaction and in turn produce significant change in the lives of severely traumatized patients.

Accordingly, I propose a synthesis of contemporary psychodynamic views on trauma and dissociation with the traditional literature on traumatic stress and dissociative disorders. Advances in the treatment of trauma and dissociation from the contemporary psychoanalytic perspective can offer new and valuable insights into the nuances and complexities of transference/countertransference patterns with patients who are survivors of the extremes of human malevolence and depravity. Likewise, the realities addressed by the traditional trauma and dissociative disorders field can eclipse the ambiguities of psychoanalytic discourse—the traumatic fragmentation process, the alterations and concretizations in personality, and the autonomous capacities of dissociative states of mind that flourish when an individual is raised in a chronically perverse developmental context.

But instead of engaging in respectful and mutually informing dialogues, a cacophony of traumatologists, psychoanalysts, lawyers, social theorists, behavioral pharmacologists, systems-theory and cognitive-behavioral practitioners, and others has perpetuated schisms easily exploited by critics who wish to discredit psychotherapy and the emerging trauma paradigms. When the professions dedicated to treating dissociative disorders are themselves composed of mutually exclusive dissociated fragments—each encapsulated in its own worldview with little recognition for the other—both the training of clinicians and the effective treatment of trauma survivors are subverted.

The primary focus of this book is articulating the dynamics of—and philosophy for conducting psychotherapy with— patients at the extreme end of the dissociative continuum, many of whom can be diagnosed with dissociative identity disorder (DID) or multiple personality disorder (MPD), atypical dissociative disorder, chronic posttraumatic stress disorder (PTSD), complex posttraumatic stress disorder, and/or dissociative disorder not otherwise specified (DDNOS). Interpersonal trauma is enacted in a social and relational context; it follows that recovery and healing are best addressed in a socially conscious therapeutic relationship, where interaction based on mutuality is internalized and where the psychology of domination is systematically dismantled. Throughout the book I emphasize the essential and reciprocal relationships between intrapsychic, interpersonal, and cultural healing practices—and their obstruction.

With respect for the dialectical interplay of psyche, culture, and trauma, I argue for an unstinting look at child-abuse trauma and neglect—its variations, its components, its effects, its most extreme manifestations, its cultural embeddedness—toward recognizing its role in driving and creating severe dissociative disorders. Dissociative reactions may be intrinsic psychological responses to trauma or psychic overload. They are not maintained, however, without the negative potentiating factors of social facilitation via denial and disavowal of violence against children along with the failures of diagnosis, recognition, and inadequate application of reparation processes.

Thus, trauma-driven dissociative disorders are cultivated and sustained at least as much by the lack of interpersonal and cultural recognition and reparation processes for child victims and adult survivors as they are by the intrapsychic coping strategies and attachment needs of victims. From this perspective, we must also acknowledge that the social structures that permit the massive abuse of children to take place virtually unimpeded also perpetuate the core cultural dynamics of exploitation, dehumanization-objectification, sacrifice, lethal competition, misogyny and the eroticization of women's subjugation, and the valorizing of domination and collusion as modes of human relatedness.

If we agree that dissociative symptoms and dissociative disorders are almost always ultimately traceable to conditions of misuse of power in interpersonal domination, collusion, and neglect along with their intrapsychic elaborations, then analysis of pathological dissociation and analysis of pathological social relations must go hand in hand. By appreciating the embeddedness of dissociative disorders in cultural contexts of violence and prevailing oppressive power dynamics, we do not necessarily lose or obscure the psyche—its fantasies and organizing principles. However, we do potentially avoid reobjectifying and revictimizing the trauma survivor and subverting his/her messages, protest responses, and unusual pleas for recognition. In this connection, among others, psychotherapy and all of the allied mental health professions have a real mandate to challenge rather than reinforce conventional social arrangements and to reenvision social justice.

POLES OF THE CONTROVERSY

Severe dissociative disorders have landed in the heart of a psychological and cultural civil war. For some people, the problem isn't an epidemic of child abuse; the real problem is "false" memories, concretization of inchoate psychic states, transference psychoses, incompetent or overzealous clinicians, or coercive social influence. People are overstimulated and underinformed where severe trauma survivors are concerned and find it simpler to ignore child-abuse trauma altogether or jump on one of the readily available bandwagons of doubt, skepticism, and incredulity; meanwhile, in an era of escalating Holocaust denial, scholars and academics ponder the questions of whether we can ever know what really happened to anyone.

It has become increasingly difficult and intimidating to diagnose, treat, and report or even investigate cases of severe traumatization and dissociation. The existence of extreme dissociative disorders challenges our basic concepts of what it means to be a human being. Once accepted into one's worldview, the extremes of dissociative adaptation seen in many chronic trauma survivors open up deeply unsettling questions about human nature—the malleability of human identity, the astounding permutations of denial, collusion, and complicity, the workings and personifications of the unconscious mind, the existence of bizarre and sadistic forms of individually and group-directed child abuse, the power of implicit and explicit forms of thought reform and mind control, and the extent of organized crimes exploiting young children as well as teenage and adult dissociative sexual-abuse survivors.

Unfortunately, those who seek to minimize the role of trauma are encouraged by a cultural backlash predominantly orchestrated by the False Memory Syndrome Foundation (FMSF) and its media and professional advocates who, for a variety of personal, professional, economic, and political reasons, marginalize discussion of the effects and extent of child abuse in the culture and in psychopathology and tend to overplay the role of the intrapsychic and social influences or clinician malfeasance in "producing" severe dissociative disorders. Some others, motivated by more theoretical and clinical concerns, also de-emphasize the centrality of trauma in order to move our field beyond simplistic archeological and reconstructive models of psychotherapy and personality, to avoid concretization of psychic material, and to conceptualize the individual as always an active agent in his/her own life and not as just a passive victim of social and intrapsychic forces. For therapist and traumatized patient alike, navigating the intrapsychic and cultural torrents to steer a safe passage between recognizing and validating one's victimization on the one hand and transcending it on the other can be a tricky business.

Insisting on a central role for exogenous trauma in the etiology of severe dissociative disorders is not to preempt or exclude from the developmental picture the important roles of intrapsychic conflict, psychosexual development, psychological deficit, fantasy, and external shaping influences. After all, what is traumatic about trauma is both real and symbolic, both intrapsychic and relational—the events themselves, the meanings and fantasy elaborations of those events, and the interpersonal and cultural responses to those events. And none of that is to deny the existence of a minority of cases of malingering, factitious, or iatrogenic versions of dissociative disorders.

LIMITS OF NEUTRALITY

Psychotherapy is necessarily a moral discourse in which ethical commitments are always enacted and validated either covertly or overtly. Therapy and psychological theory cannot be neutral, objective, or divorced from cultural imperatives. Maintaining an appreciation for perspectivism, paradox, postmodernism, intersubjectivity, and dialectical process does not necessarily mean that one does not take a stand or hold a moral position. It does mean, however, that one's relationship to one's positions and values is porous enough to revisioning and that one is sufficiently open to scrutiny and interaction to balance the need for validation with the value of healthy, respectful conflict and dialogue. At times, for example in the face of character assassination, spurious generalizations, myopic fanaticism, extreme anti-therapy rhetoric, professional and/or forensic opportunism, and radical forms of (motivated) skepticism that seek only to negate the veracity of both child and adult survivors' memory and testimony or the value of depth psychotherapy, this ideal of paradox or dialectical awareness might mean there simply cannot be real negotiation and dialogue. A transitional space of interaction and cooperation is not possible and the term "debate," which presumes a sane, respectful, and redemptive process, becomes a euphemism for ideological trench warfare and public relations hype.

The theoretical convictions, allegiances, and approaches of most social scientists including myself are doubtless related as much to personality and life experience (characterological patterns, trauma history, values, politics, ideology, social positioning) as they are to "objective" facts or truths. As a consequence, differences between advocates of opposing viewpoints will not generally respond to logic or reasoned argument. "For that very reason, they need to be discussed as problems of subjectivity and unconscious reasoning—not as issues of local politics" (Spence, 1993, p. 5). Paradoxically we need to include, within our "objective" discourse, an awareness of the "illusion of objective discourse" (O'Hara and Anderson, 1995, p. 174), which has been created by various disciplines and professions expressly to lend credibility and authority to those who are continually fighting for legitimacy. All discourse in the fields of child abuse, traumatic memory, and dissociation should be held with these thoughts in mind.

Leowald (1960) conceptualized neutrality as a love and respect for both the individual and the development of the individual; Pizer (1998) views neutrality as the therapist's responsibility to maintain an area of illusion for negotiation within the psychotherapy relationship. Both positions guarantee preservation of the interplay between reality and fantasy, protection for long periods of "not knowing," and support for the patient's capacity to face previously unassimilable traumatic realities. The intersubjective critique of the illusory and defensive aspects (viz., e.g., Orange, Atwood, and Stolorow [1997]) of the "doctrine of neutrality" of classical psychoanalysis has catalyzed appreciation of the reciprocally influencing, codetermining nature of all psychotherapy interactions: the therapist's perceptions and perspectives can never be viewed as intrinsically more real or true than the patient's.

From a relational perspective, the role of therapist is not that of neutral purveyor of expert knowledge. Rather, the therapist is a facilitator of transformative conversations, a moderator of benevolent disruptions, a coprocessor of unmetabolized pain, helplessness, and terror, and a navigator of creative and disturbing dialogues that assist traumatized patients in expanding both their imaginations and their repertoire of relatedness to self and others. At the core of this mutative process is an equal honoring of multiple narratives, multiple meanings, and multiple identities.

A DIFFERENT UNIVERSE

When clinicians spend thousands of hours with severely traumatized, dissociative individuals, their worldviews inevitably change. Those who treat trauma and dissociation occupy a different universe from those who do not. It is a consistent aim of these pages to illuminate, integrate, and *extend* the work of relational psychoanalytic theorists who have begun addressing the complex issues of sexual abuse, trauma, and dissociation. Many of these theorists, myself among them, are committed to advancing the view of complex dissociative disorders as more prevalent than is commonly believed, and also potentially more treatable psychodynamically.

Invariably, how we conceive of the patient's problem influences the solution to the problem. A delicate balance between disruption and stabilization must be continually renegotiated or the traumatized patient and the therapist will be perpetually overwhelmed or stalemated. The therapy relationship must break down old, as well as forge new, linkages between the inner world of the patient and his/her relationships with the sociopolitical world. The dissociative trauma survivor's essential individuation and differentiation from traumatic relational matrices is fostered only through ongoing challenges to the patient and therapist's unavoidable complicity with and dependence upon pathological social relations (Flax, 1996a), so that self (and society) can be reconfigured in more egalitarian and compassionate terms. In most cases, a therapist's emphasis on the patient's growth and self-awareness must be balanced with the therapist's emotional receptivity and psychological availability to the patient. Because all intimacy is perceived as threatening and potentially dangerous by severely dissociative trauma survivors, the possibilities for extended periods of agitation, psychological "disappearances," states of dissolution and deadness, treatment stalemates, or destructive acting out (on the part of patient and/or therapist) are endless.

THE TREATMENT MODEL

This book explores the effects on the patient's internal world, and on the treatment alliance, of the therapist's treatment values and goals and their communication, direct or indirect, which include

- fostering mutuality and interconnectedness
- dismantling internalized patterns of domination and complicity
- articulating and embracing of all the patient's dissociative states (in dialogue) regardless of degree of concretization or apparent threat
- encouraging restorative fantasy over repetitive (and concrete) self-defeating solutions
- fostering aggression in the service of the self rather than against the self and in the service of the perpetrator(s); this includes the therapist's supporting the patient's questioning of the authority of the therapist
- tolerating ambiguity and paradox
- processing and metabolizing fragments of helplessness, pain, dread, and terror
- expanding the capacity for freedom of association and freedom of thought—that is, restorating critical thinking
- developing more flexible psychological organizing principles, expanding and enriching the repertoire of relatedness to self and other
- developing a unified observing ego
- balancing internalized limits with internalized compassion
- developing a restored narrativity, historicity, affectivity
- facing existential issues regarding the self and human nature
- learning to live in the present, finding (and creating) joy, meaningful work, and interrelatedness in a life that is governed by neither the alternations of posttraumatic intrusions and psychic deadness nor the injunctions of perpetrators and collaborators.

The proposed treatment approach accepts the fundamental, but paradoxical reality of pathological multiplicity but consistently challenges the patient in attempts to help him/her move beyond a kind of balkanization of mind, with its polarized, warring, mutually deceiving factions attempting to dominate, eradicate, or ignore one another. The treatment approach also challenges forms of internalized irresponsibility and authoritarianism and helps develop an internal social "democracy" of self organized around authentic tolerance of internal diversity (i.e., going beyond the expert avoidance, camouflage, and polarization cultivated by most severely dissociative individuals). In this model, the internalization of new, healthy interaction patterns is as important as the internalization of new objects. These goals, like those of all relationally oriented treatments, are accomplished through immersion in (and survival of) the transference-countertransference matrix of feelings, fantasies, enactments, and memories; in this forum, polarized entanglements can lead to mutual reflection and mutually resolved disentanglements, fostering true ownership and freedom of mind.

CHALLENGES TO TREATMENT

Profound reintegration of basic attachment patterns is essential to meaningful recovery or healing. When parental, institutional, or archetypal authority has chronically betrayed a child as is the case among survivors of severe abuse, the elements of love, trust, power, and mutuality have to be reworked from the ground up. Therapists treating severely dissociative trauma survivors must be vigilant to the dynamics of power throughout the therapy relationship as these patients have experienced the most egregious abuses of power in intimate situations known to our species. Because of the ubiquity of abusive power dynamics in the lives of these patients, the clinician needs to be adept at attending to the potential replication and unconscious reenactment of the domination, torture, sacrifice, blackmail, seduction, "bait-and-switch," hostage-holding, and betrayal relational paradigms within the therapy relationship. The clinician needs to create an environment of shared inquiry, shared authority, and eventually mutual recognition and influence without negating the fundamental asymmetrical aspects of the therapy relationship (Aron, 1996). The commitment to humanizing and democratizing the therapy relationship, instead of encumbering it with the unnecessary trappings of higher authority and professional expertise (Hedges, 1997) as a vehicle for subverting old and establishing new attachment patterns does not preclude the therapist's directing, confronting, and interpreting at times. A central precept of feminist therapy (L. Brown, 1994) declares each of us an expert or source of information and authority. Often, we must help our traumatized patients who have been forced to submit to the excesses of irrational authority develop their capacities for listening to—not compulsively negating—and relying upon their own internal authority.

Because psychotherapy involves multiple parallel processes, this book is a call for an enhanced appreciation of the *complexity* of both patients' and therapists' dilemmas. The patient's challenge is to make it to therapy at all after childhood torment followed by posttraumatic symptoms, marginalization, and the unconscious lure of traumatic reenactments and self-destructive patterns; then s/he must have both the finances to afford and the will to endure the lengthy process. S/he may become the focus of the therapist's unbridled countertransference enactments ranging from fascination, rescue fantasies, denial, incredulity, and various forms of subtle or overt domination (often through interpretations) to boundary violations and distancing. S/he may become the focus of his/her family's as well as society's skepticism and derision.

The treatment of severely dissociative trauma survivors is a high-risk enterprise for therapists. Treating this highly misunderstood and difficult population the clinician faces numerous hazards, all of them leading to a high likelihood of secondary traumatization. These include the variety of aggressions, transgressions, and threats dissociative patients make toward their therapists, immersion in the traumatic transference-countertransference matrix, the hostility and incredulity of professional colleagues, increasing double binds generated by licensing boards and the legal system (including malicious lawsuits), organized antitherapy advocacy groups and skepticism salons within the society, and now the unrealistic expectations and constraints of managed care.

Both dissociative patient and therapist are caught in a sticky web of complex feelings and enactments and are enmeshed in parallel processes within the larger culture and social systems in which the treatment is embedded. Somehow, through it all, they must find ways to stay emotionally vulnerable and emotionally available in a context that is fundamentally retraumatizing for both. Most recent reviews of the issues involved in treatment of survivors of severe trauma have not taken the full measure of complexity into account.

THE BOOK

My primary intention in writing this book is to facilitate critical thinking about some of the most salient aspects of treatment for severely dissociative individuals and their therapists, and to establish a strong and lasting bridge between the contemporary psychoanalytic and the trauma/dissociation communities. My agenda is not to dictate to clinicians how to conduct psychotherapy with traumatized, dissociative patients, nor is it to establish a new list of techniques, or to push a particular theoretical agenda. Case presentations illustrate only one therapist's effort at integrating diverse clinical theories and translating them into practice. And, given the current state of polarization and the panoply of perspectives on patients' trauma memories and narratives, it is likely that various clinicians, theoreticians, and skeptics will interpret my descriptions of clinical work according to their preferred paradigms.

Every psychotherapy is unique. Every individual who is a trauma survivor is unique, and must be defined by his/her full range of adaptations, strengths, resources, and creativity more than by the nature and extent of the trauma s/he has suffered. For therapy to succeed, the therapist and patient must each find some freedom of movement within extremely restrictive and reactive intrapsychic, interpersonal, and cultural conditions. A clinician's strict adherence to dogma and party lines may obstruct effective communication and interfere with genuine opportunities for healing. A therapist's creativity and flexibility and capacity to tolerate the patient's impact on his/her psyche, open up new ways of being and experiencing for each individual patient, and for specific passages within each treatment.

The book is presented in three parts. Part One explores the issues of dissociative survival, extreme child abuse victimization, and the psychology of perpetration and complicity (collaboration). Part Two is really the clinical heart and soul of the book, applying the principles of relational psychoanalytic theorizing to restoration of the traumatized, dissociative self. Part Three introduces the multifaceted issues of the therapist as witness-participant and the therapist's survival of the treatment process. Investigations of the core dynamics of *mutual destruction* and *mutual survival* in the therapy work between therapists and severely dissociative trauma survivors track a healing journey at once grueling and inspiring.

Part One

The Landscapes of Dissociative Survival, Child Abuse Trauma, and Social Complicity

CHAPTER 1

Necessary Illusions:
The Multiple Dilemmas of
Dissociative Survival

Freeing yourself was one thing; claiming ownership of that freed self was another.

—Toni Morrison *(Beloved)*

Many people enter treatment with complex, undiagnosed, or misdiagnosed problems resulting from severe childhood trauma and dissociative adaptations to chronic and sometimes sadistic abuse. As psychotherapy and psychoanalysis have matured over the last century, a growing number of clinicians have been able to discard some of the assumptions inhibiting the profession's understanding of, and response to, such patients, and to take another look at human subjectivity in general and also at altered states of consciousness, the structure of the unconscious, legal and ethical responsibilities, and the nature of evil.

The receptive clinical posture places a higher value on intersubjective discourse, reciprocal influence, and the complicated relationships among intrapsychic, interpersonal, and sociopolitical phenomena. It makes room for a host of formerly suppressed voices of traumatized individuals to surface and be recognized. The voices echo, among other things, abject terror and helplessness, shame and the conviction that the self is damaged or evil, the

3

callous rejection of needs, feelings, and attachments, and prideful identifications with abusive perpetrators.

VOICES

"In my family I was a commodity. Everyone and everything was a commodity. I was owned—I was sold, rented, bought, traded. I never thought I could have a life of my own. I felt so intruded upon and so much hate and so much demand for service that I built a shield over myself and no can get through it anymore, not even me."

"My hurt and pain is stored in a beehive, in honeycomb form with lots of different compartments. The syrup is not golden, however, it is black and it oozes, it is disgusting. I am the one who lives outside of all of that. The others they are covered in the ooze. Me, I live in nowhere."

"I don't want to get it that this happened to me. I don't want to get it that this happens to anyone, anywhere in the world, not just in my family. I don't want to feel what I know I have to feel. I don't want to know. I want to be normal. I don't want to be an 'abuse survivor.' I want to have picnics and family reunions, pay the bills and quibble over the garbage pick-ups like everyone else. But it's not an option. It's not an option."

"They told me I liked it. I didn't like it, did I? They told me I was pretending when I said I didn't like it, and that I really did like it and want it. I pretended a lot, so I must have liked it—so maybe I really wanted it, even though I thought I didn't; and then they said I was lying when I said it hurt, so I must have really liked it but I really didn't. Do you believe me?"

"I played my part. It was the only part to play. Without it there was nothing for me. I mean nothing. I pretended to be asleep so he could pretend he wasn't doing what he was doing to me and if we both pretended then nothing happened and no one would know, especially not me."

"In order to survive I had to cling to all the wrong things and the wrong people, and now I have to unplug all of the wires and rearrange everything. But what happens when you unplug all of the wires—are you free or do you detonate?"

The child-victim's journey through the terrifying landscapes of trauma often requires, for psychological survival, the urgent mobilization of the mind's natural capacity for multiplicity in support of dissociative adaptation. Dissociation is a desperate effort to preserve life and sanity by constructing an identity to manage (for example, disown, compartmentalize, diffuse) pain, anxiety, terror, and shame. It involves the creation of self- and other-representations rooted in psychic exclusions (*Not me/Not him/Not happen*) and in identification with the only apparent objects of attachment or sources of protection—powerful others who *seem* to offer protection, escape, or some type of relief of pain or punishment. During[1] and after the trauma, the child imitates, pretends, distracts his/herself, enters altered states of consciousness; later in life, dissociative survival has to be bolstered continually by an arsenal of avoidance, addiction, and camouflage strategies.

Complicitous interpersonal and social contexts inevitably shape and reinforce the development of altered states of consciousness and the elaboration of a repertoire of alter personalities and attendant characterological patterns. The challenge to our cultural belief in a sane, just, benevolent, world and to our idealized societal self-image and the mental health professions serving it has fomented sharp divisions and bitter debates about the realities of child abuse, the veracity of patients' memories and histories, and the role and effects of psychotherapy in the treatment of trauma. Dissociative disorders are the product of a collaborative "revisioning" of history and identity by the victim, the perpetrator(s), and the colluding (i.e., invalidating, silencing, abandoning) family and social systems.

A world unready for the revelations of survivors of traumatic abuse sets up one of the primary templates for revictimization when it greets their psychic wounds with contempt, disgust, or incredulity. Any attempt to separate their adaptative mechanisms from the dynamics that spawned them runs the risk of pathologizing victims and subjecting them to another round of retraumatizing decontextualization and domination, which latter is the hallmark of interpersonal trauma. Accordingly, *recognition* of dissociative disorders must be another joint venture—of remembering, feeling, and witnessing—this one engaging the patient, the therapist, and the more benign and courageous components of the larger social system.

Part of the disturbing power of dissociation is the way it ignites parallel abusive, collusive, and revictimizing processes in every interpersonal environment, including psychotherapy. Severely dissociative patients are prone to the kind of destructive reenactments that turn those who engage with them into unwitting partners in re-creating the dynamics of their original abusive systems. Survivors of sexual abuse fear that something traumatic is about to occur, or is in fact occurring, at any given moment; moreover, their unconscious, trauma-driven preconceptions about disastrous relational outcomes disfigure the ways they anticipate and construe, as well as conduct, their own relationships (Van der Kolk, 1989; Levine, 1994).

Trauma survivors' belief systems inevitably get reinforced in treatment—not only when patients are actually mistreated, as they so often have been and still are in our mental health system, and not only because transference/countertransference pressures catalyze reenactments of traumatic relational paradigms—but also because the power of the compulsion to repeat the trauma is so intense (Van der Kolk, 1989; Briere, 1992b). As the severely dissociative patient's reality-testing fluctuates precipitously with the repetitions, the line between reality and fantasy becomes tenuous, and the "as if" or illusory quality of the transference may disappear altogether (Levine, 1990). Retraumatization will necessarily be an ongoing factor in the early phases of the therapy relationship, which will be informed and organized, like all other experience, by the memory of the trauma and its associated events. Sorting real from imagined revictimization in treatment is especially arduous when a patient steadfastly assumes the victim role or has only minimal self-reflective capacities.

Dissociative identity disorder (DID), the extreme end of the dissociative disorders continuum, is but one of the many personal and cultural passion plays of thwarted psychological liberation. It is, among many things, a complex posttraumatic stress disorder, a variable and mixed character disorder syndrome, a disorder of consciousness, and a disorder of self- and other-representation. DID is most notably an internalization of the dynamic patterns of (intimate) interpersonal violence experienced by the victim—exploitation, betrayal, subjugation, collusion, coercion, domination, blackmail, sacrifice, and forced submission to bondage (and loyalty) to irrational authority. This chapter explores the dimensions of severe dissociative adaptation, the traumatic relational dynamics that give rise to severe dissociative disorders, and the social and intrapsychic conditions that sustain them.

DILEMMAS OF DISSOCIATIVE SURVIVAL

Why? I am asked. Why do you bring that up? Must you talk about that? I asked myself the same questions until finally I began to understand. This was a wall in my life, I say, a wall I had to climb over every day. It was always there for me, deflecting my rage toward people who knew nothing about what happened to me or why I should be angry at them. It took me years to get past that rage, to say the words with grief and insistence but to let go of the anger, to refuse to use the anger against people who knew nothing of the rape. I had to learn how to say it, to say "rape," say "child," say "unending," "awful," and "relentless," and say it the way I do—adamant, unafraid, unashamed, every time, all over again—to speak my words as sacrament, a blessing, a prayer. Not a curse.

—Dorothy Allison, *One or Two Things I Know for Sure*

- *Donna's mother regularly turned her over to her father for sex from the age of four or five to get grocery money for the family, and also to pimps who paid well to use her in child prostitution and pornography. Donna was well-trained by the time she was six to initiate sexual behavior with any man, and when she began indiscriminately to approach her friends' fathers for sex on visiting their homes, her mother called her a slut and a whore and brutally beat her as punishment for acting like a tramp.*
- *Anna's father would ritualistically drown her in the bathtub until she was virtually unconscious. Then he would hug and kiss her in a theatrical display of rescue. Then he would sexually molest her. Then he would force her to get down on her knees and thank him.*
- *Craig was initiated into a sadistic pedophile group at the age of six by his older brother, who had been abused for years by the same group and had been molesting Craig ever since. The brother took him to a neighbor's garage where there was "a surprise" for him, opened the door, pushed Craig in, and locked it from the outside. In an exact replication of his brother's initiation, Craig was gagged and then serially raped by various men waiting their turns. He was told to get used to it, told that it would be his life from now on, and told that if he said anything to anyone, he, his brother, and his parents would be killed. A few years later, quite dissociatively organized, he was easily manipulated by the men in the group into "recruiting" other victims.*
- *Eileen finally managed to talk about how her father would gather her up after her psychotic mother's violent rages left her nearly unconscious. He would put her gently to bed and then begin molesting her; when she resisted, he sometimes acted as though she was hurting his feelings and sometimes as though she had badly misbehaved and had to be beaten. Eileen's father also used her body to teach his three sons about sex and urged them to have sex with her in his presence. They did so on their own as well throughout her adolescence.*
- *Brenda describes being buried alive by a group of seriously disturbed ritual abuse perpetrators and left in a box in the ground, cold and naked. The next day when they "discovered" her, they punished her for running away and*

hiding. She could choose—to be raped by the group or put back into isola-tion. Convinced that she had exercised free will when she "chose" the former, Brenda was traumatized into internalizing their edict that she belonged with them and their injunction that she obey all their wishes. As the perpetrators took over her intrapsychic and interpersonal life, she lost most of her mind with what was left of her will.

SEPARATION AND REUNIFICATION

The self-protective mechanisms of all organisms can take on a life of their own and go awry under conditions of constant bombardment: natural protest responses can devolve to autistic retreat or into addiction to self-injury; healthy detachment can calcify into heartless objectification of self and others; and restorative impulses can mutate into patterns of arrogance and domina-tion. Our innate, malleable survival capacities adjust creatively to environ-mental impingements or prolonged periods of stress and deprivation by segregating, sequestering, reduplicating, distracting, and/or sacrificing parts to protect the whole, such that when physical or psychological survival is threatened, breakdowns occur. Disunity is almost always favored over unity.

"I know there is a 'there' there but I can't get at it and it can't get to me."

"I can't be astute for too long a time. It's too dangerous. I have to keep everything ambiguous, vague, tentative, optional, conditional. I need to be able to rearrange things at a moment's notice. If I don't keep my world like that then some things could get very clear and then I might have to make judgments about things and peo-ple, like my parents. I keep insisting on keeping things in two dimensions so I don't have to deal with life in three dimensions. When you ask me to relate to you and the world in a three dimensional way then I get scared that everything could come tum-bling down all at once."

"They locked me in a huge meat freezer inside of a small grocery store that one of the guys in the cult I was abused by owned, I think. I was left there with the raw meat hanging and there were also dead human bodies or parts of bodies that they were saving for something, hanging there too. I know this sounds unbelievable. Anyway after a while I was taken out, I must have been unconscious and was given some kind of drug to make me not remember anything and then I remember these men were there and they were telling me things in my head about what to do, how to do it, how to remember, how to forget, what to remember, what to forget.

After a while, there was no me left anymore. I gave up somewhere in the freezer. . . . What they did after that didn't matter because I no longer cared. The 'mes' that got built up or created after that point were just puppets or marionettes acting on the commands and training of the men in the group. I became them, they became me."

Optimally, when threat disappears, motivations to reunify may take over. But when threat is chronic and enduring, it is entirely conceivable that atomized parts of the psyche will never be rejoined. Over time, the links in individual or collective memory that hold the map of unification erode. Then, only external recognition and intervention—building on the evolutionary-biological design articulated by Slavin and Kreigman (1992) whereby the self under siege stashes away elements for future actualization, validating human reparative potential—can bring about integration.

But as disunity qua survival strategy comes to constitute an independent homeostasis, the dissociative survivor comes to experience any break-through toward reunification of the self as a serious threat to his/her equilibrium. S/he may regard relational patterns that hold seeds of integration—insight, empathy, respect, love, compassion, encouragement to feel and reflect—as so perilous as to merit attack or avoidance; and s/he might actually seek out seemingly protective behaviors that soothe and reduce tension by sustaining psychological disunity (e.g., self-destructive acting out, substance addiction, workaholism, sexual compulsivity, involvement in abusive or duplicitous relationships, etc.).

PROTECTING DISSOCIATIVE STRUCTURES

I was very tiny when I began filling in the blank spaces, the inconsistencies. Not being able to account for minutes or hours of time, finding myself in different clothes or geographical locations, was just an accepted part of my life. I became very adept at scanning the scene and putting together what the others inside had just done or said . . . —[explaining] what my body had done while I was not there. . . . My behavior was erratic because my many selves didn't connect with each other. Because of the continual social confusion, we all agreed to try and cooperate. . . . We all learned very quickly to stick by "The Code." . . . we made some rules, such as they had to call themselves [by the same name] in public. (Cameron, 1995, p. 101)

"It is humanly impossible to become fully alive in the present without facing and owning all of the hated, disavowed parts of the self that have shaped and been shaped by one's earliest object attachments" (Bromberg, 1998, p. 6). Existing inside a dissociative labyrinth with its oblique and unarticulated grief and continuous intrapsychic pressures (e.g., cacophony of voices) is like living in a permanent state of exile from the human community. Survivors of chronic abuse are tragically impaired when it comes to trusting or even cognitively processing the reality of their own experiences (Herman, 1992; Briere, 1996). Through repeated acts of distancing, disavowal, and dissociation, they develop an idolatrous faith in eradicating their pasts (including affectivity) while losing any faith in human solidarity and redemptive (i.e., witnessed, expressed) suffering.

Trapped in guilt, shame, and relentless self-blame, they remain enslaved to the traumas and traumatizers of the past even as they seek desperately to obliterate their history (including its pain, its meanings, and its impact). The litany of inconsistencies and self-betrayals that has become part of everyday life for survivors as by-products of their fears of change and their allegiance to dissociative defenses thwarts the development of new, loving relationships. Yet anything that jeopardizes the extension of their dissociative adaptations, including any threat to their attachments to malevolent but "protective" objects, makes the prospect of dismantling their persecutory theater of mind as hard and terrifying as sustaining it.

For complex dissociative adaptations to be truly effective, they must eradicate or conceal all evidence or knowledge of dissociation. "Cloaking devices," therefore, are essential to survival (and, because exposure is so threatening to the dissociative self-organization, extremely difficult to work through in the early stages of treatment). The severely traumatized individual works overtime "to prepare for almost any conceivable emergency that would startle [some]one into becoming aware of the dissociated system" (Sullivan, 1956, p. 203). Unfortunately, his/her unconscious motivation to deflect evidence of dissociation is often further potentiated by the incredulity of society and by manipulation on the parts of perpetrators who compound their victims' self-generated shame-based camouflage with intimidation, posthypnotic suggestions, even programmed resistance techniques.

VICTIMIZATION BY CHILDHOOD TRAUMA

Self-preservation no longer existed in my head. Enduring was all I knew.
(Cameron, 1995, p. 92)

Interpersonal trauma is at its most pernicious when it is embedded in the deliberately inflicted cruelties of a dependent relationship with a betraying, irrational authority—and just such a relational history is at the core of most severely dissociative patients' experience. In many forms of child sexual abuse, the negative impact comes more from the depth of betrayal than the severity of the violence itself (Salter, 1995). As Harris (1996a, p. 169) explains,

> Incest involves a child in coercive sexuality with an adult well known and often well loved by the child in an experience that is silenced and neither narrated nor integrated for the child by any compassionate, safe adult at the time of or in the immediate aftermath of the incest.

Severe dissociative disorders arise from internalization of social paradigms of domination, coercion, and sacrifice as sexually abused children replicate, potentiate, and simultaneously attempt to transcend the profound damage sustained by their ongoing exploitation and betrayal by caretakers and authorities. The paradigms can encompass perverse sexuality (Brenner, 1996), sadism, and the perpetrator's intentional structuring (i.e., programming) of dissociative identification with evil and malevolence; among survivors of ritual abuse groups and criminal organizations trafficking in child prostitution and pornography, "a number of dissociated sexual pathways may be [observed] in the same individual, [encapsulating] aggression, childhood trauma, anxiety, and sense of self" (Brenner, 1996, p. 165).

Throughout the literature on severe dissociative disorder, childhood trauma histories are the most consistent and prominent feature of clinical reports (Ross, 1997). Childhoods marked by chronic and severe physical, sexual, psychological, and spiritual assaults correlate with diagnoses of dissociative identity disorder (DID), formerly called multiple personality disorder (MPD) (Putnam, 1989; Kluft, 1987a; Ross, 1989; 1997).[2] Most related current research is consistent with the theory that dissociative symptomatology is based on responses to chronic childhood sexual and physical abuse (Braun, 1984; Kluft, 1987a; Ross, 1989; 1997; Putnam, 1989; Chu and Dill, 1990; Coons et al., 1988), or combinations of child abuse and/or reactions to other childhood stressors such as neglect, familial loss, and witnessing violence and abuse (Irwin, 1994; Zlotnick et al., 1995).[3]

A spate of recent studies investigating the relationship between psychological trauma and dissociative phenomena corroborated these earlier findings. In a nonclinical sample, Irwin (1999) found that pathological dissociation was positively predicted by dimensions of childhood trauma, but that nonpathological dissociation (e.g., psychological absorption) was not. Draijer and Langeland (1999) found that the level of dissociation in relation to childhood trauma in a large sample of inpatients was primarily related to reported *overwhelming* childhood experiences (sexual and physical abuse); when sexual abuse was severe (involving penetration and multiple perpetrators, and lasting more than one year, etc.), dissociative symptoms were even more prominent. Highest dissociation levels were found in patients reporting *cumulative* sexual trauma (intrafamilial and extrafamilial) or both sexual and physical abuse. (In particular, maternal dysfunction was related to level of dissociation suggesting that dissociation is neglect- and abandonment-related as well.)

Chu et al. (1999) found strong associations between *any* type of childhood abuse and elevated levels of dissociative symptoms in a large sample of women admitted to a trauma disorders unit. Higher dissociative symptoms were correlated with early age at onset of physical and sexual abuse and also with more frequent abuse. (A substantial proportion of all participants reported partial or complete amnesia for abuse memories; early age at onset of abuse was correlated with greater levels of amnesia. A majority of those who later recovered memories of child abuse were able to find corroborative evidence.)

The results of a comprehensive review summarizing and synthesizing recent findings on child abuse and dissociation (Gershuny and Thayer, 1999) suggest a fairly strong and consistent relationship among trauma, dissociation, and trauma-related distress (e.g., posttraumatic stress disorder, borderline personality disorder, bulimia). Individuals who had experienced traumatic events were more likely to dissociate than those who had not, and individuals who experienced more dissociative phenomena were more likely to also experience higher levels of trauma-related distress. The authors hypothesize that dissociative phenomena and subsequent trauma-related distress may connect to fears about death, loss, or lack of control above and beyond the occurrence of the traumatic event itself.

Despite the criticisms of skeptics and revisionists (Hacking, 1995; Brenneis, 1997; Piper, 1997; Haaken, 1998), both research and clinical experience consistently show that with increased frequency, intensity, number of perpetrators, and earlier onset of abuse, and in the absence of soothing and restorative interpersonal responses (Kluft, 1984; 1987a; Briere, 1996; Ross,

1997; Strong, 1998) there is a higher likelihood of longer-lasting and serious dissociative symptomatology. Personal clinical experience with dissociative survivors suggests that the term "child abuse" may not adequately reflect the levels of torture, degradation, terrorization, and psychic invasion that these individuals have endured.

Strong (1998), summarizing the potentiating factors of neglect, complicity, and denial, reminds us that it is not merely the acts of violence and intrusion that damage victims of abuse and lead to extreme dissociative adaptations but also the dysfunctional family systems that allow abuse to occur in the first place and often remain invalidating and dysfunctional long after the acts of sexual abuse have stopped. He notes that "incest survivors may feel even more betrayed by the nonabusing yet nonprotective parent . . . who either tacitly encourages the abuse or fails to recognize and stop it" (p. 77).

"It felt like hell lying in bed at night wondering if my father would come and take me, and then if he would take me, what he would do with me. I learned to distinguish the different pattern of footsteps . . . that would tell me whether he was going to take me down to the basement and rape me, or pick me up like a sack of potatoes over his shoulder and deliver me to those awful houses where children are used in everywhich way, and where I would have to go from room to room all night, or whether I was being taken somewhere to live for a while to participate in whatever they wanted for however long they wanted. I became a vacant shell, living between dread and numbness and physical pain until I discovered drugs and alcohol at age 13. Then I could control my body and what went into it for the first time. Or at least I thought I could.

"After getting me used to being raped and molested my father and his friends, who only seemed to like abusing little boys, gathered some of the children together in one place and had us do sexual things to one another while they watched and laughed and sometimes, not always, took pictures. We had no idea what we were doing. We thought it was fun, or special, or some secret initiation, even if we also felt scared and dirty and bad; but really they were just manipulating our innocence and getting off on it. I hate them more for raping my innocence than for raping my body."

Loss of Language

Intense and overwhelming pain that is not met with human contact, compassion, and soothing (Kluft, 1987a; 1992; Van der Kolk, 1989) is one of the primary driving forces behind dissociative solutions, particularly when the traumatized child's (or adult's) need for soothing is greeted by further abuse, humiliation, and/or abandonment (including denial). And when extreme physical and psychic pain is compounded by interpersonal betrayal, social isolation, and the powerful global mistrust they engender, it leads also to the shattering of language, to the captivity and destruction of the victim's autonomous voice. The child-victim's incapacity to articulate—to witness, locate, externalize, or interpret—the traumatizing, assaultive exploitation of the self magnifies the split between his/her reality and the reality of others.

> As the content of one's world disintegrates, so the content of one's language disintegrates; as the self disintegrates, so that which would express and project the self is robbed of its source and its subject. (Scarry, 1985, p. 35)

The resulting isolation and appropriation of the victim's pain by the abuser(s) further sequesters the wounded, tortured self, and makes the individual hostage to an internalized dissociative system of perverted power dynamics. In that system, constructed under extreme conditions and elaborated during the prolonged captivity of childhood, any proximity to pain or even its relocation in memory is prohibited—and the victim's own mechanisms of denial are often lubricated by the perpetrator's conscious attempts at decontextualizing and recontextualizing his/her experiences. The language that would otherwise express those experiences is avoided, distorted, or deleted; in psychotherapy, insight alone will not be able to access what is thoroughly out of the intellect's communicative reach.

Since verbal language is either unavailable or inadequate to describe the intensity of the chronic trauma survivor's internal states, s/he is "left with a mute hopelessness about the possibility of communicating in a way that will help . . . get critical needs met. Words then seem to take on terrifying proportions; they are both too powerful and completely useless" (Strong, 1998, p. 44). In treatment, especially early on, the severely dissociative trauma survivor will more than likely fluctuate among at least three states: belief that expressing such feelings as sadness and rage will immediately lead to the destruction of him/herself, the therapist, and/or the office; use of the body as a vehicle for expressing pain through self-mutilation and other forms of self-injury, accident-proneness, or brutal reenactments of sexual trauma; and a complete sense of futility about any communication, and specifically about the therapist's ever really "getting it."

Dissociative Patterning

The natural capacity to dissociate is "the escape when there is no escape" (Putnam, 1992, p. 104). When traumatic relational events overwhelm and shatter the vulnerable self, all the mental contents that constitute one's self and one's world—including one's voice, which generates and is generated by language—cease to exist (Scarry, 1985); what remains is pure *negation*.

Dissociation, a surrealistic set of discontinuities and disparities related to identity, awareness, and responsibility, sustains the survival of the trauma-tized individual by restricting the scope of the self—that is, by excluding the insupportable from the self-system. Cohen (1996) organizes the dissociative exclusions into four essential features: *not me* (signaling the development of alter parts); *not now* (characterizing incapacity to remain in or experience the present); *not then* (indicating disavowal of personal history); and *not ever* (identifying lack of hope, even of future orientation).

Constructing elaborate dissociative defenses while keeping toxic emo-tional states at bay (Briere, 1995) isolates the survivor of chronic abuse in bondage to the past. It narrows the windows of awareness and opportunity, preventing the updating of the central autobiographical consciousness, and makes guarding against retraumatization a central organizing psychological principle of life. Since intense experience, regardless of valence, can open floodgates of affect and cognition, the individual must continually *constrict* to avoid thoughts, feelings, and situations evocative of the original trauma (Van der Kolk, 1989).

The preservation of some boundary between self and not-self prevents the complete collapse of personhood[4] (Bromberg, 1998); indeed, it restores san-ity. Dissociation hypnoidally unlinks incompatible states of consciousness, allowing them only separate access to awareness—that is, in the form of un-connected mental experiences—(Bromberg, 1994). And once separated, dis-sociated mental contents—behavior, affect, sensation, knowledge (Braun, 1984)—or interpersonal patterns (Pearlman and Saakvitne, 1995) coexist in parallel streams of consciousness without interacting and even without ref-erence to one another. In the absence of intersection (much less conflict) be-tween good and bad memories of a person or experience, the highly dissociative individual is not alerted to incongruity and thus not moved to resolve it.

The internal confusion and detectable inconsistencies that result from the strenuous psychological effort to avoid psychic conflict, pain, and disorientation must be camouflaged on an ongoing basis. Both the survivor who daily lives with this disjointed internal reality and those who get close enough to him/her to notice must continuously develop explanations to fill in the gaps. Combinations of cover stories (Waites, 1997), dissimulations, persona-restoring behavior, distractions, and evasions create a false sense of continuity for the dissociative survivor and for others not paying close attention. Intimacy of any kind is dangerous, however, and freighted with intrapsychic and interpersonal anxieties because the unremitting evasiveness, amnesias, and inconsistencies would become increasingly apparent under its umbrella.

Whereas repression maintains psychic material in the dynamic unconscious (Gabbard, 1994), dissociation preserves and suspends it in an array of parallel self-states and parallel fragments of consciousness, and they in turn can be multidimensionally sequestered, amplified, elaborated, and personified by a variety of fantasy operations. As Gabbard says, dissociation not only divides the self, it divides patterns of object relations. In patients with extreme dissociative disorders, these two primary sets of divisions intersect and potentiate one another so that tracking, "mapping," or following the lines of the polyfragmentation becomes nearly impossible.

Eigen (1996) describes the dazzling array of psychic possibilities once splitting and recombination run amok:

> Good or bad aspects of the self can be identified with good or bad aspects of the object, and good or bad aspects of the object can be identified with good or bad aspects of the self. If one adds dislocations and amalgams of affect, the clinical possibilities become mind-boggling. Ego, object, and affect can be taken apart and put together in myriad permutations. Bad ego can hate good ego, good ego can love bad ego, bad object can hate good object loving good ego, good ego can love bad ego hating good object, bad object can hate bad ego loving good object, good ego can hate bad ego hating good object, and on and on. (p. 31)

The dissociative system is like a labyrinth of mirrors and trapdoors, and the dissociative process the ultimate intrapsychic trickster. It reverses cause and effect and self and other configurations, and obscures (or lies about) the individual's connections to his/her history. Lost in time, fragmented in identity, hypervigilant to the possibility of exposure while ostensibly guarding against all manner of other catastrophes, and truly confused in all relationships though pretending not to be, dissociative survivors become the victims of their own dissociative roller coasters. Tragically, the vicious cycles involving impression-management and avoidance of feelings, memories, and detection frequently cause people (professionals included) to doubt and distrust everything severely dissociative trauma survivors have to say. And that leads to further rounds of self-doubt and invalidation for the survivors[5].

In keeping with the development of a "hot line" to a nodal memory network associated with fear and panic (Allen, 1995), highly dissociative individuals may demonstrate indiscriminate panic, startle responses, or even hatred toward any source of out-of-control feelings. Activation of any part of this emotional network can rapidly activate the entire complex, where hyperarousal, overstimulation, addiction to traumatic enactments, poor judgment, and intense sensation-seeking alternate and overlap. All such patterns move trauma survivors toward retraumatization, job and relationship loss, and eventually tortured lives of extreme bewilderment, isolation, and meaningless, nonredemptive suffering.

Although much remains to be learned, it is clear that young children have difficulty in cognitively and emotionally processing overwhelming and violent experiences and that they deploy dissociation as a way to master and contain traumatic affect and preserve some kind of meaning amidst mind-shattering events. Once the dissociative-survival process is set in motion, they lose control over personality changes and neurochemical alterations and sustain permanent damage to the integrated sense of agency.

The dissociative structuring of children's minds is very much in the hands of the perpetrators, however, when periods of disabling anxiety and isolation are *intentionally* followed by moments of pain and fear reduction and some form of soothing contact, human or nonhuman (food, drugs, sleep, blankets); when the abusive context systematically switches experiences of terror, pain, and helplessness with "opportunities" for actual or imagined empowerment; or when orchestrated guilt and shame alternate with orchestrated relief from being overwhelmed.

The pattern of breaking down and building up is one of the hallmarks of thought-reform and mind-control technology (see Chapter 8). It is exacerbated to advance and enhance the objectives of the perpetrating individuals or group by the planned imposition, under conditions of chronic and extreme stress, of trauma-shaping rape, torture, forced witnessing of and coerced participation in harming animals or infants as well as children or adults, electroshocks, disorienting or overstimulating drugs, learned helplessness paradigms, classical and operant conditioning techniques including powerful suggestion during and after the event, and sophisticated psycho-manipulation to foster identifications with abusers and extreme states of rage and detachment. Such know-how has been available to the worldwide intelligence community since the 1950s and certainly accessible to cults and criminal groups (which sometimes overlap)—yet the mental health and academic communities have been reluctant to accept the validity of survivors' reports, and have resisted integrating it into their treatment protocols.

"I saw things no human being, no person should see. The fog is what I have to keep me from seeing that again, from knowing that which I saw, or that I ever saw it. Without the fog I have no life. It is the fog that allows me to live. And it feels like what is inside that fog could kill me."

"I am not a person. I am a creation of them. I am a cube posing as a person. I've been allowed to have a life providing I play by the rules and instructions book. If I don't I can be recalled. If I am recalled, I have to be broken down all over again. That would be a pain I could not survive."

"They told me they would always be watching me, always know what I was thinking or feeling or saying. They said they had watchers everywhere, could even read my thoughts. If I ever told anyone anything about what happened I would die and the person I told would be killed. Even if the watchers were dead, they told me they could still have eyes to see me and ears to hear me. They were everywhere and I could never get away."

Losing and Finding the Self

Patients with severe dissociative disorders represent a veritable human encyclopedia of psychological adaptations to childhood abuse, including denying it, exonerating perpetrators, claiming guilt; maintaining sexual innocence, manifesting sexual expertise, using sexuality for power and control; betraying and abandoning the self; rebelling against and defying authority; feeling special, chosen, and above the rules of society (Goodwin, 1989).

Because of severe fragmentation and discontinuity, highly dissociative individuals are perpetually losing and finding themselves (their many selves). They frequently go unrecognized even in the mental health system, where some clinicians' entrenched biases interact with the patients' confusing presentations, eventuating in inaccurate diagnosis and ineffective treatment (Ross, 1997). Dissociation is an oddly invisible defense since when one alter or system of alters is running things smoothly, therapists do not see the dissociative process in operation and may therefore believe they have never seen a dissociative patient (McWilliams, 1994).

> If intimate partners of people with admitted, diagnosed multiple personality disorder miss signs of dissociation, it is not hard to see how uninitiated professionals can be even blinder. People who dissociate learn to "cover" for their lapses. They develop techniques of evasion and fabrication in childhood, as they find themselves repeatedly accused of "lying" about things they do not remember. Because they have suffered horrific abuse at the hands of people who were supposed to protect them, they do not trust authorities, and they do not come to treatment with the expectation that full disclosure is in their interest (p. 331).

The very strategies for conflict avoidance and psychological subterfuge that once saved the lives and the minds of childhood abuse survivors give rise to other thickets that obfuscate diagnosis and obstruct treatment of post-traumatic conditions. Some, for instance, expertly conceal their true anguished and archaic selves beneath compliant false-selves, studied personas of normalcy, and they can often appear as if they have sustained no damage whatsoever from the abuse (Grand and Alpert, 1993). Some patients' patterns of dissimulation and compliance allow for the creation of treatment-seeking selves contemporaneous with the maintaining of attachment to, and collusion with, abusive caretakers/perpetrators (Alpert, 1995). And some patients' oscillations among such extremes as asserting sexual expertise, asexuality, and assertion of sexual innocence, or construing themselves as chronic liars and then as honest informers, produce a continuously perplexing clinical picture. Complex issues of diagnostic comorbidity (reviewed by Kluft, 1996a; Ross, 1995b) amplify the chaos.

The isolation of a child or his/her captivity in an environment whose hallmarks are cruelty and irrational authority has a profound effect on that child's mental and emotional development. Such children live in a persecutory and amnestic structure where there is no continuity and few predictable links between events or relationships. Survivors of chronic trauma develop a strange but enduring attachment to states of *oblivion* and *absorption*. Although resignation, and an abiding sense of futility, contamination, and abandonment all lie close to the center of the dissociative self-organization, many dissociative trauma survivors can actually alternate between periods of heightened dedication to tasks, especially those that serve others, and periods of complete escape from all responsibilities. In extreme dissociative individuals, states of dissociated innocence and naiveté alternate with states of absolute corruption and cynicism. Their fortified persona-restoring functions often leave them oblivious to the reasons why they feel chronically guilty, self-hating, and why they are vulnerable to revictimization.

> Wherever evil occurs, systemic ambiguity, denial, and obscurity will attend it. This collusive trend toward concealment proceeds not only from evil's intrinsic unknowability, but also from the peculiarities of that developmental regression which follows upon massive trauma. For trauma is met and endured by a psyche that is creative in the exigencies of survival. Under threat of annihilation, the mind mobilizes primitive defenses, perceptions, cognitions, and affects . . . in an attempt to metabolize that which cannot be borne . . . these primitive defenses involve an autistic retreat from the human other, and an incapacity to know both history and agency (Grand, 2000, p. 12).

In order to perfect dissociative survival, traumatized individuals must develop their capacities for camouflage and self-deception. By replacing or displacing consciousness and memories of childhood terror and misery with more benign history, they achieve an essentially life-saving compromise-by-traumatic-necessity between surviving and abandoning themselves. The shattered psyche, relentlessly reorganizing and reconfiguring itself in relational milieus of abandonment, neglect, and incredulity, repeatedly discovers safety and protection in reenactment of the original trauma(s)—interspersed with denial, distraction, amnesia, and periods of apparent equanimity. The memorializing of the past through real and symbolic reenactment and repetition dynamics is "a desperate, convoluted attempt to maintain an identity . . . separate from and unvanquished by the original perpetrators" (Kafka, 1995, p. 141), while paradoxically maintaining, at least unconsciously, the attachment bond with childhood caretaker/abusers.

Invisibility, distraction, and ironclad containment allow unbearable suffering to be dispersed and denied in order to ward off (the continuously impending) inundation by traumatic affects and images or the threatened loss of needed attachment objects. The ability to pass as unitary or untraumatized and to shift identities based on perceived danger and interpersonal expectations is strengthened by the survivor's exposure to the cunning and duplicity of his/her abusers, whose agenda of secrecy and subterfuge becomes the victim's own. Now it automatically self-reinforces, but originally it was potentiated by double binds, forced choices, and variously elaborate setups to coerce complicity with the perpetrators' evil, thereby confirming the victim's evil and the shame, guilt, and fear that keep the cloaking devices on.

"When I go to work some real cool guy comes out and takes over and he is incredible at what he does. Not the insecure, incompetent, overly sensitive guy sitting before you. He is so masterful that no one would know anyone else is in here. The nights before work I can feel so much anxiety, all the time, from what I do not know. But then when I go to work, somehow, and I don't know how, he just takes over. Work itself is the best single reinforcer of my dissociation. When I come to therapy from work I cannot just shift out of this mode. When the cool work guy is out there are simply no feelings to feel. For him therapy gets in the way. For me, it feels like my only chance."

"There are too many of them [alters]. They're just getting in my way—why can't they just go away and leave me alone. . . . I don't want feelings, I don't want memories, and I don't want to be MPD. Can't you make it all go away?"

"Childlike voices in my head tell me, 'Please don't hurt me, I won't be bad anymore, I promise. I'm sorry I told, I'll be quiet now, I'll be good.' Angry, mean male voices in my head threaten to kill me repeatedly, saying: 'You traitor, you're nothing without your secrets, you're nothing without us, now you must pay. We can kill you whenever we want to, just remember that.' Another voice in my head keeps saying over and over that I'm just making it all up, why don't you just talk about something else and stop listening to stories about your family that never happened?"

"There are many levels of blocks to my remembering and telling you anything or to knowing my own mind and history. First there is just a big old suitcase slamming shut in my mind saying, 'Danger, Beware, don't go there!' Then there are the threats that people and animals I love will be harmed. That was demonstrated many times by my abusers. The next level is where I feel so sleepy that I cannot remember anything I was thinking about or that I was going to say. I was taught in some state and probably a drugged state, that every time I begin to think about so and so I will begin to feel sleepy, like a hypnosis thing deeply embedded. Beneath that is a layer of command poisoning. Somehow I am supposed to poison myself with something dangerous or take an overdose of tranquilizers if I am beginning to remember or talk to someone outside of the group. Alters have been trained for that. Still, beneath this level are messages to call specific people, contacts in the group, to let them know I have disclosed something and then they will take care of it from there and make sure

I never do anything like that again. Finally, or at least what I can know now is a
level of self-injury and suicide training, sort of like training to have a car accident
or to cut my wrists. You see, I am wired or programmed to die rather than heal."

CAPACITY FOR TRANCE AND
SELF-HYPNOSIS

In pathological families (and criminal systems) where children exist solely to
gratify the psychological needs of the adults, their survival depends on
somehow adjusting to a psychotic world where abusive behavior is acceptable but telling the truth about it is sinful (Summit, 1982). The child, literally
captive to the family (Herman, 1992), must accommodate to norms of assault, exploitation, and betrayal with secrecy, self-sacrifice, and self-betrayal
(Rieker and Carmen, 1986). Biologically driven to form attachments to
his/her primary caretakers regardless of the quality or price of the caretaking, s/he has no choice but to love and want to be loved by his/her abusers
(Ross, 1997). To cope, the traumatized child splits off experiences of terror
and pain. S/he invents illusions of fantastic dividedness, including imagining him/herself as existing and *not existing.*

Over time (and with reinforcement, and biochemical alterations in the
brain)[6] these sophisticated dissociative solutions develop into relatively autonomous alter personalities as well as less organized ego- or self-states generated as repositories for traumatic affects and meanings. The alteration of
memory, consciousness, and identity in ways that prevent full participation
in the interpersonal world makes room for the dissociative individual also
to "reassociate" to fantasies of more powerful self and/or more benign or
benevolent other.[7]

The roles of hypnotizability, suggestibility, and proclivity for fantasy in
the etiology and maintenance of severe dissociative disorders have yet to be
confirmed (Whalen and Nash, 1996). While Bliss (1986) emphasizes that dissociative phenomena are essentially autohypnotic, others comment on the
formidable self-hypnotic capacity of most DID patients, the utility of hypnosis in treatment, the utility of self-hypnosis for focusing, distancing, and
concretizing magical thinking (Bliss, 1980; 1986; Kluft, 1987a; Braun, 1984;
Putnam, 1989; Ross, 1989), and the fact that transient analogs of DID can be
created in normal subjects through the use of hypnosis (Carlson and Putnam, 1989). Still others find little correlation between dissociation and hypnotizability (Kihlstrom et al., 1994; Ray, 1996) or between dissociation,

abuse, and measures of increased use of fantasy and imagination (Rhue, Lynn, and Sandberg, 1995).

Whalen and Nash (1996) conclude that there is no compelling evidence to support the proposition that hypnotizability and dissociativity are overlapping (rather than independent) psychological capacities or personality constructs. And Ross (1997), going a step further, asserts that labeling DID phenomena autohypnotic is tautological—tantamount to inferring etiology from phenomenology; inevitably, a comprehensive model of DID needs to take into account much more than autohypnosis. (Those who remain outraged by the trauma-dissociation connections that ground most current clinical theories insist, to the contrary, that the posttraumatic DID is nothing *but* an artifact of fantasy, suggestion, hypnosis, and social facilitation [Spanos, 1994; Ofshe and Watters, 1994]).

Fantasy and symbolic functions in DID and traumatized patients are quite different from those in nontraumatized people (Van der Kolk, 1987a; Bigras, 1990; Levine, 1990; Krystal, 1978; Huizenga, 1990). Specifically, their uses are highly rigidified, circumscribed, and repetitive, and only minimally restorative, transformative, or interactive with other aspects of mind. In many cases, severely traumatized individuals cannot even imagine benevolent outcomes (i.e., generate restorative or retaliative fantasies); in others, imaginal/symbolizing functions are completely suppressed—or never develop at all.

Personal clinical experience shows most severely dissociative trauma survivors to have unusually restricted imaginal lives; they actually tend to fear deployment of fantasies in problem solving, as if getting too near their inner worlds for any reason could be dangerous. By extension (see Chapter 7), DID should be construed as a disorder *of* fantasy (i.e., characterized by disordered imagination and fantasy) rather than a disorder driven by or arising *from* fantasy. The fact that severely dissociative individuals have the adaptive resources to invent closed systems for surviving physical and psychic pain and impossible double binds does not make them fantasy-prone (or, for that matter, autohypnotic, or otherwise vulnerable to any/every suggestion; in fact, they are variously suggestible and impervious at once). The right question is not how much fantasy, but what kind, for what purpose, how flexible, and how effective in promoting negotiation of complex psychic realities. Furthermore, and in keeping with Ross's (1997) advocacy of a comprehensive etiological model, attributing all of the phenomenology of severe dissociative disorders to any one factor is theoretical reductionism at its most absurd.

OMNIPOTENCE

Omnipotent solutions to traumatization—*I made it happen, I made it (them) go away, I wanted it, I deserved it and the pain makes me stronger; the abuse happened to her, she is not a part of me; I am impervious to any effects of the abusers then and now, I am secretly in charge of everything and everyone, my anger is dangerous and will annihilate everyone and everything, I like being evil and I chose to be evil*—allow the developing child to hold on to elements of healthy grandiosity when all of the nurturing and narcissistic supplies essential to development are either unavailable or only accessible through submission or self-sacrifice. In abusive family systems the requisite disconfirmations of reality and other accommodations to irrational adult authority destroy the healthy self's ability to assign appropriate meanings to, and trust perceptions of, interpersonal behavior. Omnipotent defenses, including manic denial, and alterations in reality and consciousness occur because the child's interpersonal reality has been profoundly distorted and not because the patient was originally developmentally arrested, grandiose, or lost in some elective fantasy disorder, independent of malevolent social forces.

In keeping with omnipotent solutions to childhood trauma, victims commonly minimize their abuse or assume total responsibility for it and for all violent or self-destructive sequelae enacted to reduce helplessness and vulnerability. Grotstein (1999) describes how abused children see themselves as originators of the trauma in order to master it and to reclaim some sense of self-respect or agency: their love was bad (schizoid position), their hatred was bad (depressive position), or their maltreatment was otherwise their fault. Other grandiose distortions may lodge in the shame and guilt of implicit participation, survivor guilt, and/or the perceived failure to stop the abuse from happening.

As in any rigid psychological adaptation or survival, the fixed dissociative repertoire eventually becomes self-limiting and self-destructive. All desperate attempts to maintain attachments and reclaim some aspect of the humanness broken at the time of the trauma only catalyze the submergence of self in a dissociative web of internal persecution and unusual displays of pride and bravado. The adult trauma survivor will often resort to seeking sustenance for unusual defensive grandiose self-states in keeping with what was reinforced in the abusive developmental context—for example, helplessness, perfectionism, compliance, denial, and displays of arrogance, righteousness, and sexuality.

Childhood omnipotence matures into healthy self-esteem when healthy grandiosity, or "archaic expansiveness" (Orange, Atwood, and Stolorow,

1997, p. 81), is mirrored, nourished, and nontraumatically limited; when the shame and self-hatred underlying "defensive grandiosity"(p. 81) are empathically understood; and when compulsive defenses against terrible realities and the fantasies (and the conflicts) they engender do not need to be continuously mobilized (Kohut, 1971).

DEVELOPING ALTER PERSONALITIES

Putnam (1989) succinctly defines alter personalities as "highly discrete states of consciousness organized around a prevailing affect [and] sense of self (including body image) with a limited repertoire of behaviors and a set of state dependent memories" (p. 103). Binding affect, memory, and behavior into such a series protects the abused child against being flooded by painful thoughts and feelings when s/he is not being traumatized and allows him/her to function and to continue, to some extent, to develop (Putnam, 1994). Integrating cognitive and psychodynamic perspectives, Fine (1999) views alter personalities as personified adaptational strategies that may be representations of conflicts, fears, and/or wishes, ultimately representing a traumatized child's desire to not face overwhelming experiences alone. Ross (1994), capturing the essence of MPD, calls it "an auto-immune disorder in which the psyche has become confused about the distinction between self and non-self, and has learned to turn its destructive mechanisms on the self, mistaking it for a foreign invader" (p. xiv). Children build their alter personalities from the raw materials available to them, but their multiple identities are shaped as they mature by influences in the larger society: DID patients may absorb values, attitudes, and stereotypes from family, race, religion, ethnic and other communities, the media (Kluft, 1994), and even from their own individual histories in the mental health system.

Such a complex dissociative defense as the development of alter personalities is not put into place after one traumatic episode; however, the personality fracturing arising from a single event may create the preconditions— malleability and dislocations in both personality and brain chemistry. The more severe and continuous the trauma, the more challenges to the victim, the more complex the dissociative defenses must become (Beere, 1995). Some survivors' "dissociative virtuosity" (Herman, 1992, p. 102) creates barriers to communication and impermeable boundaries for the containment of traumatic affects, escape from the constraints of reality, and an alteration in subjective sense of identity (Putnam, 1989). "The patient creates her own environment based on lack of reciprocity with the external world instead of creating a dialogue with [it]" (Elin, 1995, p. 249).

Victims end up with too many identities, each and all of which are insufficient to anchor them in time, space, and relationship. Most highly dissociative individuals are quite uncomfortable about being seen switching from one to another and will not acknowledge the process even to therapists until real trust is developed (Kluft, 1994). Many actually generate strategies to mask switching from themselves, including the design of special alters to cover the multiplicity in general and the switching phenomena in particular.

As children, most traumatized, dissociative patients consolidate the idea that no one will believe the truth about their abuse and they learn to disavow and disremember (Kluft, 1994), often after letting "their initial denials . . . crumble into false confessions [of lying]" (p. 27). They become masters at rewriting history through alter personality construction, which Braude (1995) calls an *idiom of distress* serving the short-term and then long-term adaptation needs of the besieged individual who wants to reinterpret both past and present in order to harmonize them into some desired vision for life. This process may well be the source of most of the most serious and most common "false" memories in the minds of DID individuals—fabricated memories of *nonabuse* ("Nothing happened," "I made it happen," "I liked it," or "It wasn't that bad").

EXTENT OF THE DISSOCIATIVE SYSTEM

Multiplicity exists on a continuum, and according to Kluft (1988b) the degree of multiplicity experienced by any one individual depends on the amount and severity of the trauma, the degree of dysfunction, the amount and quality of the internal communication among part-selves, and the degree to which the different alters or "parts" cooperate. Networks of alter personalities can vary greatly in their size, their permeability, and in the way aggression is distributed among them to serve developmental functions, trauma containment, and the self-hatred that keeps much of the system running.

In the severe conditions (MPD/DID), the dissociative web may be so intricately interwoven that there is actually considerable overlap among the mental systems and considerable interference with one another. That is, the overall network of dissociative barriers may not be as extensive and impermeable as what the patient presents to him/herself or to the therapist. According to Braude (1995), this explains why dissociated personalities may have common memories and why some MPD/DID child states may have access to adult vocabularies and linguistic capacities, for example. Even when alters know each other's thoughts, experiences, and actions, they nevertheless are considered dissociated from one another in multiple variations of "asymmetrical awareness" (p. 43).[8]

> If one understands the process of alter formation as one of defensive reduplication and/or reconfiguration rather than division, the problem of wondering how the mind becomes divided into such complexity ceases to be relevant. The alters become different patterns of whole and/or partial copying and/or reconfiguring, which, when activated, may be more or less similar to one another, and inevitably will have a lot in common (Kluft, 1988b, p. 57).

One part-self can have a totally loving, deferential, idealizing bond with a parent and refer to him as "my" father while another calls the same man "the" father or "her" father or a "parental unit" or "that other person who does what the adults want." Some alters may hate that parent and some do not know him at all. Aggression is transformed into separate sets of homicidal and suicidal feelings through complex dissociative splits and personifications. Feelings of sexual arousal are often personified in promiscuous alters; sexual repression, sexual avoidance, and/or frigid states predominate in marital or other intimate relationships. Mystics and demons exist side by side but never interact (outside the therapist's office). Epistemological barriers can separate part-selves when they are aware of each others' existence but otherwise dissociated (for such functions as ownership, self-awareness, and capacity for beliefs about self-states' referents) (Braude, 1995). In extreme cases of possession or dissociated will, DID patients report feeling like the passive and obedient instrument of the will of another (Spiegel and Cardena, 1991), although more often guilt- and shame-ridden dissociative trauma survivors claim that their own choices governed when in fact their sense of agency had been obliterated or co-opted by perpetrators whose own perverse wills actually defined and controlled their behavior. Negotiating tangled ownership of responsibility is one of the most difficult aspects of treatment.

The degree of overtness of the alter phenomenology may depend, according to Kluft (1996a), on the resilience of the host alter, the incidence of contemporary stress in the patient's life, the influence of secondary gain, the evidence of narcissistic investment in separateness, and the extent of underlying cooperation and number of shared goals within the dissociative self-system. Personal clinical experience with DID patients who insistently deny their multiplicity and switch smoothly and seamlessly among alters shows it to be most typically submerged by those who are highest functioning and have measurable worldly accomplishments, those who have undergone extensive thought reform and suffered extreme coercion at the hands of criminal perpetrator groups, and those who maintain frequent contact with the sources of their childhood abuse. Their covert alterity is empirically predictive of excessive swings between revelation and recantation, prognostic complications, and a greater likelihood of treatment stalemates.

Kluft's (1985; 1991b; 1995; 1996a) identification of key features and functions of alters is essential to review in light of the sensationalization of flamboyantly overt multiplicity over the past decade and the professional alternation between fascination and incredulity with the alterity phenomenon over the past century.

- The purpose of alters is the creation of alternative self-structures and psychological realities to facilitate emotional survival and cope with intolerable experiences.
- They facilitate that adaptation by segregating certain aspects of experience, self, and knowledge from one another in relatively consistent and rule-bound fashion.
- The form and content they take and elaborate is influenced by characterological and cultural factors, imagination, creativity, intelligence.
- More crucial than overt manifestations to understanding alters and their defensive and developmental functions are inner beliefs, cognitive processes, and complex interrelationships.
- Alters should be construed as "reconfigurations rather than reified divisions" (1996a, p. 343), as ways the mind may be organized rather than as pieces of a pie or any other unity; because the need, incentive, and potential for reconfiguration is exponential, their number may be very large.
- When alters can accomplish their functions without emerging completely and demonstrating their separateness, they often do so, and they are usually quite muted, contrary to public (and sometimes professional) misconception.[9]

Types of Alters.[10]   The development of alters, although purely structural, self-regulatory, and adaptive, is one of the more colorful aspects of extreme dissociative living. The literature describes a wide range of different types— among them: host personalities, child alters, internal persecutors, internal self-helpers, suicidal personalities, protectors and helpers, memory trace personalities, cross-gender personalities, promiscuous alters, administrators and obsessive-compulsive personalities, substance abusers, autistic and handicapped alters, analgesic personalities, imitators and impostors, demons and spirits, personalities with special talents and skills, guardians of memories and secrets, avengers, expressers of hidden impulses, and defenders of or apologists for the abusers (Putnam, 1989; Kluft, 1984a; Ross, 1989). More unusual variations include: animal alters, cross-race personalities, babies, sadists, dead people, zombies, ghosts and other discarnate entities, specific deities, angels or religious saints, demons, mystics, healers, couriers, informers and "tape recorders," trained assassins, trained kidnappers, trained prostitutes, trainers of prostitutes and pornographic performers, time bombs/ booby traps, calendars, indexers, and file managers.

In the dissociative abuse survivor's world the rules of identity are extreme, the operating assumptions and convictions outdated but accepted uncritically, and the fulcrums are domination, exclusion, and polarization. Kluft (1996a), pointing out that most classification systems cannot reconcile the full complexity of the clinical presentations of alterity, distinguishes alters according to their genesis—in response to trauma, to various narcissistic, sexual, and aggressive conflicts, to problems in attachment, and to developmental needs, conflicts, and related deficits.

Goulding and Schwartz (1995) organize alters by roles, conceptualizing three groups—*exiles, firefighters,* and *managers.* Exiles contain needs or traumatic memories and embody sensitivity and fears; often child-identified and frozen in time, they perpetually relive the trauma as if it is happening in the moment. Firefighters, invested with a "negative specialness" that Briere (1989) calls the power to do bad, are assertive, high-energy, highly automatic, controlling parts who relate primarily on the basis of distrust and one-upmanship, act out impulsively and destructively, identify with the perpetrator, and adopt unwise, expedient protective behaviors. Managers permit the individual to function on a daily basis and maintain a façade of normalcy and unity (almost a caricature of the people they have studied in order to "pass"); devoted to work and cunningly manipulative, they actualize high ambitions, tend to be hypomanic, obsessive-compulsive, and socially ingratiating, fear psychological work and cannot tolerate intimacy, and kill off spontaneity by distracting, placating, rationalizing, and avoiding.

Frankel and O'Hearn (1996) compare fractionated internal DID organizations with the fragmented culture of Eastern European Jewish ghettos during World War II. The survival agendas designed in response to extreme and unremitting stress, both individual and social, feature help-seeking *bonding* forces—traumatized alters seeking to offload pain and find someone to improve their lives; *probonding forces* charged with communicating to outsiders about the atrocities—protector alters, whose roles include generating hope, giving comfort, and disclosing secrets of the trauma; and utilitarian *antibonding forces* mandated to prevent destabilization—persecutory alters (often bonded to the abusers), whose job is to disrupt bonding with the outside world to guard against retaliation and preserve attachment to perpetrators and perceived power. (In this model, engaging with the antibonding alters is key: clinicians can defuse the guilt/innocence split, building alliances with them by acknowledging their power in the system, and by empathizing with their isolation and intense shame.)

In therapy, particularly with higher functioning patients—and contrary to the typical focus on aggressive, acting out, and self-destructive or child alters as obstacles to treatment—the internalized collusive, complicitous, and collaborationist states are most profoundly obstructionist. More often than not the source is the worldly host personality, along with passive, vacant, technically innocent alters or clusters of self-states, whose insistent superficiality, direct and indirect camouflage of injuries, naïve protection of the perpetrators, and massive denial are unnegotiable.

Internalized complicitous "bystander" states often serve the rest of the dissociative system as decoys and deflectors, not least from psychological inquiry (for which kind of work they have very poor memories). Collaborator alters, some completely controlled by still other alters, run the gamut from direct assistants to internal perpetrators to "psychotically blind" self-states who miss the most obvious danger cues or facilitate the setting up of the entire personality system for self-destructive enactments. Most commonly, collaborator personalities are modeled specifically on a nonoffending parent or a relative who has managed to remain absolutely oblivious to family reality or who has allowed the child to be abused for conscious reasons (deflecting violence, making money, generating vicarious sadistic gratification) or unconscious reasons (reenacting of his/her own betrayal). These models of complicity (and the alter personalities based on them) tend to act incompetent or in a particularly manipulative fashion, enabling their victimized children to regard them as innocent (and sometimes even enabling others to see them as victims of their children's symptomatology).

Ross (1997) addresses these phenomena under the umbrella of "host resistance" (p. 276), whereby a conscientious, victimized, and often tearful, pathetic host personality entreats the therapist's help in learning about him/herself and getting better—but completely decompensates any time other alters speak or reveal memories. Such a host is enacting the collaborator message "not to communicate" and "not to know" entrenched in the pathogenic family system. And when that host covertly reinforces the rapid switching and acting out on the part of his/her alters, Ross (1997) concludes that the problem is not that the alters come out uncontrollably, but that the host decides to let them out, again enacting the dissimulation, avoidance, irresponsibility, and inconsistency that took place throughout childhood. Ross's worst host-resistance scenario occurs when the host purposefully renders false (increasingly horrendous and extravagant) memories to distract from the real work of therapy, such that the more s/he reveals, the less is actually known.

SHAME AND SELF-HATE

Shame makes us long for invisibility, makes us feel unloved and unlovable (Nathanson, 1992), and most of all isolates us from a feeling of belonging to the human community. In children, chronic shaming leads to chronic dissociation, and chronic reliance on dissociation inevitably leads victims back to experiencing chronic shame. In severe dissociative disorders, shame is so pervasive that the continuous psychological struggle to repress and dissociate it seriously depletes the patient's life energy (Duncan, 1993). In extreme cases it produces extreme psychological organizations—adamant self-sufficiency, spite and defiance, haughtiness and arrogance, numbness, envy, obsessional stubbornness—contrived to protect the vulnerable self from further disintegration. Chronic humiliation and scorn generate profound feelings of defectiveness, weakness, and unworthiness (Nathanson, 1987), leading eventually to a turnoff of all affects and the erection of an *empathic wall* against exposure to and being overwhelmed by other people's emotions. (Empathic walls are part of what sustains separations between alter personalities.)

Child-abuse survivors, like most oppressed groups, experience the particularly entrenched form of shame that comes out of the prolonged distress of forced helplessness and powerlessness. Victims often hate themselves for their vulnerability (and not their perpetrators), and their self-hatred can become a perverse home-base, one they are reluctant to leave in spite of its suffocating limitations:[11] even though they understand at some (entirely separate) intellectual level that they could not have prevented or changed things in any way, they feel tremendous shame for their complicity and incapacity to halt the abuse and end their subjugation. And this shame is profoundly silencing—victims feel complicated allegiance to their victimizers as a function of dynamics ranging from traumatic attachment to mind control (see Chapter 8), and they fear exposure both for themselves and for their abusers—so much so that, ironically, it makes them malleable *accomplices* in their own victimization, especially when the perpetrator knows how to manipulate it.

Imprisonment in shame and self-hatred is cemented in extremely violent and perverse offender group situations, where perpetrators force children to witness and "choose" to participate in wicked actions as a means of binding them to the abuse and to permanent belief in their selves as damaged and evil. The insidious reversal whereby victims are coerced into bearing the responsibility for causing and even desiring their own abuse—whereby the child is the origin of the adult's misdeeds and inheritor of the guilt and shame the perpetrator never seems to feel—is intrinsic to child abuse (Salter, 1995).

Not surprisingly, survivors are deeply confused as to who is responsible. With psyches already organized to internalize massive amounts of shame and guilt disowned by their offenders and by a tacitly collaborative culture, they are unconsciously encouraged to remain in the victimized position (preserving the homeostasis of the perpetrating and colluding systems).[12] Telling victims that what happened to them didn't really happen to them and that they are making it all up due to confusion, unconscious fantasy, or a need for attention solidifies the interlock between perpetrator and collaborator. Grand (2000) calls this labyrinthine system of mutual influence (including intrapsychic and interpersonal transactions) among perpetrator(s), bystander(s) and victim(s) "malignant dissociative contagion" (p. 17).

"When I cried and told him to stop my father said I was faking because he said I was a little whore and I wanted it. Then, later when I told him that he was hurting me, he said that he knew I was lying because I wasn't crying, and he kept on hurting me."

"It seemed so normal from the outside when you didn't know the whole story and all that was going on. The only explanation that I could come up with was that I was the crazy one, since they were all acting like nothing was going on, watching television, talking and eating. They seemed to be having a good time. My father was always more talkative and nicer to the other kids after he raped me. He was calmer, and he even paid attention to them a little, which he almost never did. I would be feeling so strange and sick to my stomach; and then, on top of that, I thought I must be the crazy one since they are all acting so normal. Then I'd hate myself for not being like everyone else. I always wished to be normal. Then I just stopped thinking about it."

"I can't find my self-hatred anymore. How am I going to take care of myself? I feel naked without it."

Feminist legal scholar Catharine MacKinnon (1987) articulates the societal bind that can only be managed by turning the victim into a nonperson:

> Whoever is so cumulatively violated as to be an emblem of collective violation is simply not that bundle of rights termed the individual. If it happened and it hurt her, she deserved it. If she didn't deserve it either it didn't happen or it didn't hurt her. If she says it hurt her, she's oversensitive or unliberated. If she says it happened, she's a liar or a natural-born whore. Either it didn't happen or she loved it. (MacKinnon, 1987, p. 13)

Internalized paradigms of domination blend all too well with the same cultural or familial authority that blames dissociative survivors and denies their reality. The insidious and ironic result is that the cumulative trauma of child sexual abuse and torture makes victims into the best perpetrators against themselves and powerful collaborators in their own torment and captivity— even when they begin to take some steps out of the domination systems. In the first half of treatment, and sometimes even later, advances toward autonomy and differentiation may be met with an internal backlash as though the perpetrators in patients' heads (and sometimes the ones in their lives as well) are tugging on their leashes lest the survivors think themselves actually free.

Eventually, when the illusion of power and control is broken and the truth revealed, a deeper level of psychic pain must be processed in an extended and difficult mourning (Ross, 1997). Unbearable grief emerges as the granite layers of self-hatred and shame erode. Owning this level of suffering without the anesthesia of dissociative armor is perhaps the most highly integrative (and challenging) phase in the psychotherapy of severely dissociative patients.

The compounded shame of the dissociative trauma survivor leads to psychic imprisonment and sense of exile from humanity because it is based on multiple interlocking and overlapping sources. Shame comes from

- the pain, humiliation, betrayal, and degradation endured during the trauma;
- the inability to have protected the self and stopped the traumatic event(s) from taking place, the inability to prevent their impact and avoid experiencing loss of control, and (in some cases) the inability to have preempted the abuse of others;
- the coerced violation of your own ethics or moral principles, the betrayal/violation of others in order to survive;

- the symptoms of posttraumatic stress disorder and the societal response to those symptoms, including psychiatric labels, diagnoses, and misdiagnoses;
- the fragmentation, intrusion, inconsistency, and incompleteness of memories, and the constant challenge to their reality from skeptics in media, academic, medical, and psychotherapeutic settings;
- the feeling of not being like other people, not belonging, and the loss of a sense of kinship with humanity;
- the feeling of being marked, damaged, and transparent—the feeling that others can see right through you and know what you have done or what has been done to you;
- the social stigma of being an abuse survivor and the internalization of society's contempt, incredulity, and impatience with the vicissitudes of recovery (*"just get over it already"*), and the labeling of your therapist (perhaps the only person you trust) as a quack;
- the internalization of hateful, degrading messages from the perpetrator(s) and from society's blame-the-victim/pull-yourself-up-by-your-own-bootstraps rhetoric, and the harboring of "dirty" secrets that cannot be shared;
- the harboring of hateful, vengeful, destructive thoughts (and/or part-selves);
- the perversion of your sexuality and the residue of bizarre, unusual, or utterly absent sexual needs and desires;
- the awareness that you welcomed feelings of specialness or actual privileges conferred by the perpetrator(s);
- the inability to forgive perpetrators in a culture that insists on and romanticizes forgiveness;
- the vulnerability to experiencing certain normal activities as triggers (e.g., films, holidays, gatherings), such that they cannot be enjoyed;
- the history of self-destructive acting out, and the accrued costs of the effects of trauma in terms of vocational, financial, medical, and interpersonal functioning;
- the chronic out-of-control feelings and the knowledge that other people do not walk around leaking profound losses, sensitivities, and vulnerabilities "like someone with a bladder problem—only this one's emotional";
- the psychological and physiological damage that will never heal in spite of your own (and others') best efforts.

"People around you cause you to feel that you are perpetrating on them for tak-ing the time to face something so difficult and to heal the trauma. There is this in-tense shame around that. My husband complained constantly about the distractions I was causing to our life, and that I wouldn't have sex with him whenever he wanted. He asked me to have a timeline to have the whole thing healed in six weeks. And my male therapist actually sat me down and told me that I should reach past my wounds to have sex with my husband whenever he wanted. This was a complete reenactment of what happened to me as a child because the perpetrator convinced me that I was wrong for not wanting to have sex with him."

IDENTIFICATION WITH THE PERPETRATOR

"She must love the people who hurt her, or die. This is the core problem in DID, and the primary driver of the dissociation" (Ross, 1997, p. 284). At-tachment to the perpetrator is emerging as the central issue in all treatments of trauma survivors. The abused child, trapped in an impossible situation, must bond with his/her abuser(s) in order to survive, must learn how to for-get his/her injuries and who caused them, and must internalize the abuser's power in order to maintain sanity.

The choice faced by the chronic trauma survivor is not a choice at all (Daskovsky, 1998). Identifying with one's abuser(s) against one's self is nat-urally preferred to experiencing powerlessness, mortification, and betrayal at the hands of needed and loved caretakers. Identification with the aggres-sor is a complex defense first described by Anna Freud (1936) whereby vic-tims cope with helplessness, pain, and humiliation by doing to others (or, in the case of DID, to the self and others) what is or was previously done to them. They achieve delayed mastery over their traumas—overcoming help-lessness and transforming themselves from threatened to threatening—by participating in the omnipotence of the perpetrators, assuming their atti-tudes and imitating their behavior. The child registers the parent as delu-sionally good (Shengold, 1989) and him/herself as delusionally bad, effectively intensifying his/her self-hatred while blindly obeying irrational authority and mystifying (and often eroticizing) domination.

Survivors of severe trauma, burdened by histories of conflict over loss of protection and lifelong vulnerability to feelings of abandonment, cling in masochistic desperation to the people who treat them in intrusive, neglect-ful, cruel, and seductive ways (Valenstein, 1973; Levine, 1994; Howell, 1997)—"velcroing to the abuser," in the words of one patient. In distorted attachment processes that go beyond the classical identification with the aggressor, victims with well-articulated collaborator-alters deny the extent or reality of the damage that has been (or is being) done.

DID children who have "chosen" to master their trauma by assisting in their own (or others') traumatization enter therapy as adults either completely convinced of their own guilt, shame, and blameworthiness—or convinced that almost nothing happened. Sorting out who did what to whom in past and present is not easy in the case of the child who instigated sexual contact instead of enduring helpless anticipation of it, who handed her mother the implements of torture to be used on her, who provoked the anger of the perpetrator/caretaker simply to get the abuse over with. It is almost as if what has been dissociated most profoundly is the intention, motivation, and accountability of the perpetrator/caretaker and the responsibilities of the colluding family and social systems.

The result of a prolonged immersion and dependent involvement with powerful adults perpetrating unspeakable abuses is that love, desire, and pleasure will be forever fused with fear, hatred, and pain, leading to a lifetime of bizarre relationship dynamics. Although from a legal-ethical point of view it is absolutely clear that sexual abuse and torture of children is a crime and that the adult is totally culpable regardless of the child's apparent acquiescence, the psychological reality is another story indeed (Daskovsky, 1998): the abuse may have been terrifying but it may also have been experienced as offering a moment of deeply longed-for closeness or of being needed or wanted in an otherwise globally neglectful surround; the pain of sexual stimulation may have been excruciating, but it may have also been disturbingly exciting or pleasurable in some ways, producing enormous confusion about accountability and choice.

A victim of child abuse may well feel even more shame when s/he responds to sexual arousal. And when the child-victim's desire is experienced as the basis for vulnerability, his/her entire relationship to desire itself becomes highly conflicted (Ehrenberg, 1992). When yearnings for attachment, self-esteem, and specialness foster in the child's concrete mind a level of instrumentality verging on participation or pleasure in the abuse, the victim has been betrayed by his/her own needs.

The need for secure attachment figures is part of what drives the invention of alters: if there is no one on the outside to love and no one on the inside with any power, then the DID solution is to create them (Ross, 1989; 1997). Different alters may become organized around different aspects of the aggressor—power, cunning, contempt, superiority, ideologies, and systems of rationalization. To grasp the complexity of DID is to appreciate the manifold dimensions of identification with the aggressor, the shrapnel of which process lodges throughout even the most apparently benign parts of the patient's self-system.

CONFUSION OF MINDS, INTENTIONS, AND MOTIVATIONS

Ferenczi (1933) suggests, in his justly renowned articulation of the psychological compromises of abused children ("The Confusion of Tongues Between Adults and the Child"), that the child-victim may collude unconsciously with what s/he believes to be the parent's needs and desires, which come to be experienced and *remembered* as his/her own. A child is exceedingly vulnerable to an adult's projections of guilt and anxiety, but his/her personality is not sufficiently consolidated to protest in thought or in action by way of expressing overwhelming confusion about boundaries, roles, and responsibilities—what happened, why it happened, or who made it happen. Ferenczi recognizes the double bind of the abused child introjecting both the guilt feelings of the adult and the adult as desperately needed object. To adapt, the child identifies with the aggressor and develops self-loathing; the only way to sustain attachment and please the abuser is to betray the victimized self.[13]

> The overpowering force and authority of the adult makes them dumb and can rob them of their senses. . . . When the child recovers from such an attack, he feels enormously confused, in fact split—innocent and culpable at the same time—and his confidence in the testimony of his own senses is broken. (p. 162–163)

Holding oneself entirely responsible for a negative event—blaming the self to preserve a sense of personal control and ward off feelings of helplessness and powerlessness (Janoff-Bulman, 1992)—may contribute to the development of an omnipotent fantasy of protection, allowing the victim to imagine she can sustain not only attachment and an illusion of power but also hope that s/he can prevent painful recurrences of the trauma.

Almost robotically, self-hate and self-mockery are used to redirect and cohere fragmented affects and belief systems so that the trauma survivor does not have to know him/herself as victim or his/her caretakers as abusers and betrayers. Instead, s/he muses indefinitely, and sometimes quite pridefully, on being "so bad no one could get near me," or filthy, worthless, and evil ("It's just a matter of time until you find out who I really am").

"When they yelled at me and ordered me around, inside me where they couldn't see me I yelled back at them. But when they laughed at me, when they mocked and humiliated me with hateful meanness I couldn't use my anger at them anymore—it didn't work—and so I joined them and belittled myself. I even enjoyed putting that boy down. Then when they laughed at the end like it was all a big joke, or a big pretend, or a big game I laughed with them too."

"I hate myself for letting him do that to me. I hate my body for responding. I hate that it still affects me and all of my relationships. I hate that he still has any power over me. I am so busy hating me I cannot see anyone or anything else."

"Am I so deeply ashamed of myself because I was helpless? Am I ashamed because I submitted and didn't shout or fight back. When I helped him or let him abuse me something broke in me. The first time I did that—not fight back in any way I mean—inside of me or outside—after that I know I was never the same again."

"Worse than feeling the pain itself is feeling like they got to me, like I failed for not fending them off, and worse than that is to think because of this they are inside of me and I am like them and always carrying around the dread that this could come out of me and I could do this to someone else even in the smallest way."

"After he raped me and in between the times he did, my father said to me what a worthless piece of garbage you are, you will never amount to anything. I have heard this in my head all my life. I have treated myself like garbage. And I have tried to prove I am not garbage. I don't know what was worse, what he did or what he said."

SELF-DISTRUST

The dynamics of shame, self-hate, and identification with the aggressor are fundamentally silencing because survivors of chronic trauma learn to distrust their feelings and sense of reality. They come to feel as if they have no right to feel what they feel or to know what they have known for so long. Protecting the perpetrator and protecting the self from exposure become one and the same agenda. Curiosity, self-observation, and reflectivity are suppressed and undeveloped; feelings and wishes become dangerous psychological territory instead of drivers of development. Sexual arousal, desire, and attraction become transmuted into helplessness and powerlessness, invoking major dissociative strategies and defensive patterns of mastery based on sadomasochistic solutions.

False memories of nonabuse or minimized abuse replace historical truth. Fantasies of invulnerability replace realities of helplessness. Personifications and enactments of self-hate replace healthy assertion, differentiation, and normal fantasies of retaliation. Suicidal fantasies fill the void created by the absence of soothing internal objects and privately become a perverse form of self-mothering and self-love. Fears of knowing and being known, and difficulties with regard to taking action (Ehrenberg, 1992) supplant a healthy quest for recognition and intimacy and the capacity for agency.

Survivors of severe trauma do not want to listen to themselves. They are exceedingly ambivalent about being heard and believed. To discover the historic reality of their fractured and betrayed existence, and to really know and experience its effects on their present lives, is such an overwhelming proposition that they have chosen, consciously and unconsciously (and in some cases forcibly through mind control), to collude in the silencing and "forgetting" of abusers and collaborating others. DID epitomizes the backfiring process whereby patients "originally victimized by others . . . they could not control, become victims of their own counterproductive survival techniques" (Ehrenberg, 1992, p. 6). In order to survive outrageous abuse and brutality, the chronically traumatized have lost and forgotten their voices.

If and when a severely dissociative patient comes to recognize what kind of disturbance s/he is contending with, s/he must then face degrading and invalidating media and academic portrayals of him/herself (and his/her therapist). The typical DID patient as presented in the media has thousands of alter personalities speaking in different accents, claims to have been a high-ranking member of an intergenerational cult, has no memories of abuse prior to starting therapy, seeks attention incessantly (especially from the media), and recants both her reported trauma history and her dissociative symptoms while pursuing lawsuits against her former therapists (Barach, 1999a).

Academic invalidation emphasizes severely dissociative trauma patients' fantasy-proneness and exaggerated needs to be believed, or their concretization of inchoate fantasies (Ganaway, 1994; Brenneis, 1997; Merskey, 1992; 1995), their roles as "storytellers" to the culture and their tendencies to "vivify and concretize more ambiguous struggles" and pass them on as actual traumatic experiences (Haaken, 1998), or their victimization by their therapists' spurious suggestions or countertransference resistances and enactments (Ganaway, 1989; 1994; Spanos, Burgess, and Burgess, 1994; Simpson, 1995; Brenneis, 1997).

Some academics view child-abuse survivors as victims not of trauma and neglect but of "semantic contagion" and "false consciousness" (Hacking, 1995), and label female survivors as suffering not from trauma but from memorophilia—addiction to the inspirational and seductive value of their stories (Haaken, 1998). Designated "empowered hysterics" who are mesmerizing their therapists, women have been said to be using recovered memories to escape diffuse conflicts from growing up female, misguidedly taking on the identity of multiplicity as a pitiful tool of rebellion, and all too willingly collapsing their developmental possibilities by following their therapists down the "dead-end street of messianic psychiatry" (Haaken, 1998, p. 221).

"When they made me dance on that stage in front of all those men I just took three steps backwards, and then there was some girl there and she was dancing for them, and I watched her do it from far away. Yes, this man trained me first how to act. She was supposed to go over to each man who showed her a coin and dance for him. She was not me, but I could see her. I didn't like her and I didn't like what she was doing. Even though I know she is me, she is not really me. I hate talking about this."

"I have this weird relationship with mirrors. When I look in the mirror I see this guy there, I don't see me. This is the way it has always been. I have thoughts, feelings—mostly criticisms and negative feelings about that guy but it is not me. I never knew what to make of that."

"I'm really just learning that the abuse isn't happening anymore. That's where the pain is, that's why I can feel pain. But I need you to know that there are parts of me that are still back there, like it's still happening and this therapy is hardest on them. While it is still happening they don't have to feel pain. If it's over, the hurt begins. So it's no victory at all to know it isn't happening anymore and never will happen again."

"One part is relieved I told you what happened, another part fears you're going to make me deal with the feelings too, another part of me is doubting and doing the false memory thing saying you put it all in me: you made me think it and say it, and another part of me is telling me—just wait, there is more to come."

"I hate thinking about what they [abusers] told me; it's in my head but I don't like to know it's there. I'm afraid to think about it or say it. If I say it I might become it. If I tell you what they taught me I might become what they taught me. My head is not a safe place. It can make me turn into someone else."

"The hard part about being multiple is that you can never finish your own thoughts. It's made that way you know because it's made a lot for distraction. It gets you into all kinds of trouble and it is hard to have a life this way."

ISOLATION AND NUMBNESS

Dissociative solutions to survival compress vitality and lead to a kind of living psychic death. Survivors shut themselves out and shut down by refusing permeability and they use up energy by keeping information out (Alpert, 1995). Old data, often unprocessed and unintegrated, is suspended and overvalued, and new material, particularly new relationship experience, cannot penetrate the dissociative barriers to rearrange traumatic belief systems. In severe dissociative disorders, this lifelessness is often buried beneath several layers of feigned normalcy.

Living psychic death is the goal in a way: if you're dead already, no one can kill you anymore; if you have no life energy left, no one take it from you; if your sexual arousal is either frozen or compulsively and promiscuously acted out, no one can control or violate your sexuality again. Repeating disasters, cultivating destructive relationships, and even inflicting pain on yourself to feel alive means that trying to hurt or negate yourself is actually saving yourself. Hating yourself is loving yourself. If suicidal fantasies are your internalized, comforting parents, no one can obliterate you without your being in control. The excruciatingly painful reality of isolation, alienation, and abandonment is buried deep beneath the cacophony of the dissociative diaspora.

"There is a coldness and numbness that comes from watching horrible, torture things being done to animals and children, and an even greater numbness and deadness that takes you over when you have to be participating in the violence. The worst numbness, like a soul death, is when you have to orchestrate others doing the whole thing, but by then you are so cut off from yourself and everyone else who is still human and loving and kind that you are nothing but a glove for the hands of the perpetrators and you feel you belong in Hell or that you must die for having survived."

"When they were fucking me I became them and it stopped the hurting. And it felt good to be the one hurting me, in charge of all that, instead of them. Now, even though I know it's me and that this belief is not real, I cannot find my way back to that little boy who was getting hurt. I haven't even felt sorry for him yet."

"With all your [therapist's] hard work, there's still no real danger of breaking through. Don't let yourself think that they [the alters/protectors] are worried that

you [the therapist] are even getting close. It's like they are still dancing in the ball-rooms of Berlin and you haven't even landed your troops on Normandy yet."

"You have no idea how precious it can be to not care anymore about anything."

"They didn't hurt me, I didn't feel anything they did, nothing got to me and nothing ever will; if I let myself feel things and know how much he got to me, then he wins all over again."

"I don't want to be helped and I don't want to be loved. I just want to be left alone. If I am continuously mean to you and torment you the way I have been doing in here, then I will make you hate me and then you will make me go away, and then that will be that—I won't have anything to worry about anymore—I'll be through with all of this. If I trust you I have to feel, and I don't want to feel anything."

INDIFFERENCE TO ESCAPE

The dubious privilege of having to join with and seek recognition from what passes for culture, society, and normalcy in the world of regular, nontraumatized people may come to be excruciating for survivors once their dissociative barriers have become permeable. The "normal" world—quite often hollow, corrupt, and hypocritical—may seem merely another reflection and variation of the damaging, authoritarian, and perverse familial world in which they were broken and corrupted. As child-abuse survivors ricochet between cultivating hope in some form of trustworthy social institutions and recognizing the authoritarian and duplicitous dimensions of society, the agonizing existential dilemma may seem like a bitter cosmic joke-conspiracy. Bypassing that awareness may be one of their strongest motivations for safeguarding dissociation as a buffer. Obversely, bypassing confrontation with the excruciating awareness of our failure as a species may be one of society's strongest motivations for perpetuating denial and disavowing the realities of survivors of severe childhood trauma.

"When I realized after some time in recovery and therapy that I was a survivor, all of a sudden things made sense to me, and for the first time in my life I no longer felt like an alien or a pariah. But now, when I remember things that actually happened to me that are such an extreme from what the world knows or believes or understands I feel that alienated and excluded feeling all over again, and I hate feeling that way. It's hard to get past that sense of not belonging with other humans."

"They [the abusers] stole my life and now I have to spend the rest of my life getting back my life. It's so unfair. They're not paying, I am."

"I get confused because everyone is saying how you shouldn't be a victim, and there are people who say those who are victims just want to be pitied and get things for free. They [the abusers] made a powerless object out of me. I used to think the only way to not be a victim was to pretend I wasn't one. But, the only way to not be a victim is by knowing that I was one, and then I don't have to be a victim anymore. It's paradoxical, but it's the only way."

"What kind of forgiveness can you expect when there is no articulation. Just like, sure, yeah, I forgive you, but there is no depth. The hungry ghost of my abuser just wants forgiveness but I have to do all the articulation myself and I resent that. But you know what I resent even more than that is that I have to do all of the articulation for everyone . . . my family, the world, everyone."

DIFFICULTIES OF COMMUNICATING IN PSYCHOTHERAPY

There are always surprises and double or triple meanings with severely dissociative patients. Time is never perceived in linear terms. The past is conflated with the present, and the present can actually dissolve into a full tilt flashback of the past where the patient is absolutely convinced that someone in his/her current life, often the therapist, is harming him/her when, in fact, this is not the case. The future is hopelessly nonexistent and the experience of the present is powerfully shadowed by a past that is distorted or unknown (never thought or fully known). Flashbacks, dreams, and memories of human sacrifice may come to represent symbolically either previously unformulated inchoate primitive psychological experience or the individual's perceived sacrificial relationship with caretakers and/or the larger society. Or they may not be symbolic representations at all, but rather the residue of witnessing actual human sacrifice—usually considered impossible in Western industrialized societies.

Such comments might be a test of what the therapist can tolerate—or they might be a way to avoid other issues. Similarly, depressive symptoms and fantasies can be used to cover posttraumatic dynamics—or talk about trauma can be used to avoid the underlying grief and despair; mystical experience can be intrinsic to the internal or external world of DID patients—but at the same time it can be used to camouflage dimensions of multiplicity or "spiritual emergency" characterized by the fragmentation of the self. A high-functioning adult can rapidly shift into a quivering child as a result of some unknown triggers. Or, after years of therapy, a "new face" can appear in the relationship and the patient will interview the therapist as if s/he had never before attended a session.

What is most important for the therapist to hold at all times is that s/he cannot immediately know what any dream, fantasy, or memory means either in the patient's experience or in the therapeutic relationship. For instance, in DID, a fantasy can become a compelling subjective reality on a moment's notice. Recalled history (forgotten or never forgotten) can be doubted and called fantasy. Consensually validated reality can be abruptly suspended, never to reappear. Trauma can be acknowledged, then disavowed, hundreds of times. Different alters will maintain different impressions of the past and present to such an extent that it is even difficult for an experienced clinician not to fall into the trance logic of believing s/he is dealing with an entire factionalized village. A patient can talk cavalierly, without feeling or a sense of meaning, about childhood beatings that resulted in still-visible scars, and yet become increasingly agitated and distrustful because an item in the therapist's office is not in its usual place. A child alter can express authentic traumatic affects and memories or split-off capacities for bonding, reaching, and longing, or s/he can be used by a patient's dissociative system to divert stress from the demands of an interaction that forces a confrontation with dissociative relatedness.

"Why are you pushing me to have my feelings? I hate you for making me feel. If I feel, then I will lose everything. Why do you want me to lose everything? And, If I come to like you or depend on you, will bad things happen to you?"

"You know how some people have false selves. Well we have false memories, only our false memories are real memories and we hold them as false memories. We wonder how you could ever believe us about anything. We want to discredit you for even considering believing us. But it seems you don't want to participate in our forgetting and this makes some of us very irritated with you."

"I'm angry at all of the people who left me in that abused and abandoned condition. I had to learn to say no to you and no to everyone and everything else before I could say yes, even to myself, because I was so deceived for so long about the yesses I thought I said, the yesses they told me I said—I just didn't know that I or anyone else could survive the pain of my saying No."

"I am ready to start being free. I'm scared. There are still a few parts of me who are not as ready as I am. I'm afraid they can still get the upper hand—but I know it is only if I let them. I know I need to listen to them—they are me, aren't they?—but I won't let them get the upper hand anymore. I want to show up for my life, to love and be loved in my life, to know tenderness, and yes, that too, sorrow. I am ready. Scared, but ready."

"I want to hurt you and then again I don't want to hurt you. This is why I may not be able to stay in therapy. This is my dilemma. You always told me that I could, but I have been too scared to talk about wanting to kill you for fear that I would kill you just by talking about wanting to. Like the babies I had to kill and the children I had to hurt with them, in this case you are the baby and I am the killer and I do not want to do that to anyone ever again. The more I talk about wanting to kill you, not just talking about wanting to kill you, but from the place in me that wants to kill you, the more I realize that I am not going to do that, and that this may be a safe place to be."

"This therapy isn't about my retrieving memories, this is about retrieving parts of myself. If I have to deal with memories as part of that I will and I have and I will again, but that's not really what it's all about—it never was. I need to reclaim every lost part of myself. That's what it is all about."

"I can see past all the shame I felt for so long for not having stopped him, for not having completely stopped this evil from spreading to other parts of my family. But now I realize that redemption does not come from stopping evil. By encountering evil and not becoming it, that is what redemption is all about. Not stopping it. It's about surviving it and not becoming it."

"As a child, I was gang raped. But I've used that to transform myself and I don't see it as a curse. Even though it has taken me many years to heal it—now I see it as one of my gifts. It allows me to be the healer I am because I have a place, a space inside of me that understands wounds—intimately, physically, universally. It allows me to see other people with greater compassion. With abuse and trauma you either turn it to light or you get snuffed out in the darkness."

JARED

Camouflage can break down and dissociative disorders reveal themselves in response to small triggers (a book, a movie, a therapist's inquiry) or major life crises (a death, a divorce, having a child, losing a job)—or in the presence of real love and intimacy, as was the case for Jared, a thirty-eight-year-old gay physical therapist who entered psychotherapy at the request of his partner and their couples therapist when both became concerned about his severe and unexplainable shifts from tenderness and timidity to cruelty and sadism.

Jared had long ago figured out that keeping emotional intimacy separate from sexuality staved off some of the intrusive posttraumatic symptoms—anxiety, depression, memory failure, difficulties managing anger, voices arguing in his head—he had been masking all his life with workaholism, substance abuse, sexual compulsivity, and massive denial. Jared had always resisted falling in love because the unpredictability of spontaneous emotional exchange threatened the control that was so pivotal to sustaining his equilibrium. Jared's dissociative condition began to surface when he entered this first healthy, nonexploitative romantic relationship.

At first, Jared presented in individual therapy like many high-functioning DID patients who are not in an acute psychological crisis—depressed but with an affable, compliant, and gentle demeanor that alternated with a very good sense of humor and an extreme avoidance of any real intimacy or vulnerability. He was aware that he used entertaining people as a way of managing anxiety and controlling interpersonal situations, but his ability to reflect on the meaning of this was initially quite limited. As time went on, Jared's charming style began to show gaps. Intermittently, when anything emotional would emerge in a session, and when humor and evasion could not be deployed to manage the tension, Jared would become quite remote; it sometimes appeared as if there was no one there.

At other times, there seemed to be a sarcastic, hostile, or menacing presence operating from behind his affable persona that would seek out opportunities to make derisive remarks about his partner, people in general, and at times in a very covert way about me as well. This hostility occurred in such a camouflaged and confusing manner that I was often left wondering if what I believed happened actually happened. That is, I became hesitant to confront Jared or even bring these comments to his attention because I came to doubt my own sense of reality. Somehow Jared had me wondering if I was being unfair to him and taking things he said out of context or simply misunderstanding him.

When I eventually questioned Jared directly about his hostility, especially toward me, he adamantly denied any such feelings and attempted to change the subject. Caught in a complex, emerging multidimensional transference/countertransference matrix, I found myself alternating between feelings of protective affection and chronic irritation and anger deriving from an uneasy sense that I was being toyed with. Tracking the sequences of what led to what became almost impossible, because of the increasing rapidity of shifts in Jared's states, his investment in camouflaging his dissociative disorder, and my own intermittent bewilderment.

After a few months in treatment when his awareness of his dissociative process was growing, and when memories of possible sexual abuse by his father, his grandfather, and an extremely sadistic pedophile group were just beginning to emerge, Jared began showing increasing hostility toward his partner and to some extent toward me as well. He seemed to look for opportunities to provoke conflicts and assault his partner's deepest vulnerabilities, and he tended to act most maliciously when his partner was having the hardest time emotionally. Jared was angry at his partner for relentlessly loving him, fighting for him, and threatening his fragile equilibrium; he was angry at me for "penetrating" his façade (an offense he experienced with all the associations of a survivor of sexual abuse) and for evoking overwhelming pain and anxieties.

Jared began to increase his use of alcohol in order to manage his anxiety and also to subdue the cruelty he was inflicting and the guilt and upheaval that followed. His escalating attempts to provoke his partner into rejecting him temporarily succeeded when he engaged in an outside sexual liaison on the day after his partner lost his job and was in deep distress. Jared immediately reframed the episode as a function of his own need for space, whereupon his partner, disgusted and completely exhausted, agreed to a separation. But he also confronted and named the passive-aggressive setup and the cruelty underlying it, marking the first time in Jared's life that someone close to him (whom he loved and who he knew loved him) had forcefully exposed his self- and other-destructive patterns (in words rather than in actions).

In a reversal of intention and responsibility typical of severely dissociative individuals early in treatment (and also of perpetrators, for that matter), Jared then claimed that it was his partner who had broken up with him and not the other way around. He felt no overt, conscious guilt. He believed the cover story he had concocted to mask his dissociative split and the evidence of his strong identification with sadistic perpetrators, whose representatives in his system could usually tell the other alters what to think when he was under stress and they got the upper hand. (Those perpetrator-identified alters had taken him over completely during an earlier such period and, in classic DID/PTSD fashion, sponsored self-destructive enactments involving drug use, prostitution, and ultimately infection with HIV.)

Now "abandoned" by the one person in his life who had loved him as close to unconditionally as he had allowed, Jared was thrown back into feeling states related to his parents' leaving him alone with his grandfather for long periods of time; he was enraged, lost all sense of control, and began to become undone. He was desperate to avoid the avalanche of memories that were about to surface and the implications of the mounting evidence of his personality changes and behavior. Part of Jared's stress came from the fact that he was surrounded by three relationships where his behavior was consistently monitored and compassionately confronted. In the past, Jared had managed to live a life of interpersonal hit-and-runs where confrontation and honest feedback were avoided at all costs; he had shed old relationships like reptiles shed their skin and he moved on to the next one without integrating the meanings of each experience. Altogether overwhelmed by the compassionately aggressive intervention, Jared was struggling with the *sadistic voices in his head* that insisted that his partner and both therapists were monsters. He was experiencing these three relationships as he had experienced serial rape throughout his childhood in the sadistic pedophile group (his involvement with which had not quite fully surfaced in treatment). Yet he also experienced them as the kind of family intervention he had always longed for—so he alternated between anger and gratitude. Because of his growing capacity to hold both emotions in one consciousness Jared was able for the first time to question the dominating, sadistic voices.

Thus on the verge of some of his greatest breakthroughs in therapy and in intimacy, Jared urgently and abruptly left town. The degree to which the self-destruction to which he turned was an act of will or an unconscious reenactment of submission to perpetrators—and/or an expression of the magnitude of the threat of therapy—remained ambiguous. He returned to the environment where he had prostituted during his last acting-out episode, and was paid well to participate in an orgy that turned out to be far from innocuous. His sadistic alters had believed they were in control, but in fact had fallen prey to a group of vicious men who had spent time in prison and had lured Jared to be bound and gang raped. In his retrospective accounts, Jared described how the child part of him was brought out to endure this violation while the sadistic part watched. At the time, however, he hid out for a week using alcohol and drugs to numb the pain of the internal injuries he had suffered and to recover and create a narrative for what had taken place. Meanwhile, his various alter personalities fought and vied for power.

Jared emerged some two weeks later with several different stories: cruelly, he boasted to his partner of how well he was doing and of how many new boyfriends he had—only to initiate another contact later the same day, during which a gentle, scared Jared recalled only that he had needed to get something out of his system and that he never wanted to do "that" again; when asked what "that" was, he became evasive and disoriented. In another, more childlike voice he shared with his partner his intense fear of losing control and his embarrassed confusion as to why they were not together anymore. He was battling a blank memory for the events of the past month and a nagging feeling that he had done something terribly hurtful and wrong.

With the support, dedication, and perseverance (not to mention unresolved masochistic issues) of his partner, and with an individual therapist and a couples therapist skilled in the treatment of dissociative survivors, Jared remained in treatment, where both clinicians welcomed feedback from him about how they might have handled the crisis situation differently, engendering real trust and mutuality by taking his criticisms seriously as no authority figure ever had before. Unlike some dissociative patients who use their therapist's errors and imperfections to solidify distrusts or evade responsibility, Jared began to exchange his lifelong blaming, externalizing, and avoiding stance for ownership of his multiple self-states, abusive actions, and internal conflicts.

The point at which a dissociative trauma survivor's world is finally recognized and challenged is often when the opportunity for growth is most seriously sabotaged. The threatened dissociative system mobilizes a takeover by its most pernicious and ultimately self-destructive forces in a desperate effort to restabilize and camouflage itself, in spite of the best efforts of clinicians who are sensitive to clinical issues of timing, pacing, unconscious anxiety over loss of protective object relations, and preservation of functioning. Jared let himself fall apart, successfully confronted his multiplicity, and eventually faced some of his tortured past. Instead of enacting another macabre narrative with his body and his partner as instruments, he revealed and played out his identities and stories inside the container of psychotherapy. Jared was lucky (and courageous). Many dissociative survivors do not make it to this point.

CHAPTER 2

Unfathomable Realities, Discredited Testimony: Child Abuse, Victims, and Perpetrators

Try thinking without apology with what you know from being victimized. Give up the Olympian partiality of objectivity and try for a fairness and an authority that neither dominates nor submits to your material or your audience. . . . Look for the deepest meaning in the least elevated places. Be more radical than anyone has ever been about the unknown because what has never been said is probably what we need most to know.
—Catharine A. MacKinnon

CHILD ABUSE AS A MODERN CONSTRUCT

The concept of child abuse is a relatively modern idea, although historically there has never been a shortage of atrocities against children. In fact, the record is replete with documented accounts of adults inflicting harm on children in the name of good (Weiner and Kurpius, 1995), sometimes in the name of God, and almost always without guilt and remorse. As the psychohistorian DeMause (1974) notes, the further one goes back into history, the lower the level of child care, and the higher the numbers of children abandoned, beaten, terrorized, abused, and murdered. From infanticide to child labor, from incest to child prostitution, and from child pornography to snuff films, the abuse of children has been an enduring outrage.

But whereas today we identify child exploitation and maltreatment as a social problem, it was a convention if not a norm in cultures where children existed solely to serve adults and the primary mandate of those adults was child control and the management of child labor, not child protection. Most of the 2,000 references in the Old Testament to children cite child sacrifices, stonings, beatings, or the rule of strict obedience to all wishes of parents and other adults; there is nothing empathic concerning the needs of children (Weiner and Kurpius, 1995).[1] And in the United States, it was not until 1871 that laws were passed against the abuse of children, following extensive publicity about a single case.[2] Only recently has child abuse been identified as a source of other social problems with enormous institutional costs—legal, medical, educational, criminological, and in terms of the perpetuation of dysfunctional parenting patterns (Briere, 1996). And it is just within the past thirty-five years, since publication of a 1962 article by Kempe and colleagues, "The Battered Child Syndrome," that recurrent waves of collective consciousness and moral outrage about child abuse have emerged. Unfortunately, recognition and public shock are consistently undermined by social counterforces of denial, minimization, and incredulity.

Because of its far-reaching social implications, including legal and moral accountability and responsibility, the phenomenon of child abuse has become part of the controversy related to trauma and dissociation, with various factions declaring child abuse over- or underrated, too politicized or not politicized enough, and/or culture-bound or transcultural. Some minimize abuse and its effects, suggesting that fondling is the most prevalent form of child sexual abuse, that many victims seem unscathed, that children lie and are suggestible, that they have memory problems, or cannot tell reality from fantasy. A few even contend that what others term "sexual abuse" may actually be pleasurable or beneficial, or meaningless (Loftus and Ketcham, 1994; Ceci, Huffman, Smith, and Loftus, 1994; Gardner, 1992; Wakefield and Underwager, 1993).

Debunking the etiological links between childhood sexual abuse and severe dissociative disorders, critics argue that patients shape their experiences and their memories to correspond with the theories, expectations, and explanations of their therapists and the popular culture. Spanos (1996) insists on the undocumented hypothesis that DID is iatrogenic. Frankel (1994) believes that patient pressures have produced an all-too-linear clinical oversimplification such that "blame has displaced shame as the predominant . . . psychodynamic force" (p. 86). Brenneis (1997) reduces the posttraumatic ramifications of child abuse to allegations of invasive therapy, unconscious mutual influence, falsely recovered memory, and the by-products of patients' confabulatory cognitive styles.

Clinicians engaged in the treatment of severely dissociative trauma survivors, however, believe child abuse to be seriously underreported and to encompass bondage situations, exploitation for profit—child pornography, child prostitution—torture, ritual abuse, human experimentation, and mind control as well as forceful acts of penetration in intrafamilial contexts, and in all cases the extensive silencing of victims (Gelinas, 1995; Cozolino, 1989; Ross, 1997; Putnam, 1989; Enns et al., 1995; Bloom, 1994; Robbins, 1996; 1997; Finkelhor, 1994; Sinason, 1994). According to Fergusson and Mullen (1999) in their extensive review of the literature, child sexual abuse "has become one of the defining cultural themes of our age, so much so that it is all too easy to lose sight of the individual victims . . . in the midst of the sound and fury generated around the topic" (p. 1).

How Many Victims?[3]

We will never know the complete truth about the scope or the specifics of child abuse and neglect, nor, probably, do most of us really want to. If we are motivated both to look and look away, we mostly find ways to look away, even as some of us dutifully conduct research or actually listen to in-depth narratives of complex child abuse involving scores of people and perpetrator groups around the world. But do we really fathom the experience of the completely helpless child-victim surrounded by pure malevolence? Do we really bring our hearts and minds into direct contact with it, or do we make sure we don't have to hear more than we have room for? When there is a possible or documented case of a false allegation, it becomes a media sensation. The legal system is in a primitive state where protecting children from adults is concerned.

Perpetrators are experts at subterfuge, and at silencing and blaming the victim. Adult survivors of child abuse are dissociative and frightened. Children cannot find ways to tell, and when they do they are often dismissed. At the slightest hint of false allegation, a case becomes a media sensation. Judges and lawyers are not necessarily enlightened, and the legal system lacks the muscle and sophistication to ferret out and cope with injustice to children or their built-in limitations as witnesses in their own behalf. Clinicians are divided and increasingly wary of dissociative trauma survivors and the legal risks associated with a controversial patient population. Finally, complicity is rampant in our culture.

Child physical abuse and neglect entered the public discourse in the early to mid-1960s, and child sexual abuse was not widely discussed until the late 1970s. Persistence by a relatively small number of professionals and by the feminist movement, along with increased media awareness, has brought it out into the open, but the level of denial in many sectors of society still remains high. Reluctance to believe that anyone, especially people who appear normal, could abuse a child sexually leads to questioning children's credibility and motives, to shifting blame to the child. Historically, when children have reported abuse they have been not only disbelieved but also punished for the outrageousness of their suggestions (Oates, 1996); even today and even by professionals, what children may have experienced can be labeled the product of a vivid juvenile imagination. Period.[4]

As Fergusson and Mullen (1999) indicate, "the Achilles heel of nearly all theory and research into [child sexual abuse] is that the measurement, description, and diagnosis . . . rests upon the potentially fallible memories of childhood experiences" (p. 98). Because of the inherent constraints on empirical investigation (and the social, political, and economic stakes) it is likely that uncertainty and ambiguity will continue to plague the field for some time to come.[5] Attempting a difficult balance, Finkelhor (1998) recently identified two questions that merit top spots on the research agenda: which investigative procedures, standards (medical, ethical, child-welfare), and policies maximize the likelihood of accurate and efficient confirmation or dismissal of abuse allegations? and which confirmation procedures (investigative, therapeutic, criminological justice, case-management) maximize the security, mental health, and sense of justice for victims and their families and the rest of society? The gravity and enormity of the issue is best captured by Whitfield, who compares the estimated number of children who were sexually abused during the time of the Vietnam War with the number of Americans killed in that war (1995, p. 51):

> About 50,000 names are etched into the Vietnam War Memorial. If we made a memorial to children who have been sexually abused, it would be more than 1300 times the size of the Vietnam memorial. If we included other forms of child abuse it would be more than 7500 times its size. But these are not lives lost in

military combat. These are souls lost in a betrayal and wounding that is so deep that most are unable to heal and reconnect with self, others and God without long-term recovery.

ORGANIZED CHILD ABUSE

In the past ten years, there has been a vehement media and academic backlash against any serious consideration of ritual abuse.[6] Even when the authors of the recent backlash literature contribute important information or perspectives, they privilege their viewpoints over all others, and they write scathingly about anyone—patient or therapist or law enforcer—who continues to believe in the possibilities of organized child abuse based on patients' memories and testimony. With the additional onslaught from the False Memory Syndrome Foundation (FMSF) and false memory movement, exploration of the issues by patients and therapists has been seriously inhibited.

All of the backlash books (and many articles as well) bear a striking similarity. They usually begin with some potentially rebalancing perspectives on child-abuse trauma, dissociation, memory, cultural reactions, and collective human experiences. By the time they reach the subjects of MPD/DID and ritual abuse—at about the halfway or three-quarter mark—the tone drastically shifts to contentious, polarized, and scathing critique. Often they associate DID and ritual-abuse accounts with UFO abduction stories or use other sensationalizing and discrediting tactics. In many of these accounts, retractor/recanter testimonies (usually of ex-psychotherapy patients pursuing lawsuits against their former therapists) are naïvely and indiscriminately elevated to extremely high levels of credibility.[7] Attacks or criticisms of feminism are usually part of the package as well. So are emphases on the breakups of families and the innocence of parents, and ditto the systematic minimization of the sexual predator/sex offender problem. Backlash authors usually claim to be truer champions of child protection than therapists and social workers. Yet they are often either nonclinicians or therapists who have never spent time with patients with DID. Egregious overgeneralizations[8] are part of the rhetoric too, such that psychotherapy in all its complexity and diversity is referred to as the "memory industry" (Jenkins, 1998, p. 185) or "RMT" (recovered memory therapy) (Ofshe and Watters, 1994).

While our cultural window on organized child abuse was briefly opened in the mid- to late eighties, the backlash has virtually silenced most other explorations and considerations. Any patients alleging organized child-abuse experiences run the risk of being dismissed as incredible or subjected to disparaging interpretations of the reasons for the presence of such grotesque material in their psyches or therapy dialogues. Any clinician willing to consider organized child-abuse allegations as real is almost immediately marginalized and discredited or labeled a conspiracy theorist, drawing "deeply from the tainted well of American paranoid theory" (Jenkins, 1998, p. 176).

We cannot address the psychology and etiology of child abuse without first surveying the commoditization of children in organized crime, syndicated sex rings, and sadistic ritual abuse.

THE COMMODITIZATION OF CHILDREN

The issue of child prostitution is a global problem of immense and disquieting proportions; no nation or region of the world is untouched (Otero, 1996; Muntarbhorn, 1996). Crewdson (1988) found that child prostitution is not just an urban problem in the United States and that arrests for juvenile prostitution have proliferated even in small midwestern cities and communities. Calling child prostitution "one of the most fundamentally outrageous issues that the world faces," Joseph P. Kennedy (1996, p. 1) acknowledges that many children as young as six or seven are being drawn or taken into prostitution rings in many cases to serve Americans who have the money to travel overseas and take advantage of young children.[9] In some cases children in prostitution (including reports about child victims from the United States) are being tattooed by members of organized crime syndicates that control them like property (J. P. Kennedy, 1996; Muntarbhorn, 1996) or cattle. The use of children as sex slaves and instruments of crime is an ultimate form of debasement and betrayal. Kennedy describes child prostitution as an attack on humanity that focuses exclusively on destroying the next generation. Victims of child prostitution are subjected to psychological and physical danger that leaves permanent scars (not to mention the undermining of their basic dignity and human rights). According to Muntarbhorn (1996), the sexual exploitation of young children has become more insidious because children are increasingly being sold and trafficked across all international frontiers.

Sex with children is a commodity with an exceedingly high exchange value. Its political economy is based on two triangulated systems of relationships: the "procurement triangle," comprised of sexually abused children, men in power, and men who get the benefits of power through procurement; and the "blackmail triangle," consisting of child victims, men in power, and men who get what they want through blackmail. "There is supply. There is demand. The biggest single problem is bringing the product to market without getting caught" (Robbins, 1996, p. 316).[10]

Pedophile rings are known to operate from North America and other Western industrialized nations with tentacles spreading throughout the Third World. In a recent case described by Muntarbhorn (1996), an American group used a so-called children's shelter as a front for pedophilia; the organizer was arrested and imprisoned. According to Muntarbhorn, connections have also been documented between American rings and European pedophiles, particularly with respect to child pornography, which is now proliferating, primarily due to computer bulletin boards.[11] In recent months Australian investigations discussed by Muntarbhorn also found a number of prominent male sex offenders involved with an "international boys' association," which was essentially a front for pedophiles to gain access to young boys from Thailand and the Philippines.

> Given the low cost of labor generally in Asia . . . what has emerged in the tourist boom is the black market for children to become prostitutes and be at the whim and call of wealthy westerners. (p. 27)

Many who investigate child prostitution in the United States and abroad (Crewdson, 1988; Muntarbhorn, 1996; Boonpala, 1996; Saikaew, 1996; Dimenstain, 1996) comment that children's parents and / or other family members may often be involved in supplying them to the prostitution and pornography trade, corroborating personal clinical and consultation experience with dozens of survivors of organized child abuse.

Crewdson documents an interview with a pedophile (1988, p. 102):

> . . . after paying . . . the hundred dollars that we agreed would be given to Yvonne's father, I had this eight-year-old to myself for about six hours. I wasn't sure I could go through with actually paying someone to have sex with their daughter. It was obvious Yvonne had been rented to several other men. The first thing she said to me that night was, "What would you like me to do?" When I was unable to take Yvonne home that night because I didn't have a car, Yvonne's father phoned my motel room and said that since I was keeping her overnight, it would cost me another hundred dollars. The next day, when her father came to pick her up, the first thing he said was, "Did you cooperate?"

CHILD SEX AND PORNOGRAPHY RINGS

Child pornography includes every conceivable lewd and perverted sexual act imaginable.[12] Child pornography is created not only for profit and for the private use of collectors obsessed with increasing the size of their collections (and sharing them with comrades in deviance), but also for demonstration and training purposes with captives—for arousing their curiosity, lowering their inhibitions, binding them by means of blackmail ("Would you like your mother to see this picture?"), and adding financial incentive (Lanning, 1984; Burgess and Grant, 1988). Even the adjunctive use of pornography in the context of child sexual abuse intensifies effects of the victim's shame, humiliation, and sense of powerlessness, because it generates a permanent record that one patient described as "having pieces of yourself stolen and trapped in hell forever."

A sex ring involves multiple victims and, often, multiple abusers; it is usually formed to turn a profit and often engages in child pornography (Burgess, Groth, and McCausland, 1981). Burgess and her colleagues (1981; 1987; 1988) have identified three types: "solo rings," where one adult is sexually involved with small groups of children and there is no transfer of children or photographs to other adults; "transitional rings," which involve multiple perpetrators with several children; and "syndicated rings," involving multiple perpetrators who form a well-structured organization for the recruitment of children, production of pornography, delivery of direct sexual services, and establishment and maintenance of an extensive network of customers.

The Burgess group (1981; 1987; 1988) studied eight sex rings, and in all cases the adults were "legitimate" authority figures —among them a scout leader, a neighbor, a school bus driver, a coach, a teacher, an apartment manager, a grandfather. Hunt and Baird (1990) studied ten sex rings: two fathers and one uncle were the offenders in three cases and child-care providers were the perpetrators in the other seven. Their operational descriptions and investigation of response patterns and psychological disturbances in child and adolescent victims are especially important to the field because their research encompassed large samples of documented sex-ring victims.

All sex rings use a combination of shaming and fear to entrap children. The victims are compelled and isolated by threats and no-exit coercion into continuing and keeping the abuse secret. Their terror is unusually intense, pervasive, and long-lasting; the violations leave them unable to follow their

own instincts for guidance in any adult-child relationships, and so traumatized that they develop massive, rigid defenses and a correspondingly inflexible interpersonal presentation that adversely effects their credibility as
victims (or as witnesses). In keeping with the usual profile of severe dissociative response to chronic trauma, both exposure and disclosure of sex-ring
abuse trigger the breakdown of the entire defensive structure of child or
adult survivors and consistently set off intrapsychic land mines in the form
of suicidal, homicidal, or sexually compulsive acting-out behavior.

The adults in organized child abuse indoctrinate child-victims through an
elaborate socialization process that locks them into patterns of learned maladaptive behavior and into distorted belief systems whereby initially
shame/pain/guilt-inducing activities are normalized (Burgess et al., 1981;
1987; 1988). Sex-ring leaders use drugs, alcohol, intimidation, money, trance-
inducing music, theatrical displays, and "games" to coerce submission and
maintain group cohesion. Perversions of Ring-Around-the-Rosey, Hide-and-
Seek, and Musical Chairs lower children's defenses and encourage competition, then engineer their participation in ganging up on the "loser"—usually
a setup involving a particularly vulnerable or particularly resistant child or
one with no registered identity, easily used for sacrificial demonstrations—
who must then endure group sexual violence (which is also sometimes
filmed). War games that mandate "punishment" for prisoners become channels for sexual degradation, sadism, and humiliation, including urinating
into the mouths and faces of one another, for the gratification of the adult
perpetrators—many of whom also eroticize the surprise, betrayal, and mortification the victims experience when they discover that playing an innocent children's game has dire consequences and that their failure to play by
the "rules" has even more dire consequences.

In Hunt and Baird's (1990) study, children reported being shown "snuff
films" (scenes documenting rituals of real mutilation and actual murders)
and photographs of themselves and family members made to look muti-
lated. They reported witnessing the murder of other children and the mutilation and murder of animals as examples of what could happen to them if
they told anyone about the sex ring. Children have been threatened with
death by guns, knives, poison, and fire; told that they could be killed by animals or that other members of their families could be murdered; made to
have sex with animals and to do so on film. One patient reports having been
forced as a young girl into lewd positions with a horse and a cow, which
were later sacrificed as part of a film with a revenge theme; another was

forced to appear as if she had borne a litter of pups after being raped by a dog. Other patients have described being thrown into fighting rings with mistreated dogs and other abused children—all of which was filmed and later sold.

A male DID patient in his mid-thirties has just described a model of brutal sexual abuse climaxed by exposure to the murder of other children. He would be drugged, stripped, raped by multiple perpetrators, degraded and humiliated, forced to walk on all fours like a dog to be alternately kicked and verbally denigrated. Following this ordeal a child or young infant would be sacrificed in ritualistic fashion. He would be told that the sacrifice was a gift for him.

Therapist: Why are they killing children?
Patient: For the big ZAP.
T: What is the big zap?
P: It's when the natural drug in your body pops through your mind and goes ZAP and there's nothing else like that.
T: You mean like a drug rush or adrenaline rush?
P: Yes, a rush, that's why they do it. But this is more than adrenaline rushing going on. Killing is the biggest ZAP they can get. Children are the best for that.
T: Why is that?
P: They are the freshest and most innocent and there's the most energy and power there.
T: Where did you get such an idea from.
P: Everyone knows that.
T: Everyone?
P: Everyone in that place knows that. They think everyone else is stupid and worthless anyway. And they laugh because no one believes this is going on so they know no one will stop it.
T: What do you think?
P: No one stopped it then and no one is stopping it now, so they must be right.
T: And then when this zap and killing is over?
P: Everything fades from there, I don't know, I just go away.
T: Go away to where?
P: I don't know. Just away, into the blackness.

T: Why do you think they do all these things, besides the rush?

P: They do it because they wanted to, they do it because they could, they do it because they are glad it is not them that is dying and I am just like them in that way because I was glad it wasn't me that was dying—that made me just like them.

T: This is one of your biggest confusions, isn't it, because all of this left you with the guilt and shame for all of this cruelty and with a deep confusion about whether you wanted to be part of this or not.

P: I was glad it was not me they were doing that to. They said it could have been me if I didn't help.

T: Then it seems to me like fear of death is part of what motivates this kind of abuse and your complicity?

P: They control life and death so I can't see that they are afraid of it. Sometimes they want death to happen in a certain way—to be done with quickly, and sometimes they want it drawn out. They have a lot of superstition and obsessions about death. They have to be in control of it, so I guess they must be afraid of it, and me too, but I never thought about it that way before . . .

[later in the same session . . .]

P: Sometimes they make pictures and films of this stuff.

T: What gives you that idea?

P: There are cameras in the room, off in the corner. Sometimes I can hear the sound of them clicking.

T: What are these movies for?

P: They'll be shown on special news shows like on television, to let the people know what's happening in the world.

T: Special news shows? What do you mean?

P: News programs, like you would have on Walter Cronkite or something.

T: But who would be watching?

P: The other people who live in the red world.

T: Who are they and what is the red world?

P: Special people . . . the red world is the place you go when this is happening. Some people live in that world all the time and these are the news reports they want to see to know what is going on. The red world is the place where there are no rules and you can do whatever you want to whoever you want.

T: How do you know about this?

P: The people in the red world told me. And they are going to be very very angry at you and me because I told you this.

T: How do you know what they would feel about that?

P: They told me, they showed me. You or I could die for this, you know.

T: What did they show or tell you?

P: Can we stop talking about this right now? I think I've said too much for one time and I need to stop.

T: Of course. I can see you're scared, and intimidated, and maybe even more than a little overwhelmed and that you're trying to protect both of us right now. This material is so difficult for you to talk about and feel safe at the same time; since there have been threats and intimidation, it's essential that you be in control of how much you tell me, if you ever tell me anything else, and when you tell me.

P: Good, I'm relieved, I'm glad you can see that I am also concerned about your being hurt. Not just me. We got to see others being hurt and killed and that's one of the ways they let us know what will happen but I don't want to talk about this more now, OK?

Sex-ring leaders exploit the children's peer network to coerce adaptations that perpetuate sexually aggressive and sadistic behaviors. The adults in power reinforce the "privilege" whereby older children abuse the smaller and weaker ones; they take advantage of the children's needs for attention, approval, and affection to foster group cohesion. A business ethic comes to prevail among the child-victims, who are locked into secrecy with escalating penalties for daring betrayal: they begin to pressure one another; their extortion increases as each victim (now victim-perpetrator) gains more resources, and diminishes only when a member can supply the ring with a new child—which is an incentive for children to recruit their own younger siblings.

Hunt and Baird (1990) point out that therapist resistance to even acknowledging that adults join together in groups for the sole purpose of exploiting children sexually stands in the way of their identifying and treating the survivors. When clinicians can assimilate organized victimization and then negotiate the tricky balance of maintaining sufficient emotional distance from the nightmare while maintaining sufficient emotional connection to the patient, there still remains the undoing of the effects of mind control or brainwashing (e.g., belief in the magical or supernatural powers of the perpetrators; institutionalized terror of mutilation and annihilation as a result of witnessing the dismemberment of living things)—which is one of the toughest clinical tasks in the treatment of sex-ring victims (Hunt and Baird, 1990).

ORGANIZED SADISM AND RITUAL ABUSE

Operationally, the leap from syndicated sex rings to sadistic ritual abuse is incremental, involving more drama and more theological dogma, an increase in the levels of violence, sadism, and secrecy, a more elaborate hierarchy, greater use of coercive influence, threats, and thought reform technology, greater crossover with the snuff-film industry, some crossover with political mind-control and human-experimentation groups, and a greater role for the ritual sacrifice of animals or human beings.

Ritual abuse is one of the extreme ends of the child-abuse continuum. The term now refers to the cruel subjection of victims to combinations of repeated physical, sexual, psychological, and spiritual abuse—often within a religious or pseudoreligious context (Sakheim, 1996). Goodwin (1993b) recommends emphatic addition of the word *sadistic* instead of the misleading *satanic*. While many people dismiss accounts of severe sadistic ritual abuse and torture because insufficient scientific or forensic evidence has been gathered to validate the phenomena,[13] the literature on child abuse reminds us that we must make room for what we do not know, for what we most fear, for what our patients across the country are telling us, and for what is clearly within the realm of already documented or increasingly visible criminal exploitation of children.[14] Clearly, violent, multiperpetrator, sadistic abuse does occur and some unknown segment of child-abuse survivors has endured torture of incomprehensible dimensions; partial if not complete dissociative amnesia is the likely result of such repeated acts (Briere, 1996).

> A ritually abused patient has just described a scene of horrific child torture, sadistic group sexual abuse, and human sacrifice that took place on Halloween.

P: There were several children killed in this one ritual because it was such a special night. Three, I think, in different ways.

T: Where did these children come from?

P: They're disposable children. Children are disposable, you know, don't you?

T: Disposable children? I never think of human beings as disposable.

P: I don't know, do they grow children just for this or do they steal them from people to torture and kill them? I don't know. Children are disposable you know, at least to these people they are. They grow children to kill like people grow farm animals to kill. Their births are never registered and they never attend school so there are no records and no one ever knows, and where they come from it's so rural there is no way anyone can know. Everyone's disbelief makes it feel that much more crazy. I feel sick to my stomach. I wish I were making this up.

T: Where are they keeping these children and who is keeping them?

P: Like I said, they are kept like on farms, in cages, or in basements and cellars—my grandmother had hidden rooms beneath her house and people were kept there, and some people have to watch over them and feed them, or not feed them and make sure they don't get away, but like I said they're like farm animals . . . they belong to the group and they are sold or killed and we're not supposed to have any feelings about those children because they won't be around for that long and because we should be happy that we are not one of those. If we don't act right we could become one of those. You live with that threat of being one of them and then you hate those children, not the abusers, but the children, for existing and reminding you that you could have it worse. So when you have to hurt those children it's easier. Do you understand?

Finkelhor and Williams (1988) propose three subclassifications of ritual abuse: cult-based, whereby sexual abuse is only one component of a child's total immersion in rituals and beliefs; pseudoritualistic, whereby sexual abuse is primary and cult rituals are secondary; and psychopathological ritualist, whereby an adult, operating alone or with others, abuses the child in a ritualistic fashion in keeping with the dictates of an obsessive or delusional system. A complex combination of abuses obtains, ranging from psychological and physical maltreatment to torture to religious oppression (Charles, 1995), and meeting several perpetrator needs simultaneously—sadistic gratification, the furthering of religious beliefs, the control or silencing of victims (Cozolino, 1989; Finkelhor and Williams, 1988), economic advancement, and the perpetuation of the malevolent system by enlisting the terrorized individuals, bonded with elaborate displays of group loyalty, to perpetrate against others. Often the abuse takes place within the context of religious ceremonies where group-specific obsessive-compulsive rituals are enacted, often quite theatrically; survivors' accounts indicate that more bizarre and extreme displays of blood and gore, together with mockery of mainstream practices, generate greater deference among group members toward their leaders.

Jones (1993) describes ritual-abuse cults as trauma-organized systems in which traumatization (and breakdown of the child-victim's personality for brainwashing in accord with the group's agenda) is intensified through the repetitiveness of ritual action (e.g., drumming, chanting, praying, posturing, etc.).[15] The repetition functions to justify the abuse by positioning it in some overarching framework. Although such justification processes are common to all forms of child abuse, they are institutionalized in ritual abuse; in many cases, rationalization systems are passed down intergenerationally in families that "pass as normal."

The abusers' instinctive (and studied)[16] techniques involve the use of trauma and violence to disrupt and empty the self of its own organizing fantasies and structures of subjectivity and to destroy the victim's critical thinking abilities. Into these wounds the cult or perpetrator group interposes its own organizing structures of subjectivity and meaning—its beliefs and ideologies paired with soothing food, warmth, clothing, drugs, grandiose beliefs in power, and fantasies of protection by the group. All of these things the beleaguered and confused child desperately takes in for lack of anything else to organize meaning and reality, and, most important, to stave off the state of annihilation produced by chronic assault and the resulting disorientation. Central to the successful breakdown of the personality prior to its reshaping is the inculcation of the belief that the child-victim has always been this way or that s/he has chosen his/her actions and attitudes. This is one of the most insidious aspects of organized child abuse and one of the most difficult aspects to resolve in treating survivors of ritual and sadistic abuse, where one is likely to encounter "cult" alter personalities who insist they were born from the earth or from a serpent's egg or that they are and always have been the child of the Devil, that they have chosen of their own free will to be who they are, that since God (or Jesus) failed to protect them, they deserve what they get and belong to the group, or in Hell, and so on.

McFadyen, Hanks, and James (1993) isolate entrapment and secrecy as core dynamics in ritual abuse. Bentovim and Tranter (1994) add that breaking down the fragile sense of morality of the child by forcing him/her into sexual activities is a powerful factor of induction into assuming an abusive role toward others. Overall, in organized sadistic perpetrator situations, the strategic use of coercion and trauma cultivates loyalty, cohesion, identification, guilt, dissociation, and silencing. Group practices are organized around indoctrination rituals, the acquisition of power, and the prevention of disclosure (Sakheim, 1996).

Cozolino (1989) has speculated that acts particular to ritual abuse may be contrived to bind the child to the group by severing his/her ties with mainstream belief systems; they also completely and deliberately undermine the child-victim's capacity for believing in the possibility of rescue, forgiveness, and redemption, in a redemptive divinity, in a just and sane world. Nurcombe and Unutzer (1991) contend that many of the severe and persistent traumas inflicted by ritual-abuse groups are purposeful attempts to induce dissociative reactions in children to ensure their compliance and cooperation—and indeed clinical evidence shows that dissociative states once induced may then themselves be systematically shaped by the groups to further control the dissociative identity-formation.

Jones (1991) suggests that the most fundamental concerns for clinicians treating ritual abuse survivors are: the significant and long-lasting distortion of the victim's attitudes, beliefs, allegiances, and fundamental personality structure, making adaptive recovery extremely difficult; the even more profound psychological damage inflicted by premeditated and sadistic activities conjoined with sexual abuse; and the utter demolition of the victim's self-esteem through the systematic degradation of the child.

> A woman with DID and an extensive history in the child-abuse criminal underground has just been describing her early training to tolerate gang rapes for the purposes of pornography and prostitution. Her shame, like the shame of all the other survivors of organized child abuse, is intense and survivor guilt is embedded in every level of her dissociative self-system. The experiences of chronic helplessness, becoming an accomplice, and being a perpetrator completely obliterate the self, making the victim/survivor (when s/he is allowed to live) a pliable puppet to the totalitarian regime of the cult or crime syndicate. Numbness and self-obliteration are preferable to thinking about what is going on.

> P: They told me I didn't feel any pain and that it didn't hurt, and when it did hurt that it was my fault. Over time I struggled less and it took less time to get me under control and so it seemed like what they were saying was true. After a while I never thought it hurt, so after a while I never thought it happened. But with the other kids, the ones who were supposed to live—sometimes they would cause too much

bleeding and the child would die and this would make them really mad—and they would do strange things to try and save the child, like hanging her upside down and things like that.

T: What about these other children?

P: The other ones who they called "nobody's children" lived in different people's houses. In the basement of some people's houses—in this country anyway, other places it is different and they can keep more children in one central place but here they don't do it that way. And sometimes these people would have real children living upstairs with them. I'm sorry I shouldn't have said real children like these others weren't real, but that's how they used to talk about them, like they were nobody's children, the kind of children who belonged to no one and who you could do anything you want with, and you were supposed to be glad you were not one of them, and they told you that you could become one of them at any time.

T: So you felt terribly guilty that you were glad to not be one of those children.

P: Yes, it was awful but we learned not to think about them, their rocking and their headbanging, and the vacant look in their eyes after a while. Sometimes we even hated them and the men liked that we felt that way and encouraged that, but then sometimes we had to make them do things and get them to cooperate and I hated having to be nice to them, that made it all harder. Then you had to feel something.

T: And feeling anything was dangerous.

P: Very dangerous, it could make you make a mistake. Or make them make you hurt them more.

T: So any act of kindness was prohibited.

P: Once they shocked the metal on the cage because I held one girl's hands, and we both went flying across the room with her in the cage, and I never did that again.

T: Any softness or caring would just cause more pain.

P: In that place all you care about is stopping the pain.

T: And that's the double bind of guilt isn't it, because you can't help but try and survive and yet your self-preservation feels like the worst thing, like a betrayal, and yet you can't help trying to get away from the pain and to survive.

P: You're trapped but that's not what they tell you and that's not what you think about at the time; even now some parts of me think about it the old way, like what kind of person am I to let that happen. Like it's all my fault and I wanted these things to happen so I wouldn't die.

T: Of course the complicated questions are who is letting what happen to whom. Who is really responsible for all of this. You're carrying a lot of guilt and shame over it and have been your whole life.

P: Right, I can think about that now, but back then it was not possible. Mostly I survived by not thinking about anything at all. And eventually it took a lot of drugs to help keep that going. . . .

T: Where did those children come from?

P: I don't know, but they always had plenty of them, but never too many in one place—except in some places with big houses in other countries where they keep many of them in rooms and cages—like I told you, it's done differently in different places. I think that many of them were just raised for this.

T: Raised to be used, raped, and then killed? Is that what you mean.

P: Yes, like they were nobody's children—to use up. We couldn't have any feelings about all of this, and I feel a little nauseous now, but I can't feel a whole lot about this yet. I don't understand why people don't believe this. Where do they think all the missing children are going to and where do they think these people get the children to sell and kill and use in their films from?

T: I don't think a lot of people know about this or can stand to know about it or to believe it. Or they say there simply isn't evidence of this sort of thing. Like you said about yourself, they just don't think about it. It's too awful.

P: Right. We just don't think about it. But it's still there. No one wants to believe this stuff and they, you know the ones who are doing all this, they know this real well. They laugh about it sometimes. Mocking everyone. They think they control everything. Sometimes it seems like they really do.

Dissociative Patterns in Victims of Organized and Ritual Child Abuse

Many patients who claim to come from intergenerational, intrafamilial cults describe specific child-rearing practices that involve the suffusion of pain and fear into the sensory and psychological experiences of infants and children from the earliest points in development (e.g., starving, burning, beatings, sensory deprivation, overexposure to severe heat and/or cold, sexual molestation, and the neglect of infants). Such patterns establish dissociative imperatives at the earliest age, disrupt normal integration of self- and other-representations, and create a storehouse of rage that can be harnessed and directed by the leaders of the group. The very youngest personality is split into cult-identified and noncult sectors, and the resulting dissociative structures are molded so that cult-compliance can operate outside the full awareness of the other aspects of personality (Young et al., 1991; Smith, 1993) (see Chapter 8). Development proceeds along parallel tracks. Many patients speak of radical splits in their dissociative identity systems between "day" selves and "night" selves and insist on keeping these separate long after their involvement in perpetrator groups has ended. (One patient commented that when the leader of her perpetrator group would enter her house during the daytime to train or punish her for some transgression reported by her parents, the interpenetration of day and night worlds threw her well-compartmentalized dissociative system into complete chaos.)

Children (or camouflaged alter personalities of the child) adopt the doctrines of, and allegiances to, the cult in the absence of their own now dismantled belief systems in order to restore their psychic equilibrium and ward off further disintegration. Their attachment is completely trauma-based, embedded in the trance logic of posttraumatic suggestions and meanings, and often buried under drug-induced and hypnotically created amnestic barriers. The victims internalize the perpetrators' messages that their own selves are no longer their possessions but property of the group—sacrifices, gifts, obligations—in exchange for keeping them alive. When the children see themselves acting contrary to their internal senses of morality or core goodness they become convinced that what they have been told is true (i.e., that they are intrinsically evil, and the cycle of self-fulfilling prophecies built into the trance logic of the dissociative self-system is reinforced). The signs and symptoms of ritual abuse in children are described in great detail in Gould (1992).

In therapy, survivors of ritual abuse consistently attest to the same see-sawing manipulations—likened by Ross (1995a) to the use of rat psychology on humans—designed to inculcate in them feelings of specialness and feelings of abject helplessness, in every possible combination. Their reports are consistent with reports in the clinical literature (Charles, 1995; Gould, 1992; Greaves, 1992; Sakheim, 1996), and also, tellingly, with recently released CIA files documenting the experimental use of hypnosis on unwitting subjects to create "Manchurian Candidates"—dissociative alter personalities who could be programmed and managed for espionage activities (Ross 1997).

The systematic abuse of attachment speaks to the depths of the wounds of the perpetrators, which compound profound betrayal, sacrifice, torture, and abandonment—namely, Magid's (1988) "evil self"—with severe problems of drive regulation and object relations. Such individuals construct coherent, cohesive, relatively conflict-free identities around delineated cores of negative or evil ideals and ambitions "whose execution—while reinforcing the structural cohesion of the individual self—is inimical to the lives of others" (p. 100). The need to feed their escalating maniacal grandiosity with enactments of wholesale revenge and destruction, often dressed up in ego-syntonic ideologies, takes on the powerful driving forces of an addiction, requiring ever increasing doses of violence and hatred.

The perpetrator's maniacal and insatiable greed must constantly be reworked to keep disintegration anxieties at bay; the terrors, the poisons, and primitive agonies—the "bad stuff"—must continually be ejected outward into an external container and this container must be systematically attacked to ensure that this "badness" does not take revenge on the perpetrator's self (Grand, 2000). According to Grand, such splitting and projective identification allow the acquisitor to pursue nonhuman fusion with immortality while the victims serve as the repository for disavowed, evacuated dread about extinction.

An extremely articulate female patient began to have a second wave of memories about her involvement in the snuff-film industry as part of larger childhood involvement in criminal cults and ritual abuse. She began to put diverse fragments of memory together in an effort to integrate this aspect of her severely traumatic childhood experiences. Telling me that she now often had to hide her fear of cameras from other people, she described how she worked in all aspects of the snuff-film industry from procurement to accounting, from stage management to filming, from costuming to lighting, and from courier/distribution to actor/killer. When asked if she was ready to talk about it, she said that she indeed felt ready to put these pieces together and have someone else know about them. However, she stated quite clearly that it was okay for the pieces she would tell me to go together in *my* head just as long as all the pieces did not go together in *her* head. "It's the programming," she said, "that's how it works. The pieces have to stay separate."

P: The procurement was simple. It always involved sailors, prostitutes, and dancers and I was trained to seduce them into different places promising work, sex, drugs, thrills and stuff like that.

T: The procurement did not involve children?

P: No, they were not procured in that way. Children were part of the accounting system part of it. They were sold or given as part of payment between people involved in this film business. Like in exchange for films or money or for blackmail and stuff. The procurement I was involved in was with adults or teenagers who didn't know what they were getting into, and filming their face up close with the surprise and horror when they realize they were being killed was a big part of the whole thing. Filming the surprise of the victim is a big thing with them. That's their game. They even have special language for it, special words that stood for things.

T: Words like . . . ? Can you remember anything?

P: Yes, one word pops into my mind. Caper, like referring to what happens. And transaction. That was a code word that could mean something else if people heard you talking about it.

T: The word "caper" has a lot of connotations, doesn't it?

P: Exactly. You see that. You see that weird sense of humor, the pulling one over, the getting-away-with-it thing that is so important to these people. And the mockery too, which is a big thing and is used as a theme in some of their movies besides.

T: I don't understand what you mean about accounting.

P: That was actually a big part of my job. There was a ledger with names of people, money, services, children who were kidnapped or bred or bought who were traded and logs were kept of all of this in secret places. It is like a business, like any business except for what it is and how sick it is.

T: How are you feeling telling me about this.

P: I am numb in order to get all this out but I am relieved to be saying it, and I have a headache. But I can keep going.

T: You said you were involved in all parts of this. Were you involved in the filming?

P: Not very much, they had special people for that, but I was involved in the backstage stuff. Lighting, costumes, rope cages where people would be trapped hovering above another scene of death and torture and their faces would be filmed as they witnessed horrible things and

as they began to know it was going to happen to them, there were lots
of close-ups on that kind of thing. And there were themes, you know.
Story lines and plots. And I was used in the story as a child, like the
role of the innocent . . . there is always the innocent child.

T: And what happens to that child?

P: Sometimes the innocent is also the killer. Well someone is set up to
do something to that innocent child and then the child turns on
them and hurts them when they don't suspect that's what is going
to happen. Tricks and deceptions and playing with real and fake innocence are some of the main themes they do in those films. When
it's a kidnapped child, then the innocent gets to be the one who gets
killed.

T: So they are always playing out and filming these themes of betrayal,
sacrifice, deception, and corruption or destruction of innocence.

P: Yes, that's the main theme and there are so many variations. Foiled
rescues is another big theme for them. Like someone is set up to believe they could be saved and their hope or desperation is filmed and
then the rescue is foiled and when they realize they are going to die
and not be saved there is a close-up of their face because the people
who like these films want to see that face when it's tricked or giving
up hope or lost. That's their favorite thing . . .

They also prey on young runaways and prostitutes and erotic
dancers. Especially the ones whose disappearances would not be no-
ticed. You know drifters and people like that, there are thousands of
them. There was this young erotic dancer who was lured into their
game with promises of money and films and stuff. She thought she
was in control and they knew she was not. She acted tough and cool
but she was really naïve. I got attached to her. I was like her assistant
in the early phases. I don't know if I knew what was going to happen
to her. But they let her dance and they got her into cutting herself and
bleeding a little bit at a time with each performance and filming so
she was like getting used to this kind of thing and thought she was
cool and in control. Like just a regular S and M type film thing. But
then one day after a while they cut her so bad she was dying while
she was dancing and being filmed and at first it was like she was
partly drugged and did not get the trick and then she got it and they
do that close-up on her face as she is realizing she is being killed and

tricked and can't do anything about it. This is like the kind of things they do. Do you understand?

[Later in that session. . .]

I also was a courier and had to bring these films from one place to another or be part of trades and distributions. Sometimes I didn't know what I was carrying from one place to the next.

After killing someone they, you know, they usually dismember bodies and stuff like that. You know, like in the films they may have corpses with limbs cut off just for background decoration to make a scene. To have an effect. Everything is for effect. They keep the bodies and parts frozen in meat lockers in different places for when they need to use them. Some of the people involved have these big or little grocery stores. Anyway, sometimes I was a courier and had to bring these films from one place to another or be part of trades and distributions. Sometimes I didn't know what I was carrying from one place to the next. It's all organized like on an underground network. They all know who they are. Nobody else seems to know who they are. You have to understand these people are into very strange jokes with one another. Or maybe it was to prove something else, like they really did it, but one time they didn't put a film in the film thing, what do you call you know those metal flat silver circular tins. They would put some part of a person, like a tongue was cut out once and when I delivered it to the person who was supposed to get the film, and it was like a big joke between them that there was a tongue in there instead of a film.

RITUAL ABUSE, EVIL, AND EVERYDAY LIFE

Ritual-abuse patients share one further disturbing common denominator—the inextricability of normal everyday, "good citizen" lifestyles with organized sadism. One patient's father preached on fundamentalist Christian television during the day and engineered satanic brutality in the evenings to rid his daughter of demonic possession. Other patients have named teachers and school officials, medical professionals, clergy, and local police officers as the perpetrators in sex rings or ritual-abuse groups and cults. In one family the physician-father's access to drugs facilitated the victims' injection with all sorts of chemical agents designed to intensify their experience, ensure their compliance and silence, and totally confuse them. With the help of the patient and his mother, this same doctor-abuser shot up his two other children before leaving the house for extended periods of time to keep them completely unconscious (i.e., "switched off").[17]

Regardless of the tactics deployed or the ideological underpinnings, ritual abuse and systematic torture—conflating sadism and megalomania—always also involve economics.

> Religious beliefs, including those associated with Satanism, may be a thinly disguised pretext for giving torturers a sadistic thrill. In instances in which cults produce pornography, peddle drugs, or engage in other illegal activities, the thrill of making money and creating extensive criminal networks is also an obvious motive. In such cases, the loyalty of the individual to the group is intensified by reminding the member that she or he has engaged in criminal acts, is now—though secretly—an outcast from normal society, and would be tried for heinous crimes if the cult activity were discovered. (Waites, 1993, p. 207)

Ritual abuse should probably be reconstrued as intricately woven into the fabric of the power and economic bases of child-pornography, prostitution, drug-trafficking, and the snuff-film industries as really a means to an end rather than an end in itself (Blume, 1995). (Trauma, sexual abuse, torture, and mind control are used to cultivate and then manipulate the dissociative structures of children in quest of "a cost-free, compliant labor force to drive such high-profit criminal activities as drug dealing, pornography, and prostitution" [p. 134].)

Before we can expect a significant shift away from skepticism, denial, and avoidance in the mental health professions, law enforcement, and the media, we must wait for one or more legal convictions for satanic abuse or ritual murder, or for forensic documentation of organized child abuse or ritual abuse—or for the discovery and details of a confiscated "shipment" of children across state lines by an organized perpetrator group to be made fully public without minimization. And yet, "In the long run, perhaps it is not the incredulity but the frightening plausibility[18] of secret cults that makes them so insistently denied" (Waites, 1993, p. 203).

By way of demystification, Ross (1995a) calls for ongoing research to systematically investigate and document the extent and effects of ritual abuse; the life experiences, memory functions, symptoms, and treatment trajectories of dissociative survivors alleging participation in satanic cults are a topic that should be studied experimentally just like any other subject area.

RITUAL ABUSE AND HUMAN HISTORY

DeMause (1994), who has continually attempted to raise society's awareness about the collective use of children as "poison containers" for the deposit of adults' and society's wounds, concludes that the bizarre dramas played out in contemporary and historical cults seem to serve certain psychological meanings and functions. Sadistic individuals continually defend against primitive annihilation, disintegration, and fears of engulfment by reenacting rituals that reassure them of their potency and separateness; individual and collective fantasies of restoring potency through sexually abusing, torturing, and killing children have motivated people since the dawn of time. The *universal psychodynamics of cultic torture* and sacrifice, which transcend time and place (DeMause, 1994), include

- regression due to fears of individuation;
- refuge in trance states;
- merging with the leader in defense against engulfment;
- projective identification to relieve intolerable feelings;
- deification of the terrifying leader as a defense against helplessness;
- totalitarian organization of the cult hierarchy;
- torture and sacrificial rebirth rituals reenacting childhood traumas to recapitulate the drama of absolute power over absolute helplessness.

The megalomaniacs driving child-abuse cults around the world are attempting to resolve primitive psychological agonies and profound spiritual wounds through extreme omnipotent enactments that turn them into "gods." By spellbinding groups of people in ritual settings, by exercising high-level Mafia-type authority over major business operations, and by controlling large populations with continuous access to the management of their life, death, and reproduction, these people ward off their own apocalyptic anxieties by living out an archetypal demonic existence.

The centerpiece of victimization in ritual abuse—coercing the victim into colluding with his/her own exploitation and in the abuse and betrayal of others[19]—was also a pivotal strategy and organizing principle of the slavery system. Both worlds involve the stealing, trafficking, and breeding of victims (for profit); the destruction of the victim's sense of self-worth and autonomy; and the dismantling of all attachments that do not advance the economic (or pseudoreligious) status quo. Both worlds involve torture, sexual abuse, death threats, isolation, breeding experiments, manipulation of attachment bonds, starvation, a rationalizing and righteous spiritual system, coerced compliance and rewards for identifying with the master against the other slaves.

Nathanson (1992), discoursing on shame and the enslavement of people of African descent in the American South, could be referring to ritual abuse:

> Can there be a greater source of shame than to be declared so much less than human that one is only a piece of property. . . . People removed from their own cultures and turned into beasts of burden and creatures designed to fulfill the fantasy needs of fellow humans who now claimed to be their owners. (p. 462)

Ritual-abuse cults, like all absolute authoritarian systems, pervert loyalty and deploy death/pain threats and death/pain-avoidance strategies to motivate and manipulate victims' compliance. Whereas slaves were forbidden to read, cult victims are prohibited from interacting with or internalizing alternate sources of information—but in both cases the objective is destruction of critical thinking capacities and forced dependence on the "master" for structuring meaning. And in both settings, thought-reform techniques are used to mystify, confuse, and disempower; both systems reinforce dissociative adaptations whereby a victim must hide any knowledge of a sense of the self-as-sacred lest it be discovered, assaulted, and appropriated by the perpetrating system. Considering slavery as a subset of sadistic/ritual abuse renders the latter more comprehensible and affirms its linkage with, rather than isolation from, the realities of our history.

The Nazi Holocaust is another example of large-scale ritual abuse, though it is not often conceptualized this way. The death camps incorporated all of the elements, however: economic exploitation, spiritual assaults, torture and child abuse, death rituals and child murders, bizarre dismemberment and human experimentation, prostitution, the manipulation of dependency, filming of bizarre killings and experiments for the entertainment of the perpetrators, the turning of victims against themselves and against one another, the destruction of hope, organized deception, and the fostering of incredulity and collaboration among large masses of humanity.

As the Nazis did, ritual abusers brutally impose on their victims delusional ideologies whose grandiose coercive pressure eliminates the possibility of escape, rescue, or any kind of witnessing. The victims have no right to protest or speak up. By virtue of their contamination by the "secret order"

(Laub, 1995), they accept subhuman status as their real and rightful identity. What Laub describes as the core assault on the individual's sense of reality in the case of Holocaust survivors applies equally to survivors of organized child abuse:

> It was not only the reality of the situation and the lack of responsiveness of by-standers or the world that accounts for the fact that history was taking place with no witness: it was also the very circumstance of being inside the event that made unthinkable the very notion that a witness could exist, that is, someone who could step outside of the coercively totalitarian and dehumanizing frame of reference in which the event was taking place, and provide an independent frame of reference through which the event could be observed. (1995, p. 66)

Ritual abuse, then, is by no means a recent or an esoteric phenomenon. It should come as no surprise to students of history, psychology, and economics. Cruelty has particular power in societies that profess democracy and deny their own authoritarian elements because, by splitting it off and denying it, we collectively empower and collude in its proliferation. It is important that we do not make the mistake of dissociating evil, of splitting it off from the family of human experiences. We can learn a great deal by studying the behaviors and effects of organized violence and thought reform as practiced in destructive cults—microcosms, crucibles, extreme manifestations of ourselves—yet, thanks to an ongoing culturally sanctioned decontextualization process, we cannot seem to make room for what thousands of people have been trying to tell us.

Ritual-abuse survivors are never surprised to be disbelieved by outside cultural authorities. Their perpetrators told them it would be that way should they ever try and testify on their own behalf and betray the group. Society's unwillingness to suspend disbelief compounds the overriding sense of alienation from, and abandonment by, the rest of humanity already instilled in survivors of chronic trauma first by their supremely marginalizing experiences and then by their dissociative adaptations to them.

THE PERPETRATORS[20]

Serious abuse is seldom ambiguous and serious abusers aren't merely normal parents who have fallen on hard times. They are criminals knowingly engaged in criminal behavior, which is why they typically blame the child and hide the

brutal results. Giving them the benefit of the doubt, letting them off with warn-
ings, propping them up with social services in the name of family values tells
them they can escape responsibility for their crimes. Violent people take such ac-
quiescence for approval, and escalate the abuse.

—Richard Rhodes

In order to understand the dynamics of child abuse and its psychological effects, particularly the ways in which offender psychology is internalized by child victims, we must know about the perpetrators. Who are they? How do they operate? What makes them do what they do? Child molesters actually come from all socioeconomic and educational levels and share few characteristics aside from their predilection for deviant sexual behavior (Myers et al., 1989; Salter, 1995). There is no profile of a typical child molester (Myers et al., 1989), no pathology discernible by generic psychological tests or clinical interviews (Salter, 1995). The most chilling aspect of this species of deviance is its invisibility (Salter, 1995); the most striking diagnostic characteristic of sexual victimizers of children is their apparent normality (Herman, 1990).

Recently, the U.S. Department of Justice (Greenfield, 1996) issued a report entitled "Child Victimizers: Violent Offenders and Their Victims." Mixing the responses of a nationwide sample of state prisoners with homicide data assembled by law enforcement agencies, the study reveals how different the victimizer of children is from the victimizer of adults. First, the *vast majority* of inmates whose victims were under eighteen had committed some form of sexual assault or molestation. Typically, perpetrators (97 percent of whom were male) knew their child-victims: about half were their parents. Indeed, nearly a third of those serving time in state prisons for violence against children had victimized their own child(ren) or stepchild(ren). One-fifth of all violent offenders serving time in state prisons reported having victimized a child (which translated in 1991 into about 61,000 child victimizers incarcerated in state prisons).

The victims of nearly two-thirds of rapists and sexual assaulters in state prisons were children. Victimizers of children were more likely than victimizers of adults to have had *multiple victims*,[21] and substantially more likely to have been physically or sexually abused themselves as children; however— and notably, toward deconstructing the myth that all perpetrators are abuse survivors—*the majority*, regardless of victim age, had *no* such history. Perhaps the most disturbing statistic the study documents is the contrast between median sentences for offenses against children—eleven years—and adults—fifteen.

Salter (1995) reports that incest offenders typically receive shorter prison sentences and are released on probation more often than other child molesters, despite the finding that about half of a sample of incest offenders had also molested children outside of their own families (Weinrott and Saylor, 1991). Salter (1995) concludes that child victimization is a highly addictive, tenacious, and repetitive problem, and, further, that it is frequently a progressive disorder: the offenses grow more intrusive, more intense, and at times more violent as time goes on; escalations can involve the types of offenses, types of victims, and numbers of victims.[22]

THE CHARACTERISTICS OF SEXUAL PERPETRATION AGAINST CHILDREN

Contrary to what society likes to comfort itself by thinking and contrary to what many abusers claim when confronted with undeniable evidence, sexual perpetration against children is not an impulsive act or momentary aberration (Pithers, 1990). Sexual offending is carefully thought-out, well-planned, and well-camouflaged behavior. "It is easier to accept the notion of error rather than evil, and coldly plotting the sexual molestation of children strikes most people as something very close to evil" (Salter, 1995, p. 38). The capacity of sexual offenders for denial, rationalization, and minimization of their deviant behavior is confirmed by Salter's (1995) finding that the population she has interviewed seem rather proud of their ability to manipulate their victims into remaining attached and loyal to them. Salter notes that frequently child abusers target their victims by calculating their probable vulnerability relative to other children, recognizing that those already being abused by others are better prey than never-molested children.

The manipulation of children's trust and betrayal of their attachment needs are such powerful guarantors of compliance that many (especially intrafamilial, nonsadistic, and/or lone operator) offenders often need not resort to anything else. (When the extremes of complicity and subjugation are involved, however, perpetrators resort to coercion, terrorization, and insidious forms of thought reform and mind control. See Chapter 8.) To protect themselves against the legal and social consequences of disclosure, they deploy threats, promises, and bribes, and, most commonly, exploit the victim's naïveté and goodwill (Salter, 1988; 1995; Howitt, 1995). Other documented methods used by perpetrators to gain mastery include the imposition of their adult authority and superior physical power and the isolation of the victim from others (Howitt, 1995). Sometimes, in preference to convincing a child that secrecy is best for him/her and for the family, an offender may not even raise the issue, lest it attract the child's attention to the inappropriateness of what is going on. In response to inquiries, abusers variously claim that "nothing" is happening or reframe the assault as somehow helpful to the child, or at least neutral. (One DID patient's mother who handed her over to pimps at night on a regular basis in exchange for money and protection would tell the bewildered girl the next morning that she had been in her own bed all night long.) Postevent suggestions become powerful organizers of victims' memories and self-reflections.

It is imperative that clinicians become well-versed in the dynamics of sexual assault and relatively fluent in the perpetrator psychology because thinking errors (Salter, 1988; 1995) that permeate the deviant sexual behavior pattern of perpetrators at every stage are often internalized by the child victims and maintained unconsciously into adult life. *Content* thinking errors among sexual offenders include palliative comparisons to minimize their behavior, reframing the abuse, and self-statements that blame the victim (Salter, 1995). *Process* errors described by Salter (including research by Yochelson and Samenow, 1976) and reflecting research by Howitt (1995) include

> *I can't*—to disguise refusing to do things they do not want to do or to justify why they cannot resist their impulses;
> *victim-stancing*—whereby the offender claims and believes that s/he is the real victim (one of the most prevalent sophistries in the false memory controversies);
> *exculpatory rhetoric*—denial, minimization, scheming, dissimulating, and believing in one's innocence;
> *lack of time perspective*—failure to take into account the future consequences of present behavior;
> *deficit in empathy*—inability to put oneself in another's position, including the failure to consider injury to others;
> *pathological entitlement*—conviction of his/her right to have whatever s/he needs; and

superoptimism—the belief that s/he will not get caught or punished, amounting to a type of omnipotent logic and grandiose thinking that enables a separation of actions from their consequences or effects.

Consistent with their well-developed denial systems, child abusers make idiosyncratic distinctions in degrees of blame that are often unintelligible to an outside observer and sometimes even accept incarceration rather than admit to the full extent of the charges against them (Salter, 1988). Within the context of perpetrator thinking errors, Salter (1988) has articulated a spectrum of denial, whose components include denial of the acts themselves; denial of planning and fantasy; denial of responsibility for the acts; denial of the seriousness of the behavior or its effects; denial of internal guilt; and denial of the difficulty of changing abusive patterns. An offender will often insist that he has suffered more than the victim,[23] readily listing the costs of disclosure and public censure—his standing in the community, his job, his freedom, his family—and evidencing little internal guilt (Salter, 1988, p. 108). "Genuine contrition in a perpetrator is a rare miracle" (Herman, 1992, p. 190).

From a clinical standpoint, the most important areas of investigation involve our learning how perpetrators affect victims' identity, memory, dissociative organization, and alterations in consciousness. Toward advancing such study, some clinicians/researchers have attempted to identify different types of sexual offenders.

Finkelhor and Williams (1992) categorize five distinct kinds of incesting fathers:

1. *the sexually preoccupied*, whose clear and conscious sexual interest in their daughters, often from birth, has always contaminated their relationships;
2. *the adolescent regressives*, who appear to be developmentally arrested in early adolescence and become sexually activated when their daughters reach puberty;
3. *the instrumental self-gratifiers*, who demonstrate significant recrimination for their fantasies and behaviors—rationalized in spite of their guilt, sometimes by mentally turning their daughters into adults— and who struggle sincerely to redirect attention toward their wives;
4. *the emotionally dependent*, who target their loneliness and frustrated marital needs toward their daughters; and

5. *the angry retaliators*, embittered men with elaborate justifications for their acting out, who often blame others.

Larson and Maddock (1986) classify four family abusive styles based on underlying purpose of the abuse:

1. *affection-exchange*, whereby sexual abuse stems from the offender's need for affection;
2. *erotic-exchange*, typical of a family that sexualizes everything and all sex in the family as normal and legitimate;
3. *aggression-exchange*, whereby sexual abuse is an extension of physical abuse and part of a system of punishment and humiliation; and
4. *rage-expression*, characteristic of highly violent and sadistic families.

Salter (1995) identifies sadistic, nonsadistic, and power/control abusers, and also distinguishes the use of force (by sadists and power/control types) from the use of "grooming" to obtain victim compliance. In each paradigm of abuse and perverted desire, the perpetrator has his own preferred relationship with his victim(s), ranging from a need to see (or fantasize) him/her as sexually desirous to a need to exercise absolute control over every aspect of the victim's life, and beyond that to the need to incite complete terror and submission in order to achieve sexual arousal and psychological stabilization/inflation.

In sexually abusive family systems the child-victim is often parentified and triangulated inappropriately into parental roles either because the parents are absent, intoxicated, or have otherwise abdicated their parental responsibilities (Alexander and Friedrich, 1991; Weiner and Kurpius, 1995). The role of substance abuse as a disinhibitor, a motivating force, and as a factor in memory distortion among perpetrators should not be underestimated (Araji and Finkelhor, 1986). Intrafamilial, sex-ring, and ritual sexual abuse often takes place under the influence of mind-altering substances and often involves the forcible intoxication or drugging of children to obtain their compliance, profoundly confuse them, and disable their memories.

Notably, child sexual abusers have been shown to demonstrate significantly more learning problems, cognitive defects, and neuropsychological impairment than normal (Langevin and Watson, 1996; Langevin, Martentette, and Rosati, 1996).[24] In general the research points out that pedophiles show language-based cognitive impairment that obstructs comprehension, information retention and retrieval, and application of new learning to therapy situations and to their lives over all. (The investigators caution, however, against making conclusions about the etiological significance of their findings: there could be a bias in the sample of offenders who are caught [that is, the brighter ones may get away], or perhaps sex offenders are no different from other criminals, who may also show more cognitive defects than the population at large.)

MOTIVATIONS OF PERPETRATORS

> *Two or three things I know for sure, but none of them is why a man would rape a child, why a man would beat a child. . . . All the things I can say about sexual abuse—about rape—none of them are reasons. The words do not explain. Explanations almost drove me crazy, other people's explanations and my own. Explanations, justifications, and theories. I've got my own theory. My theory is that rape goes on happening all the time. My theory is that everything said about that act is assumed to say something about me, as if that thing I never wanted to happen and did not know how to stop is the only thing that can be said about my life. My theory is that talking about it makes a difference—being a woman who can stand up anywhere and say, I was five and the man was big. So let me say it.*

> **—Dorothy Allison,**
> *Two or Three Things I Know for Sure*

Pedophilia must always be mentioned as part of the complex intersection of motivational variables, although Howitt (1995) cautions against regarding theories of pedophilia as sole explanations for why some adults sexually abuse children.25 Those who find children sexually arousing may be stirred by masturbatory fantasies encouraging such thoughts, the misattribution of affectionate feelings to sexual ones, or the message of child pornography that children are suitable sexual partners. Other theories of pedophilia argue that individuals who molest children do so because of their inability to establish normal adult sexual relationships.

Araji and Finkelhor (1986) contend that a variety of *disinhibiting factors* must be considered in understanding the cycle of child abuse that leads some adults to disregard or circumvent cultural norms and values about appropriate sexual behavior—for example, lack of impulse control, senility and mental retardation, disinhibitory effects of drugs and alcohol.

Externalization has been proposed as one of the primary privilegers of perpetrators or as a relational backdrop when the parent assaults the person of the child in an effort to avoid the narcissistic pain of accepting or struggling with devalued aspects of the self (Novick and Novick, 1994). Children's natural individuation and autonomy drives are experienced by such parents as hostile acts worthy of retaliation or as commodities to be appropriated or managed, since externalization is intimately linked with the inability to tolerate the separate existence of the other. The lack of empathy and the profound narcissistic deficits of most child victimizers lead to the use of the child as a repository of primitive agonies and disowned, hated, and humiliated self-representations.

Reenactment theory is another source of explanation of sexual victimization against children. Reenactment can refer to the direct or referential replication of the abuse that offenders suffer or have suffered (Howitt, 1995), although the theory that a history of childhood molestation leads to pedophilia may be untenable to the extent that many abusers falsely claim to have been violated (Freund, Watson, and Dickey, 1990).[26]

Another study (Federoff and Pinkus, 1996) was also unable to support the "abuse-to-abuser" hypothesis, but it did not rule out the possibility that there is a specific subgroup whose offenses parallel their own victimization histories (e.g., in terms of the ages at which they were abused and the ages of their victims). And while the research of Lisak and colleagues (1996) did find a clear link among convicted perpetrators between abuse and abusing, they concluded that the vast majority of their sample of men molested in childhood did *not* go on to become child molesters themselves. While direct or concrete reenactment theories are appealing in their simplicity, they seem to represent only a moderate element among diverse, complex psychosocial motivational factors. Perhaps if concrete, referential, symbolic, and interactional forms of reenactment were considered together, the motivational construct of reenactment would have greater explanatory power.

Addictiveness is motivating by definition. Salter (1995) understands the sexual abuse of children as a way for some adults to self-regulate, self-soothe, and, in some cases, provide self-coherence, by meeting their need for affection, for power or sensation, or for control of another's suffering to alleviate psychic deadness or psychotic anxieties. This conceptualization is consistent with what DeMause (1991; 1994) proposes concerning regulation of primitive emotional states and disintegration anxieties. The extremes of addiction in relation to child abuse occur when the perpetrator's (conscious or unconscious) shame about illicit and destructive activities evokes his/her anxiety and psychic disequlibrium leading to cravings for further perpetration as a desperate means of self-control. Escalations of this kind of cycle, particularly with sadistic pedophiles, can lead to brutal sprees of perpetration and serious, life-threatening injuries, and in some cases "unintentional" death of the victim.

Fetishism,[27] combined with the dynamics of malignant narcissism and sociopathy, also mobilizes sexual predation. Many abusers target children who remind them of themselves or who have other specific characteristics (Howitt, 1995). Some researchers have called this motivational factor emotional congruence (Araji and Finkelhor, 1986), referring to the most commonly cited theory about the origins of pedophilia—that sexual abusers choose children for sexual partners because children have some especially compelling emotional meaning for them. (Araji and Finkelhor describe, for example, arrested psychosexual development and emotionally immature patterns of male socialization that may encourage tendencies toward sexual dominance and narcissism whereby perpetrators seek sexual relationships with children with whom they identify.) For some offenders, the direct (or symbolic) replay of their own child abuse may be a dissociative strategy to avoid their own pain and remembering; when addictive and reenactment imperatives intersect, the victimizer maintains his/her own mental stability through the fetishistic, violent, or primitive envious exploitation of children's innocence, vulnerability, and capacity for unconditional love. Like other fetishes, child-abuse victims can provide the perpetrator with fantasies of protection, security, empowerment/omnipotence, revenge, and so on.

Many child sexual abusers are compulsive record keepers (Crewdson, 1988; Howitt, 1995), maintaining meticulous notes about each of the children they abuse, citing what was done to whom and where, the child's reactions, and so on. Lanning and Burgess (1984) describe one case where a perpetrator kept precise records on the average number of sex acts per child (64.68), the average duration of each relationship (2.2 years), the average age of each victim (10.89 years), and even the amount of sperm ejaculated by each boy he molested.

Relative *immunity* from consequences is surely facilitating, if not motivating of the choice to violate children in support of omnipotent, paranoid-schizoid modes of existence. When silence and disbelief are dependable social reactions, victimizers can take for granted that they are unlikely to be prosecuted. "Just as bacteria flourish when exposed to situations ideally suited to their growth needs, so torture thrives within environments that meet the torturer's needs" (Simpson, 1996, p. 203).

In *Psychopathic Sadism.*   Something essentially human is missing in many perpetrators, particularly in their relationships to children—an absence of normal attachment and healthy identificatory processes. Finkelhor and Lewis (1988) hypothesize that most child victimizers have severe deficiencies in empathy and show no protective feelings for children; pervasively deny that children occupy a special status and thus require special treatment; disdain childlike emotional characteristics (e.g., neediness, ignorance, spontaneity); lack interest in children and feel inadequate in caretaking roles.

Bollas (1995) expands on the lack of a "logical emotional link" (p. 189) in the more severe cases of torturers and psychopathic sadists and on their eroticized exploitation of basic trust and their need to merge sex and death—the killer's eroticism, whereby "a traumatized soul bearing a deep wound . . . [and] an envious hatred of life mutating into an envious identification with the anti-life . . . feels condemned to work his trauma upon the human race, trying to bring others to an equivalent fall" (p. 184).

The purely sadistic and ritual abusers and megalomaniacal perpetrators, extreme psychopathic sadists who achieve positions of power and whose histories emerge during the treatment of severely dissociative patients, are not likely to give interviews to researchers like Salter (1995) or Howitt (1995). This subgroup of perpetrators shows proclivities that go beyond sadistic sexual abuse to forcing the participation of children in the abuse and torture of animals and other children, embodying bizarre eroticizations of death, dying, and dismemberment. These are the people involved in the snuff-film industry, ritual abuse, and organized victimizer groups, people who take particular pleasure in using torture, terror, and trauma to induce children to engage in behaviors that forge identificatory links with their own malignant universes. These most pathological of malignant narcissists create miniature versions of themselves in their child-victims' minds and demand precise mirroring through repetition and participation in all the perverse acts that organize their representational worlds.

The destruction and perversion of innocence (along with the mortification of the child) is eroticized and reenacted as the extremely sadistic perpetrator concretely and psychologically penetrates the child-victim with his/her own deep psychospiritual wounding, temporarily alleviating the mounting annihilation anxieties and the chronic threat of destabilization. Once penetrated by and merged with a completely demonized psyche, children become the containers for the perpetrator's living hell as well as for some of the culture's most extreme (and extremely disavowed) shadow elements. Even as this subset of profoundly disturbed patient-survivors has been surfacing in the offices of therapists who treat severe dissociative disorders, the corresponding subset of perpetrators has not been documented, studied, or consistently arrested and incarcerated.

Grotstein (1984) highlights the chronic fear of being someone else's prey as the source of the individual's becoming a predator him/herself: in order to reify his/her manic defenses and ensure his/her psychological safety, s/he reenacts a traumatic fantasy on a passive victim. Grotstein describes willful sadists and murderers as wishing to inflict pain not so much for the joy in seeing the victim suffer as to see the look of agony in the victim's face, which reestablishes contact with their own suffering selves one step removed, by means of projection. (Survivors confirm that this sight of agony is a key element in torture, snuff films, and human sacrifice situations.) The perpetrator's manic defense operates to deny and translocate the victimized self into another victim: "Evil, having been deprived of its prenatal innocence, seeks to regain it by stealing it from the unborn child, the special one, the ego ideal, the one who does not have to experience demoralization through the act of living" (p. 222).

> After he beat me, he tied me up and raged at me for the audacity of resisting him. His eyes were wild and on fire, like he was possessed. Any movement unleashed more violence and ranting. His hatred is beyond description; it cut through me like a knife. I had to learn to be completely still, but if I closed my eyes or tried to go away, you know, to dissociate, he would bring me back and make me face him so he could watch me struggle. Each of my pleas for some humanity from him were met with more abuse, making me have to face that there was no humanity left in him. Facing that was worse than the pain and fear.
>
> **—Anonymous**

Psychopathic sadists "have to continually punish the victim to prove to themselves that they are in control, that it is not themselves but someone else who is the victim. The compulsive component of this behavior is crucial to its identification" (Howell, 1996, p. 440). Howell believes that the addictive need of the psychopathic sadist for power over the lives of others comes from the dissociation of vulnerability and dependency. Howell (1996) also describes the psychopathic sadist's continuous and compulsive need to "put one over" on other people, which she equates with Meloy's (1988) concept of "endogenous deception" (p. 120). The experiences of exhilaration and contempt that follow the successful exercise of manipulation in response to internal pressures themselves become addictive; deception is ultimately necessary for the maintenance of psychic equilibrium, and not just for the usual instrumental reasons.

Sadistic ritual abusers are masters of deceit both in the contexts of the traumatic scenarios they engineer and in relation to the outside world. Specifically, they are masters of the psychological reversal: they want to control the victim's pain and escape from pain and interpretation of pain, but they do not want the victim to understand clearly who is actually inflicting the pain. The victim comes to believe that s/he is simultaneously special and worthless; is causing the pain and sexual violence; wants the pain and sexual violence; has forgotten the pain and violence and who caused it; should be ashamed of what s/he has done; is a liar who makes up stories to get attention or to get others in trouble; is victimizing the perpetrator by having rebellious thoughts or actions and should therefore feel guilty; is voluntarily one with the will and mind of the perpetrator; has false memories of abuse instead of false memories of nonabuse; is evil, whereas the perpetrator is good; is not believable, whereas the perpetrator is; and so on.

Gender Conditioning.

> The more messages males get from the culture that female children enjoy sex with adults, and/or that they deserve it because they are inferior creatures, and/or that they are not really human, the more men's internal inhibitions will be undermined. (Russell, 1996, p 182)

Social conditioning to gender roles and values lies beneath all theories of perpetrator-motivation. Indeed, the preponderance of perpetrators (particularly those who prey upon women and children) are men.[28] Russell and Finkelhor (1984) and Russell (1996) argue that patriarchial societies' sex-role socialization practices contribute to males' willingness to abuse females in general and children in particular, including

Elevating and emphasizing development of masculine qualities like dominance, fearlessness, competitiveness, toughness, and so on, that make way for predatory sexuality;

Encouraging males to split off feelings of tenderness and respect from sexual desire, allowing for their treatment of women (and children) as objects to conquer and control;

Endorsing hypersexuality as proof of virility, such that males may define all affectionate contact as sexual;

Identifying as preferred partners for men those who are younger, smaller, weaker, more innocent, vulnerable, dependent, all of which qualities are highly compatible with sexual interest in children;

Teaching men to take the initiative in sexual situations, to perceive resistance as a cover for sexual desire, and to overcome it, habituating them to coercive sexuality (Briere, Smiljanich, and Henschel [1994] refer to this as conditioning associations between sexual arousal and subjugation);

Conferring economic power on males, which reinforces their feelings of superiority and entitlement and serves to insulate them against punishment;

Exposing men to pornography, which may undermine their inhibitions and strengthen pedophilic and sadistic desires in those who already have them and arouse responses in those who do not through the laws of social learning;

Eroticizing children (particularly girls) in the media, again reinforcing emergent patterns of desire or disinhibiting some men from acting on them; and

Institutionalizing in the legal and law enforcement systems the prevailing social skepticism that men will only rarely be held accountable for incestuous abuse (Russell, 1996).

According to Melamuth, Heavey, and Linz (1996), sexual aggressors are most likely to score relatively high on measures of hostile masculinity and impersonal sexual orientation, which correspond to power and sexual motivations. They conclude that those factors in conjunction with opportunity-predictor variables can explain and predict the acting out of sexual aggression; their work demonstrates that sexual aggression may be expressed in behavior and underlying characterological patterns that are not overtly aggressive, and that sexually aggressive behavior should not be considered an isolated response but rather a way of conducting social relationships, particularly with women, and dealing with conflicts. Lisak, Hopper, and Song (1996), also addressing the convergence of gender and perpetration, document a combination of gender rigidity and emotional constriction in male perpetrators as compared with nonperpetrators.

THE WEB OF PERPETRATION

The perpetration of violence, torture, and sexual abuse of children is a multilayered, complex phenomenon, always involving the complicity and silence of many nonoffending adults (see Chapter 3). While some professionals have continued to explore the patterns and psychodynamics of child sexual abusers, some social critics like Kincaid (1998) are concerned that excessive emphasis on sexual abuse and sex predators will make innocent people (men) fearful of bathing or photographing their naked children, in addition to distracting from more important social issues and further reinforcing the sexualization of children. He encourages us to "stop looking for monsters and their victims. If we look, we'll find them. If we don't we won't," and concludes that "Such activity . . . really is a fraud, making all of us pay heavily for nothing" (p. 285). Others, like Jenkins (1998), contend that our notion of the sexual predator or sex offender is (merely) a socially constructed concept and that as such it changes with the causes, panics, and moral anxieties of each passing decade.

To date, our knowledge of child abusers derives primarily from the very small minority who get caught or come in for treatment. The proposed taxonomy that follows mines the raw material of which victims' often fragmented and variously ambiguous narratives are made, in the belief that the collective experiences of survivors are vital to expanding the scope and texture of our understanding of perpetrators' patterns. Beginning with the least destructive, those patterns are analyzed in ascending order of severity; each succeeding category incorporates the characteristics of the preceding ones.

PARASITIC PERPETRATORS

Least violent and at times nonviolent (viz., Salter's [1995] "grooming" offenders), parasitic perpetrators eroticize and prey upon children's innocence, sweetness, natural sensuality, and purity. If they suffered the traumatic loss of their own innocence in childhood (among other psychological disturbances, and not necessarily through sexual abuse), they may seek reparations through merger with the innocence of their victims; at the same time they enact their own traumatic loss by corrupting children's emerging sexuality, usually under the guise of "special relationships." Parasitic perpetrators wish to avoid harm to their victims at all costs—that is, to preserve the very innocence they feed on; indeed, due to an absence of empathy, they may not believe they are causing any damage whatsoever, and often they get their victims to internalize their beliefs. They may eroticize and exploit the children's spontaneity and mischievousness and may even create fantasied romantic attachments with them to alleviate their own emotional voids and to coerce compliance from needy, lonely victims.

Parasitic perpetrators are highly addicted to having children to molest since without victims they are almost like diabetics without insulin; they become depressed or agitated and, in some cases, disorganized unless they have a steady supply of psychological innocence to self-soothe and to self-regulate. Consequently, they position themselves to have access to prospective victims (e.g., by career choices, by marrying women with children; some commit incest instead). More apt than other types of perpetrators to get caught because they rarely resort to threats of harm or violence to ensure silence, they are also vulnerable to blackmailing and setups by sociopathic types. They may collect child pornography but they rarely traffic in children; if they are addicted to alcohol and drugs, it is only to manage their intermittent guilt and shame. Parasitic perpetrators, unlike others, do see their child-victims as separate from themselves; however, they have obvious boundary difficulties, deficits in empathy, and problems with entitlement. They leave their victims deeply mixed up about love and abuse, affection and sex, innocence and corruption. Abusers in this group are the most likely to benefit from treatment, when, as Salter (1995) indicates, such treatment is directed at teaching them empathy for their victims and correcting their cognitive distortions.

Narcissistic Perpetrators

These abusers are defined primarily by their lack of self-other differentiation and their tendency to enact their own self-hatred and primitive grandiosity through molestation, shaming, humiliation, hate, or vicious acts on children. Externalizers par excellence, narcissistic perpetrators are threatened by any demonstration of their victims' independence, so they can become enraged and punitive in the face of evidence of autonomy or separateness; protests or struggles against the abuse, particularly indicative of just such separateness, are quick to incite further cruelty. They are most interested in exploiting the children's innocence and availability as receptacles for their own toxicity, fear, and projected emotional pain. Children's natural mischievousness and spontaneity stir their envy and intense anger in connection with their unconscious recognition of their own limitations and their corresponding psychic scarring; many mothers who sexually and violently abuse their children fit in here (as do Munchausen mothers, who generate medical crises in their children).

The self-hate and masochism of narcissistic perpetrators is often masked behind their cruel treatment of the victims from whom they do not experience themselves as separate. Some, believing they own their children, may sell them into prostitution and pornography in exchange for drugs or money; many patients report having been handed over by their fathers, stepfathers, and so on, to cover their losses at cards. Others raise their children to be the perfect "mistress," sex slave, or puppet, mirroring the perpetrators' omnipotent (e.g., restorative) fantasies and regulating intense needs for power and control. In the most severe circumstances, adults moving in and out of psychotic states of dissolution torment and torture their children by way of establishing some kind of self-cohesion and psychic equilibrium; in the absence of access to children, they may become depressed, disorganized, or overtly psychotic.

Their narcissism may allow this group of perpetrators to avoid detection and to present to the community (or the rest of the family) a completely different façade from the one they show to their children in private; the severely deranged among them may appear eccentric or unusual to the neighbors or relatives, but rarely do people suspect what goes on behind closed doors. Despite their cruelty, they are not driven (as the sadistic offenders are) by the primary desire to do harm. The harm they inflict is, in fact, secondary to their need for externalizing the hatred and pain that threaten to destabilize them psychologically. (This distinction may not matter to victims on the other end of their cruelty and machinations.) If and when they are caught, narcissistic perpetrators are likely to deny their actions or the impact of their actions, blaming everything on their victims and manipulating the victims' belief and perceptual systems even into adulthood. Left with intense shame, self-hatred, and deep feelings of unworthiness, victims of these perpetrators find themselves unlovable unless they are abused; fearing any kind of dependency, they may grow up to disparage their own vulnerability, and may even engage others in perpetuating their residual core confusions between love and hate, feelings and actions, loyalty and self-destructiveness. Survivors of this type of perpetration develop unusual fears and behavior patterns regarding feelings of anger, aggression, and hate.

PROGRAMMED PERPETRATORS

Survivors of organized child abuse often fall into this category of highly dissociative individuals whose drive to commit sexual or violent acts against children is a function of training and largely an artifact of their histories, which latter they may or may not recall or reveal for some time in treatment, even as they struggle with unconscious guilt and shame for what they feel they have done. For the most part, they do not make reenacting their abuse on children a habit or even a pattern; desperation to avoid intimacy (i.e., to avoid exposing themselves to others, and to themselves) can cause them to behave extremely inconsistently and hurtfully in their adult relationships, however. Their guilt/shame leads to chronic addictions to drugs and alcohol, sexual compulsivity, and suicidality (signaling impulses to both punish themselves for, and prevent themselves from repeating, their crimes).

Vulnerable throughout their lives to the reactivation of their programming—which might even have included training as assassins, depending on the nature of the organization to which they were captive—they tend to be highly self-defeating and self-destructive. Some of their dissociated states of mind or alter personalities may still have implanted belief systems about child abuse that are completely contradictory to the convictions they hold more consciously. Not at all incidentally, they are programmed to have no memory for their "crimes," so they are unable, if caught, to endanger their own perpetrator-programmers.

SPECIFIC-TRAUMA–REENACTING PERPETRATORS

A relatively common kind of perpetrator (when symbolic and concrete reenactment of prior trauma are considered and included in one category), trauma reenactors can be divided into masochistic and sadistic types. All tend to retain conscious beliefs in their own innocence, and their abuse reenactments involve considerable mimicry, imitation, and repetition. Those in the masochistic subgroup are usually highly self-destructive, suicidal, and addicted to drugs; they often engage their child-victims in performing sexual acts (or acts of compliance and obedience) to which they were subjected, and these sometimes include violent acts upon themselves as well. More apt to get caught (and, in fact, to unconsciously set themselves up for suspicion or detection) than their sadistic counterparts and more apt to experience guilt and shame, masochistic reenacting perpetrators are not necessarily moved to cause pain or suffering; rather, they play out the boundary violation, exploitation, and seduction/betrayal aspects of child abuse trauma. In most cases, this subgroup can more accurately be located in this sequence between parasitic and narcissistic perpetrators.

Unlike masochistic reenactors, the sadistic reenactors enjoy having control over others and externalizing pain and suffering. Eroticizing hierarchy (and at times, terror and mortification of the victim), they may be drawn to the military or to authoritarian religious and political movements; professionally, they hold positions of relative power (judge, lawyer, doctor, police officer, etc.). They are likely to seek opportunities to enter trance states from which to enact sadistic violence on children in order to release the accumulating tension generated by their own split-off traumatic affects. They are cunning and rarely ever caught. Their sadism is a lifestyle that has found expression throughout history in politically oppressive regimes. They may be among the consumers of sadistic child pornography and snuff films. As a group they are vulnerable to influence by more seriously disturbed perpetrators described below and may devolve into more malignant varieties.

"CEO" Perpetrators
(Vicarious, Culturally Sanctioned)

Interested in power and money, like high-level pimps, and not necessarily in violating children, these profiteers are products of both our societal and criminal hierarchies; they play an abuse-supporting rather than an abuse-enacting role. They may be in economic, religious, and political positions of power, and their exploitation of subordinates—particularly women—dovetails so smoothly with cultural norms as to mask their destructive impulses. Or they may be underground cartel leaders, sociopathic CEOs, whose organizations directly and indirectly support and profit from organized child abuse—or they may hold government or law enforcement positions where they take money from others in order to guarantee noninterference in criminal activities. What they want is power, and accordingly they are involved both in blackmailing actual child abusers and coordinating related "delivery" services; they may also traffic in arms and in drugs.

MIND-CONTROL PERPETRATORS

Highly sadistic and utterly callous, these perpetrators are interested in the conquest of the human mind and in maintaining complete control over individuals and groups (sometimes nations), and also in economic exploitation—that is, not just in inflicting harm. They often have leadership roles in cults or mainstream religions, military intelligence, or underground criminal groups. Early incarnations of this species could be found in the more perverse elements of the Church's colonization of the indigenous people of the Americas, who combined religious indoctrination with slavery and sexual exploitation to exercise complete psychological, spiritual, and economic dominion over vast numbers of people; more recent versions surface in documented accounts of CIA mind-control projects (Weinstein, 1990; Bowart, 1978; 1994).

A highly educated segment of the perpetrator population, they have access to mind-control technology and cold, scientific attitudes toward human beings, using children like laboratory rats for medical and psychological experiments in shaping and managing dissociative response patterns. They leave victims feeling completely dehumanized, psychologically and spiritually raped, desolate, and with absolutely no sense of free will or agency. Often employed by highly secretive subgroups hidden in mainstream organizations, they are almost never caught; indeed, their existence is largely ignored, denied, or disbelieved.

RITUAL-ABUSE PERPETRATORS

Not only are these offenders highly sadistic but their brutality is also often combined with complex religious and superstitious beliefs. Their sexual abuse of children reflects extreme power and control themes and enactments. Moreover, they have eroticized, and become highly addicted to, combinations of sex and death (in fantasy and reality), and various forms of extreme mortification of children. If they come from families where perverse belief systems were passed down intergenerationally, they may be highly dissociative and able to successfully lead double lives.

Their primary imperative is the corruption and destruction of children's innocence and purity, expressed in human and animal sacrifice and dismemberment, enacted in order to obtain power. They seek to sever the victims' internal relationship with their own sense of core goodness and their relationship to hope, faith, and belief in a benevolent, redemptive deity. Their interest in conquest resembles that of mind-control perpetrators—and many ritual abusers do, in fact, engage in brainwashing and thought reform—but their goals are predominantly religious and spiritual; both economic and psychological opportunism are secondary. Also involved in the snuff-film industry and in blackmailing less sophisticated child abusers into committing more heinous crimes, they concretize fantasies of conquering God and evidence a raw, unmodulated hunger for power and dominion over their entire environment. They have a paradoxical relationship with hierarchy, debasing culturally and institutionally sanctioned models, on the one hand, and eroticizing extreme patriarchal and demonic variations on the other.

Having experienced the extremes of hatred during their own childhoods, they have committed themselves quite consciously to lifestyles of destruction and contemptuous mockery of cultural norms and mainstream religious traditions. Hence they are highly retaliatory, and leave their victims in abject devastation, indoctrinated with hateful, fear-based ideologies and phobic of (or contemptuous of and/or enraged at) mainstream religious traditions. Higher-level ritual abusers are not primarily dissociative, but rather consciously malevolent, essentially warped at their core, cunning, and rarely if ever caught. They exhibit such extreme psychological malformation that our current classification system for psychiatric disorders cannot explain much of their behavior: they appear to be so profoundly spiritually wounded that no category can contain them. Unlike the pure sadists, some of these individuals can move comfortably and without detection among various social milieus—between the "day world" that they so contemptuously mock, and the "night world" where they feel they really belong (and where they believe they rule). Their existence is currently denied by most mental health and law enforcement professionals.

PURE SADISTIC PERPETRATORS

The primary distinction here is the unmitigated intent to harm—the demonstration of unbridled sadism, independent of revenge or retaliation or, most important, ideology or doctrine. Driven by the pure joy of doing harm, sadistic perpetrators are not interested in corrupting children as much as they are in torture and the abject destruction of innocence. Their lust to destroy, like the disturbances of ritual abusers, defies psychological explanation. Their violence takes the form of sexual torture because that targets the greatest vulnerability in and elicits the most power over their victims. Addicted to sex-death enactments, sadistic perpetrators are often involved in the snuff-film industry, dismemberment rituals, and intermittent human sacrifice. They often become highly dependent on or addicted to opiates, amphetamines, tranquilizers, and/or other mood-altering substances to sustain their fragile psychic equilibrium in between sprees of destruction.

The Third Reich (among other fascistic movements of the past century from South Africa to Guatemala) permitted many such individuals to rise to positions of prominence. Giving new meaning to the concepts of hate, greed, and envy as they devour all life forms in their path, they desire to dominate others at the very deepest fathoms. They are consciously and willfully parasitic and must feed off the pain and suffering of other human beings— mostly children—in order to sustain their own psychological survival. No single organized group can accommodate too many of these highly feared (and sometimes revered) individuals; they simply do not and cannot share power. Unable to move around fluidly, they usually live in some controlled habitat or restricted-access environment, and often require drugs to maintain their psychological equilibrium.

Megalomaniacal Perpetrators

These are the ultra-perpetrators, a rare breed that combines the sadism, power needs, complete lack of conscience, and extreme psychopathy of all the others—with the added dimension of social acceptability. Unlike the pure sadist who cannot be out in the world for any length of time in a conspicuous or public role, the megalomaniacal perpetrator (e.g., Hitler, Mengele, Saddam Hussein, Papa Doc and Baby Doc Duvalier, Pol Pot) can function in diverse social settings and move easily between conventional and criminal worlds. But like the pure sadist he is committed to wreaking havoc and inflicting harm, taking pleasure in extreme forms of power and domination over others. Unhampered by the pure sadist's limitations, the megalomaniacal perpetrator is able to split off from his overtly destructive aspects, gain social approval, and function successfully for long periods of time in the normal culture—especially if the social and political conditions are conducive. The ultimate cult or cartel leaders, megalomaniacal perpetrators are evil incarnate, and their extensive networks almost always engage in the wholesale exploitation, abuse, and slaughter of children on a vast scale.

KNOWING AND NOT KNOWING

What makes people (mostly men) abuse children? We can develop theories based on economics, psychodynamics, PTSD, reenactment, gender, spiritual deficits, addiction, and chemical dependency models. We can conjecture. However, for all of our scientific advances we do not fully understand this disturbed side of humanity or our collective role in producing thousands, perhaps hundreds of thousands, of sex offenders and child-abuse perpetrators. The analysis of perpetrator dynamics clearly reaches the limits of psychology's ability to explain human behavior; in fact, we have no precise nomenclature to describe many of those who abuse children. What is clearly needed, alongside an integrated approach to understanding them is an equally sophisticated multidisciplinary approach to the problem of collusion, individual and cultural, in the social facilitation of child abuse.

The exploitation of children's dependency, emotional vulnerability, and nascent sexuality as organizing principles for stabilizing disturbed psyches and dysfunctional families, or as a "cash crop" in the criminal subcultures of Western industrialized and third world nations, mirrors the profound greed and indifference of a society endowed with the resources to reverse it. Because our own constructs of sexuality are destructive and revolve around shame, guilt, misogyny, fear of the body, and, most important, the eroticization of hierarchy, they manifest themselves accordingly in the objectification of women, the sexualization of, and violence against, children, in denial and dissociation about the effects and meaning thereof, and, finally, in assaults on those who bring the bad news. We cannot look forward to an end to the child-abuse epidemic until we see a transformation in society from glorification of hierarchy and domination (lip service to human rights notwithstanding) to authentic commitment to social justice and the mental health and well-being of all citizens.

CHAPTER 3

Child Abuse and Cultural Ambivalence: Complicity, Incredulity, and Denial

Our culture has enthusiastically sexualized the child while denying just as enthusiastically that it was doing any such thing.
—James R. Kincaid

Child abusers, like others who commit crimes against humanity, rely on the convenient incredulity of the rest of us—on our incapacity to imagine the darker regions of human possibility, or our desire to disavow them, or both.

BARRIERS TO RECOGNITION OF DISSOCIATIVE DISORDERS

Public and professionals alike resist the idea that abused children develop real symptoms like multiple personality disorder: in the face of incomprehensible evidence of bizarre sexual abuse, sadism, and torture of children it is easier to blame and diagnose the victim than to confront (much less empathize with) the adult who has abused the child (Miller, 1984). One of the toughest challenges in treating trauma and dissociation is to integrate what we know (and don't know but can imagine) about both traumatic realities and intrapsychic fantasy. The landscape of trauma/DID treatment is a minefield of clinical recognition errors on both sides of the reality/fantasy fence where posttraumatic states and traumas are misconstrued as unconscious fantasy, and concretizations of fantasies are remembered as traumatic events.[1]

Relational psychoanalysis makes room for ideas about multiple self-organizations, the actual influence of real interpersonal events, and the dynamic interplay of psychic structures along with (and often theoretically more important than) classical notions of hierarchical renderings of conscious and unconscious mind. From this viewpoint, in other words, psychic structure is figured in terms of associative-dissociative processes; the common appearance of dissociative states in the course of intensive psychotherapy in general and in work with survivors of severe trauma in particular should not be the least bit surprising (Davies, 1996a).

At the crossroads of trauma theory and relational psychoanalysis there is a transitional theoretical space for understanding the panoply of dissociative voices emanating from the psyches of the severely traumatized. When the therapist learns to recognize and speak the often paradoxical language of multiplicity (for example, regarding alter personalities as both subjectively real and objectively illusory/delusional; regarding psychic material as both symbolic and posttraumatic), the clinician can enter a transitional space (Winnicott, 1969) where the traumatized patient's world becomes manifest, articulated, and knowable. In this milieu of transitional experiencing, theoretical absolutes and ideological autocracy about what is and isn't real or fantasy are simply impractical.

The elliptical idiom of multiplicity has blocked the appropriate recognition and legitimization of severe dissociative conditions, partly because of a historic unfamiliarity with the phenomenology of posttraumatic states in the helping professions and the mass media alike, and partly because of the complexity and magnitude of the symptoms of severely dissociative patients, their difficulties with close relationships, and their easily misunderstood character pathology. Indeed, DID patients are particularly vulnerable to misdiagnosis and to becoming revictimized by therapists and other mental health caregivers (Herman, 1992; Putnam, 1989; Ross, 1997).[2] In addition, skeptics misunderstand and misrepresent the dynamics of entitlement among DID patients as part of a cultural dissociation process that not only marginalizes and dismisses them but also—by ridiculing and pathologizing their survival strategies and isolating the effects of victimization from the cause—subjects them to a kind of collective revictimization.

This severely traumatized population has been noted to be among the most frequently involved in sexual boundary violations by therapists (Smith, 1984; Van der Kolk, 1989; Hedges, 1994; Salter, 1995). Further, and for a variety of reasons including unconscious reenactment and secondary gain, some severely dissociative patients are convinced to display their bizarre symptoms and unusual histories on television in a perverse circus atmosphere that does little to educate an already confused and overstimulated public. Survivors of sexual abuse, socialized to comply with the irrational demands of authority figures in exchange for nurturance, care, and protection, may not question the behavior of an exploitative therapist or media investigator (Pope and Brown, 1996). The average DID patient spends six to seven years in the mental health system diagnosed with schizophrenia, depression, bipolar disorder, borderline personality disorder, even premenstrual syndrome (Carlson et al., 1993; Kluft, 1987a; Putnam et al., 1986).

MIXED MESSAGES FROM THE MENTAL HEALTH PROFESSIONS

Dissociative identity disorder is so controversial in part because of disagreement about its etiology; from there follows disagreement about its status as a legitimate psychiatric diagnosis, about its treatment, and about its relationship with other disorders (Ross, 1997). The most recent schisms in the field reflect fascination with the question of whether increased diagnosis of dissociative pathologies echoes a change in the epidemiological prevalence of such disorders, overdue public acknowledgment of what has always lived secretly among us, or the iatrogenic suggestions of the psychotherapy professionals gone astray (Davies, 1996a).[3]

Specialists who have continued to explore the phenomenon of DID and its posttraumatic origins are accused by hostile colleagues of gullibility, incompetence, misdiagnosis, overdiagnosis, and faddish preoccupations (Ross and Gahan, 1988; Kluft, 1994), of using contorted logic and contradictory definitions, and of engaging with their patients in a "hoax" or a "tango of suggestion" (Piper, 1997, p. 53).[4] Multiple personality disorder has been deemed an iatrogenic creation (Merskey, 1992; Fahy, 1988), the cocreation of patient and naïve therapist (Victor, 1975), a product of social learning and role playing (Spanos, 1994), an outgrowth of patient compliance with therapist countertransference enthusiasm and feminist agendas (Ofshe and Watters, 1994; Loftus and Ketcham, 1994), a consequence of the concretization of the patient's inchoate psychic states or therapist's avoidance of painful or primitive transferences (Ganaway, 1994; Hedges, 1994), a result of masterful malingering, or a borderline psychopathology run amok.

Goodwin and Sachs (1996) respectfully attribute some of the skepticism with which severely dissociative patients' narratives are received to doubts about the trustworthiness of reconstructed memory, subject as it is to distortion and to contamination by fantasy and imaginal processes, exaggeration, cognitive confusion, erotic transference, drugs and hypnosis, and the conscious and unconscious masking of other trauma. But responsible clinicians must not be seduced into *dis*belief by those vicissitudes of memory, must not look away from the repugnant by dismissing it as implausible, must not back away from witnessing the histories even of those whose chronic exposure to extreme trauma generates alternating revelations and recantations and erratic symptomatologies.

Perlman (1999) reports how the experience of treating heroin addicts who prostituted their children for drug money reminded him that accounts of the misuse of children in profitable organized sex rings and the torture and brainwashing of children in sadistic ritual-abuse groups were not at all deniable. McWilliams (1994) points out that we already have plenty of evidence for the existence of malevolent subcultures that

> operate like factories for dissociation. . . . For every destructive cult that has been identified—the most notorious of recent years being David Koresh's Branch Davidians—there may be several that operate in complete secrecy. In an era that has seen the crimes of the Nazis, the Ku Klux Klan, the Mafia, and more isolated groups like the Manson family, we cannot afford to ignore any evidence that evil is being propagated in organized ways. (p. 326)

Greaves and Faust's (1996) conclusion supports keeping a wide-open mind:

> Every hypothesis and observation about child sexual abuse is partially true: (1) It actually happens; (2) It is overreported; (3) It is underreported; (4) It is exaggerated in importance; (5) It is diminished in importance; (6) It is lied about; (7) It is covered up; (8) It is denied altogether. (pp. 596–597)

And McWilliams (1994) wisely champions a nonideological clinical stance:

> I recommend that whatever the reader's bias, he or she try to comprehend the phenomenon of dissociation with an "experience-near" sensibility; that is, from the standpoint of empathy with the internal experience of the person who feels and behaves like a composite of many different selves. (p. 328)

The violation of children in both the family[5] and the culture can be conceptualized as a continuum beginning with benign neglect and mild narcissistic appropriation and extending through malignant narcissistic misuse and physical abuse, severe and willful neglect, emotional abuse, abandonment, and betrayal, to outright exploitation—the selling, humiliating, and trafficking in children; the sexual, fetishistic use of children; sadistic abuse, ritual abuse, human laboratory experimentation, torture, sacrifice, and sexualized murder for the snuff-film industry. The depth of the severe dissociative disorders calls attention to how victims internalize violent belief systems and relationships with disturbed caretakers, to their patterns of identification with aggressors and collaborators, and to the insidious exercise of mind control. The extreme alterations imposed on normal psychological and physiological processes by exposure to chronic violence, neglect, and terrorization, must not be underestimated.[6]

LOCATING DID IN DIAGNOSTIC SPACE

First reported almost four centuries ago (Bliss, 1986), multiple personality disorder was resurrected with the rediscovery of dissociative conditions in the mid-1970s by a few trailblazing pioneers (such as Wilbur, Caul, Greaves, Bliss, Allison, Kluft, Braun), who shifted paradigms and found new ways to listen to their patients instead of boxing them into rigid, preexisting rigid categories (Fine, 1996). Pronouncement of MPD/DID continues to elicit reactions from fascination, concern, and outrage, to incredulity, and to evoke sharp attacks on those who suffer from it as well as on those who treat it (Kluft, 1995).

Despite the ambivalence attending its reception, DID is solidly in the mainstream of American psychology and psychiatry[7] (Kluft, 1996a). In the professional literature, DID has had many names: multiplex personality, double existence, dual personality, double personality, plural personality, dissociated personality, multiple personality, split personality, and multiple personality disorder (Brenner, 1996). Kluft (1996a) notes that the reified term "personality" has long been a problematic one. The name was changed from multiple personality disorder to dissociative identity disorder in an attempt to circumvent the argument that the disorder cannot be real because it is not possible to have more than one personality (Ross, 1995b).[8] *Dissociative identity disorder* deemphasizes the notion of proliferating personalities and highlights the patient's inability to integrate various aspects of identity, memory, and consciousness (Cardena and Spiegel, 1996). But clearly, as Brenner (1996) states, the condition is experiencing an identity crisis of its own.

DID seems most functionally associated with Herman's (1993) Complex PTSD and Herman's (1992; 1993) and Van der Kolk and Fisler's (1995) proposed DESNOS (Disorders of Extreme Stress Not Otherwise Specified). The first model integrates complex and unusual variations of PTSD with specific characterological and relational patterns, including the development of identity-formation paradigms under conditions of domination and subjugation, and vulnerability to repeated harm and revictimization. DESNOS can account for the sequelae to prolonged victimization and repetitive trauma in captivity under conditions of terror, torture, and strong perpetrator-attachment bonds, all characteristic of DID. Classification based on severe and unusual posttraumatic etiology would institutionalize a coherent diagnostic vision for reparative clinical, political, and social decision-making; moreover, because it emphasizes unequivocally the role of the social context, such a schema depathologizes responses to extreme violence and trauma. The unusual, perplexing, and often provocative characterological features of DID would be understood to be secondary to the traumatic interpersonal and dysfunctional cultural environments that nourish them.

Unfortunately, the validation of posttraumatic foundations of DID and its rightful locus in the *Diagnostic and Statistical Manual* is a politically charged and controversial one, as are most correlates of trauma, dissociation, and multiplicity. The evidence adduced here supports the linkage of dissociative and posttraumatic stress disorders (see Pitman, 1993; Brett, 1993) with DESNOS, and the establishment of DESNOS as a diagnostic syndrome distinct from, if overlapping with, PTSD and dissociative disorders.

PUBLIC AND PROFESSIONAL REACTIONS TO
DID PATIENTS' ALLEGATIONS OF RITUAL ABUSE

Nowhere is the polarization around child abuse, dissociation, and MPD/DID more extreme than in the debates about sadistic ritual abuse and organized evil, where there seems to be no middle ground (Charles, 1995). It is generally agreed that a good part of the polarization arises simply because of the extreme nature of the allegations involved in ritual abuse, which are startling, disturbing, and quite difficult for most people to believe or even comprehend unless they have a very good grasp of the dark side of human history (see Newton, 1996, for example, for a review of the history of human sacrifice). And it is generally recognized that some patients confabulate, or pick up material from other patients and the media, or willfully lie, and that some patients demonstrate primary process thinking and incorporate satanism or ritual abuse into their manifest delusional systems; always, there are likely to be elements of idiosyncratic distortion (Sakheim, 1996). And always in the patient population there will be those who are confused, delusional (or cultivating primitive transferences), suggestible, and extrinsically influenced, those who are malingering, elaborating for secondary gain, and camouflaging other trauma—along with those who have indeed experienced the extreme brutality and dehumanization that is sadistic child abuse.[9]

While Lanning (1992), for one, counters reports of organized sexual abuse with the fact that the FBI has not found evidence to support them, rejoinders by Noblitt and Perskin (1995) and Newton (1996) remind us that—given J. Edgar Hoover's record (of denying the existence of organized crime and suppressing evidence of Ku Klux Klan terrorism, for example)—that comment says more about the FBI than it does about child abuse. Ross (1995a), however, recommends separating the forensic and clinical issues altogether, espousing an approach that transcends the debate over whether ritual abuse is real or not and focuses on treating the patient. For Ross, neither believing nor disbelieving is the appropriate clinical strategy. And either extreme can lead to retraumatization.

While this middle ground is an important fundamental posture, psychoanalytically oriented therapists working intersubjectively or relationally cannot hide in the safe cognitive-behavioral crucible; they will have to enter the fray with their patients and confront the questions of belief, denial, incredulity, and confusion. In both their own private reveries and what they share of their countertransference experiences toward making interventions and interpretations, such clinicians will acknowledge and struggle to balance their willingness to believe with their desires to look away and deny. Discussing feelings and deconstructing doubts and fears free of absolutes promises not just the eventual reconstruction of elusive history but also transformation: the process will subvert authoritarian paradigms of coercive control—domination and silencing—and help the patient find his/her own voice and, regardless of how the facts turn out, a new and reparative relationship experience.

While acknowledging that incompetent therapists exist, that people are open to suggestion and influence, that memory is fallible, and that some individuals would rather believe they were victimized by a cult than by a beloved parent, it is still impossible to rule out the existence of organized, economically and psychospiritually motivated criminal behavior by groups of exploitative adults and sadists. Aside from the fact that the subject of ritual abuse is exceedingly controversial, our information being largely supplied by survivors whose testimonies have become increasingly marginalized by the onslaught of the false memory movement, we must, as Waites (1993) points out, balance what we know about the psychology of rumor with what we know about the psychology of denial.

> We recoil from what our preconscious perceptions tell us is happening. We reassure ourselves that such things only happen in fantasy. We hope for the best. We don't allow ourselves to ask too many questions. We get irritated when someone reminds us that there may be a problem. We wonder if they are trying to call attention to themselves or sensationalizing or are morally rigid and trying to get someone else in trouble. (Goodwin, 1994, p. 480)

As Goodwin points out, human beings are always hoping for evidence that things aren't as bad as we have suspected. Consequently, the most extreme cases are the least credible. That is, while child abuse is almost never admitted by perpetrators, victims' allegations (or even some admissions of severe child abuse) are almost never believed (Goodwin, 1994).

Yet it is unlikely indeed that the organized child pornography/prostitution industries are completely monitored by our law enforcement systems; it is also unlikely indeed that all the organized child abuse alleged by thousands of patients to thousands of therapists in this and other countries is fabricated or confabulated. Our legal and child protection systems have a long way to go before clinicians can dismiss the collective accounts of multiple perpetrator abuse and networks of child trafficking.[10]

The battle over the criminological evidence of ritual abuse may be obscuring a more basic reality: there is something fundamentally flawed in our society's ability to protect children from intra-and extrafamilial abusers. In the years to come, as denial recedes and tolerance for knowing about atrocities increases, more evidence is likely to surface about the widespread sexual abuse and sale of children. The bulk of the evidence will probably always be buried in the psyches of victims, however, and for the perpetrators, there is no better place to hide their crimes. As Nachmani (1995) reminds us, being a victim often means having no witnesses, having no capacity to witness, and having no narrative.

COLLABORATION, COMPLICITY, AND COLLUSION[11]

In 1909, it was estimated that gonorrheal infections afflicted from eight hundred to one thousand girls in Baltimore alone. . . . Chicago's county hospital maintained a ward for children with venereal diseases, "one of the most pathetic sights" in the city, which over a twenty-seven month period was used by six hundred youngsters under twelve years of age. . . . In 1915, in a case study of sixty-six little girls diagnosed at the St. Louis clinic, researchers briefly considered the idea that infection might be spread by rape or sexual assault. . . . Lacking other hypotheses, the writers of the article traced the contagion to badly designed toilet seats. (Jenkins, 1998, p. 31)

Collaboration takes overlapping forms in abusive family, mental health, and social systems: simple ignorance; selective inattention; turning a deaf ear to the protests of victims; not confronting explicit acts of domination and perpetration; denying the extent, the intent, the consequences, or the meaning of various abusive behaviors toward children; ignoring the connections among pornography, prostitution, and child abuse; ignoring or distorting statistical data on child abuse; unquestioning identification with the existing family or societal institutions, arrangements, or customs; publicly declaring an accused perpetrator innocent when aware of his/her guilt consciously or unconsciously; producing or supporting extremely biased television documentaries on child abuse, DID, or psychotherapy; allowing one's children to be used sexually by family members; spuriously generalizing about children's suggestibility, memory problems, or tendencies to lie in order to discredit them; diagnosing and pathologizing the sequelae of abuse without linking them to the external events that precipitated the need for extreme psychological adaptations; valuing personal anxiety reduction above all other ethical or moral principles; punishing children for revealing sex crimes; failing to adequately investigate child abuse charges; selling or handing over one's child directly for abuse; exploiting the abuse of others for psychological, spiritual, or economic gratification; blaming the victim and minimizing (or contemptuously mocking the extent or continuation of) his/her pain; refusing to invest in or to orchestrate reparation processes; pressuring victims to give premature forgiveness to their perpetrators; and supporting elaborate coverups or strategic manipulation of appearances for the sake of avoiding criminal prosecution.

All of these patterns characterize severely dissociative patients as well as members of abusive family systems and our society as a whole. From this point of view, as well as from a feminist perspective, the problem of child-abuse trauma and perpetration cannot be located in the individual alone, but must simultaneously be located in the social, power, economic, and gender arrangements of the dominant culture. Any analysis of child abuse that focuses solely on the perpetrator and not on the colluding systems runs the risk of perpetuating a kind of collective dissociative consciousness where parts of a whole are separated and treated with unequal attention. Talking about child-abuse victimization without simultaneously discussing collusion is like believing that Holocausts happen because a few powerful individuals make them happen. The malignant creativity of many child abusers may involve elaborately playing on the naïveté, denial, and incredulity of society, but the ready availability of such a willing and cooperative audience meets them halfway.

The Matrix of Complicity: A Classification System for Collaborators in Child Abuse

The diabolic is an arena of disorientation and confusion in which truth is lost, becoming unrecognizable even when seen. This arena is the perpetrator's cloak of invisibility, the evacuation of the victim's mind, the bystander's refusal to acknowledge sin. . . . In this obfuscation of truth, evil eludes accountability and justice. Secrecy, concealment, denial, ambiguity, confusion: these are Satan's fellow travelers, requiring elaborate interpersonal and intrapsychic collusion between perpetrators and bystanders. The operations of silence potentiate evil and remove all impediments from its path. (Grand, 2000, pp. 10–11)

Collaborators come in many forms, ranging from true innocence and ignorance to opportunism and an educated and fully aware cooperation with the perpetrator. This list is formulated in order of increasing *conscious* awareness and interaction with the perpetrator.

Innocent Collaborators.   Innocent collaboration exists everywhere. We all participate. We watch the news and hear of atrocities from child abuse to war, and—in our innocence, ignorance, or inexperience—we choose to disbelieve or discount them. Near universal denial, facilitated by mass emotional withdrawal and intellectual dismissiveness, ensues; the victims, thus abandoned, are revictimized by the larger group, whose collective attention could stop such crimes and whose inattention (disregard, disbelief) constitutes at least passive cooperation with the perpetrators—unintentional collaboration. In our innocent denial, we become part of the problem.

Innocence can be deadly. For many patients over the years, the misdiagnoses arising from innocent collaboration by dedicated professionals biased toward regarding claims of abuse as fantasy led to the administration of shock treatments and improper medications, to prolonged hospitalizations, even to suicide. Institutionalized silencing and subjugation have pernicious consequences for dissociative patients isolated in states of traumatic bonding and captivity to perpetrators. Wholesale failures to validate their past and current experiences not only drive the survivors further underground but actually reinforce everything the perpetrators ever told them would happen if and when help was sought.

"Switched-off" (i.e., Unwittingly Permissive) Innocent Collaborators. Characterized by a mix of vague awareness that something is wrong and specific ignorance born of a kind of ingenuous or preoccupied lack of imagination, this subset of innocents cannot conceive of what that something might be. They are enablers.

For example, a divorced mother may notice that little Jimmy has become depressed, even morose. She observes the bruises on one of his wrists after his uncle took him to the park and assumes he got them while playing. She works long days and she does not stop to connect the recent changes in her son's behavior with anything beyond the changes that came with the end of her marriage two years ago. Even as Jimmy becomes quieter and moodier and she does start to think about ways to cheer him up, she *literally* cannot imagine any cause but the divorce, having no life experience from which to draw a different conclusion; she opens dialogues with her son, but he cannot seem to tell her what is wrong. Tired and overwhelmed, she accepts with relief when her ex-husband's brother offers to help. Unconsciously, she opts out of the problem, and, unknowingly, she sends Jimmy off for the day with the very source of it, the uncle who is sexually abusing him.

In such unwitting collaborations, the evidence is there but the ignorant, unreflective individual lacks the wherewithal to recognize, much less stop, the violation or the perpetrator. Teachers, clergy, and medical and mental health professionals who overlook certain symptoms and patterns or fail to pursue the veiled comments of children or patients similarly cannot conceive of the dilemmas of abuse victims and/or choose to banish their own anxiety about the unknown.

Narcissistic Innocent Collaborators.　Narcissistic innocent collaboration is not uninformed. It is distinguished by an element of gain that supports the individual's pathological narcissism.

- A news reporter may have a vested interest in disbelieving a child-abuse story if disproving the allegations would advance his career. He might choose to pursue only leads that would validate his cause and to disregard or dissociate information inconsistent with it.
- A male judge may directly or indirectly discourage or disallow children's testimony against their fathers in custody disputes or women's delayed-recall testimony against their fathers. Although he is technically innocent, his resistance to accusations against men may lead him to believe only the expert witness who confirms that the legal system treats men unfairly. As a consequence, he could unintentionally remand a child to the custody of an abusive parent and/or authorize the release of a perpetrator instead of punishment.
- An academic might make the opportunistic decision to omit from her dissertation medical reports citing scarring on children's genitals because they conflict with her hypothesis that child abuse does not exist.
- A mental health professional whose ideological allegiances or defensive biases run counter to the trauma-based conception of pathology

may persist in negating the reality of severe dissociative disorders, traumatic memory, or organized child abuse, or the extent and damage of child sexual exploitation. When faced with a highly dissociative patient who presents with intimacy problems, addictions, and various cover stories, such a clinician may never adequately assess, inquire, or consult and may subtly quash the patient's efforts to bring his/her sequestered, traumatized subjectivity to the foreground by reinforcing behaviors and reflections consistent with a more optimistic view. Survivors of extreme childhood abuse, accustomed to self-sacrifice and to praise or pseudo-acceptance for participating in conscious and unconscious compliance and collusion, may for a time feel quite at home with this kind of arrangement.

Narcissistic collaborators are "innocent" because they mostly believe in the opinions they advocate; they cannot see the extent of the harm they do because they also cannot see the existence of a problem or their tacitly complicitous roles. Nevertheless, their reverse-witnessing not only abandons the victims of child abuse to their atrocities but also damages their hopes of recovery. These opportunists use the current controversies around trauma, memory, and dissociation for their own gain and in the process collaborate with perpetrators who count on such voices to protect them; because they are often respected and well known, they are often heard over the victims themselves.

While one perpetrator may molest dozens of boys in his lifetime, the written word of one narcissistic innocent can convince hundreds of thousands of people to believe that perpetrators do not exist, to ignore the call of abused children and adults, or to denounce those who work with trauma survivors; thus, they can leave legions of other children vulnerable to perpetration.

Dissociative Denial Collaborators.   Unlike those whose denial is born of ignorance, these collaborators do have awareness or knowledge of heinous acts.

For instance, a mother may notice her seven-year-old daughter's unusual ability to describe sexual acts and highly sexualized behavior, and, as time goes on, she may also observe mood changes and chronic fatigue. Then, up late one night getting a glass of water, she sees her husband—from whom she has slept separately for the past few years—entering their daughter's bedroom. She hears her daughter cry, but assumes, during that first moment of conscious awareness, that he is disciplining her for some reason, and does not interfere. However, after several replays of the same scene, she knows the truth. Still, she does not act. She cannot act without putting something shameful under public or personal scrutiny. Instead, she chooses to sacrifice her daughter for her own comfort. She begins to create an elaborate internal system of self-deception and denial to support her collaboration, convincing herself that nothing really wrong is happening inside that bedroom every night, or the system of cover stories and confabulations that generate false memories of nonabuse becomes so entrenched that the mother eventually persuades herself there was no way she could have stopped the abuse. Over time, her denial devolves into full-blown dissociation whereby she believes the abuse never took place. In this scenario, the child is not only violated by the perpetrator but also variously abandoned, blamed, sacrificed, and victimized by the collaborator. In extreme (and virulently narcissitic) variations of this type of collaboration, the "nonoffending" parent, in the face of substantial evidence confirming the perpetrator's deeds, will testify against the victim (his/her son or daughter) and may serve as a character witness for the perpetrator in a court of law or on television documentaries; such collaborators may even become leaders in pro–false-memory, or anti-psychotherapy advocacy, groups.

Therapists who have been exposed to training on child abuse, dissociation, and trauma but choose to overlook the signals because doing otherwise might produce psychological discomfort or intimidating dilemmas (clinical, legal, and ethical) may intensify their patients' symptoms by disavowing, denying, or dismissing their causes and effects. Such professionals also fit the profile of dissociative denial collaborators. At times, elaborate theories (alternatives to abuse hypotheses) are necessary to sustain some professionals' dissociative-denial complicity.

Associative Denial Collaborators.   Associative denial collaborators, by contrast, have suffered child abuse themselves. Regardless of their personal experience and their recognition of heinous behavior, they elect to deny the actuality of the abuse to which they are witnesses.

When those with "unconscious" personal experience of child abuse see abuses of their own children, self-preservation will force their memories into deeper sequestering. To acknowledge abuse of their sons or daughters would be to unlock their personal histories—and where that means too painful a journey, denial of their children's abuses joins their own.[12] Many women with this background continue to partner with men who abuse their children.

In cases of "conscious" memory of childhood abuse, the internal emotional support mechanisms are very often broken, so normal, healthy reactions to abusive situations (e.g., recognition, protection, aggression) are not in the repertoire. As they could not rescue themselves, such survivors cannot rescue their children. A mix of helplessness, apathy, derealization, or shock recapitulates the futility they learned from their own traumatization; they abandon their children to denial systems they create, reasoning from experience that they can do nothing in the face of such malevolence.

Similar forms of this pattern of complicity can take place when mental health and medical professionals or teachers with their own conscious, partially conscious, or dissociated histories of child abuse systematically veer away from the kinds of recognition and interventions that would assist victims and survivors. Such gross inaction, misrecognitions, and omissions perpetuate the cycle of betrayal, submission, and futility.

Programmed Dissociative Collaborators. Programmed collaboration takes place largely within organized perpetrator groups, be they criminal child-abuse syndicates or cults. Varieties of mind control combined with repeated abuse train victims to dissociate from the abusive acts, to assist the perpetrator(s), and often to turn against other victims—all at the very real risk of death or further victimization if they resist.

Further programmed to forget both their abuse and their participation in the abuse of others, victims live mostly dissociative lives outside as well as within the cult or perpetrator group systems. While victims are aware of their collaboration in the moment, the self-states in which their awareness is lodged are so strongly associated with the perpetrators (and, correspondingly, dissociated from normal waking consciousness) that separate part-selves capable of contrary thought or action do not exist. They are completely broken to the will of the perpetrators and cannot act independently, due to their violent associations to protest, escape, or autonomy responses.

Vicarious Sadistic Collaborators. Vicarious sadistic collaborators enjoy seeing (or imagining) other people suffer. Becoming collaborators makes them essentially vicarious perpetrators. A mother who consciously knows that her son is being raped repeatedly by his father and grandfather does nothing to stop it because she derives some perverse pleasure from knowing about it. At times, she may even assist the perpetrators by bringing her son to a preassigned location (their bedrooms, a private meeting hall). She does not want to perform, watch, or otherwise participate directly; her satisfaction comes from vicariously experiencing what the perpetrators are doing. Thus, she seeks to live on the edge of such perpetration, supports it to feed her own needs, and ultimately sacrifices her child to those needs—consciously and with little regret. The line between perpetrator and collaborator is tenuous here. The collaborator becomes highly dependent on the perpetrator, who needs to exercise no mind control because the control mechanism—the collaborator's addiction to his/her perversions—is already intact.

Vicarious sadists have little or no sense of separateness from their victims (which may suggest, in some cases, that there is also an element of vicarious *victimization*). They actually believe they have the right to sacrifice children for the sake of gratifying their own perversions; indeed, they find deep satisfaction in the element of sacrifice itself. (Ritual-abuse survivors have described mid- to high-ranking female cult members in such terms—women so victimized by the system in which they were raised that they sold out completely to it rather than struggle dissociatively to preserve separate innocence and the hope of recovery.) Adroit manipulators of and in the world around them, vicarious sadists live easily within the web of cover stories that enable their addictions to flourish at the children's expense. Many of them look like model citizens and show no signs of disturbance other than inordinate power/control needs, which may well be camouflaged behind socially sanctioned roles.

Sadistic Collaborators.   For the sadistic collaborator, however, indirect or vicarious contact is insufficient and unsatisfying. S/he has a more powerful addiction to causing and witnessing another's pain and fear. The sadistic collaborator is apt to be a high-functioning, highly visible member of society, and is always severely, perhaps malignantly narcissistic. Adept at hiding his or her collaboration, s/he enjoys the excitement of living a secret and forbidden life. S/he collaborates out of a pure, undisguised sadistic need.

For example, an uncle may not only bring his nephew to a pedophile group to be used for sexual acts, but may actually set up the meeting himself as well as stay to watch without participating. Or a judge who has knowledge of just such a group may exercise his legal influence to protect it; in exchange, he is allowed to watch films of their activities.

In organized groups there are always those who play solely the role of sadistic collaborator. They most often hold exalted positions in the hierarchy in keeping with their power in the outer world. In cases of isolated perpetration, the sadistic collaborator has a no less pivotal part. A father may bring his daughter to a group of his friends, witness her rape with conscious intent, no guilt, and defined enjoyment of the brutality itself. There are no boundaries between the perpetrator and the sadistic collaborator; one is the mirror image of the other. They are equally destructive and particularly difficult to locate, document, and incarcerate outside of war settings.

VARIETIES OF DENIAL

We live in a culture that would absolutely fall apart if the truth were told.

—**R. D. Laing**

Ambivalence.   Ever since Freud recanted his proposal that traumatic childhood sexual abuse was the cause of hysteria, the psychiatric establishment has betrayed ambivalence about it (Van der Kolk and Van der Hart, 1991), and the relationship between trauma and psychiatric symptoms has been a politically charged issue. In cases of posttraumatic stress disorder, especially those arising from family violence or failures in child protection, is society responsible for the individual's suffering or is the victim's personality or inherent inferiority to blame?

Historically, the case against the victim has dominated the literature. The effects of child abuse—seductive behavior with clear origins in the abusive relationship—were almost always confused with the cause as evidence that the child had initiated the incest. Children were described as acting-out, provocative, "willing participants" (Mohr, Turner, and Jerry, 1964) and the majority of pedophiles as harmless individuals whose victims were known to be aggressive and seductive (Revitch and Weiss, 1962). Not long ago, incest was thought to be as rare in North America as one in a million (Weinberg, 1955/1976; Weiner, 1962). As late as the end of the 1970s clinicians were still being taught this information as a basis for understanding child sexual abuse (Summit, 1988).

Kinsey et al. (1948) concluded that incest was to be found more in the imagination of therapists than in the lives of patients, and that there was no logical reason for children to feel disturbed by sexual abuse—in spite of the fact that they documented a 24 percent rate of sexual abuse of females and an 80 percent rate of affirmation that victims were frightened by it. In fact, Kinsey et al.'s (1953) reversal of blame onto the victim is unnervingly similar to the contentions of the false memory backlash movement that the emotional reactions of parents, teachers, and police to the discovery of child sexual abuse disturbs the child more seriously than the abuse itself. Reversals of this kind have dominated the psychiatric literature until the last decade and a half, and advocates of the false memory syndrome have lately revived them. Our collective ambivalence about naming abuse as abuse, holding perpetrators accountable, acknowledging direct effects on the victim, and supporting therapists in the work of diagnosing and treating victims of childhood trauma continues to this day.

Media management of these subjects at once echoes and sustains society's ambivalence toward child abuse. During the last decade, for instance, when national newspapers and television reported on the discovery of the largest child pornography "sting" operation of its kind in U.S. history (Taylor, 1996; Stout, 1996)—45 arrests, 70 more expected; operation in 36 states, generating some ten thousand dollars a week; a client pool including, among others, police officers, ministers, printers, laborers, and a psychoanalyst—the story was almost immediately dropped after its initial broadcast. No analysis was offered and no linkage made with the child-abuse problem nationwide, and, while there was commentary on the possible violation of the civil liberties of the pornography consumers, there was none at all about the violation of the rights of the children. In fact, there was no mention whatsoever about the known or probable effects on the lives of the children involved, nor any articulation of just how the seven- to-nine-year-olds depicted in photographs or videos having sex with one another and with adults were "being sexually abused in unthinkable ways" (Taylor, 1996). Explicit exposure of the unthinkable, however horrifying, and follow-up stories, too—what happened to those children, where are they now, how was their compliance enlisted—could have educated the public to the dynamics of child abuse instead of reinforcing the convention of mystifying it.

Legal Dilemmas.   In every state, the law requires various professionals to report suspected child maltreatment to the police or child welfare authorities. Penalties have been established for failure to comply and the laws usually provide civil immunity for people who make mistaken reports in good faith. It is incumbent on clinicians to understand the statutes, know when to take action, and know whether or not doing so would be in the patient's best interest. While most support mandatory reporting laws in principle many question whether the reporting itself actually results in greater safety for children (Melton et al., 1995).[13]

The inadequacy of our bureaucratic responses to child abuse is well documented. The legal system, for one, has failed to respond adequately: few cases are referred to court and the process is painfully slow when referrals are made (Bishop et al., 1992; Jellinek et al., 1991); we often allow the government to point the finger of suspicion even in the absence of the resources to follow through. "Thus, inquiry and identification are a threat and a promise; if the promise cannot be kept by appropriate and sustained services, there is the threat of more risk of violence to the vulnerable child" (Solnit, 1994, p. 37).

Getting clinical services to those in need is also an underestimated problem. McCurdy and Daro (1993) found that about 40 percent of families in which child abuse or neglect is substantiated receive no services at all. A *New York Times* article exposing the failures of the collapsed child protective service system in New York City (Alvarez, 1996) cited serious acts of omission, narrow and incomplete research, lack of follow-up investigations—a "litany of inattention and ineptitude." This particular "child protective" bureaucracy did not adequately investigate to determine if children were in immediate danger in 13 percent of the cases; did not bother with face-to-face contact with children in 20 percent; did not bother to review previous reports of abuse in 40 percent; did not pursue abuse reports within twenty-four hours as required in 10 percent; and 18 percent of cases considered closed involved children still in potential danger. Case workers in child protective services in the United States will readily acknowledge that the state of national protection of children is mediocre at best. But child protection is not a national priority, and cultural denial about abuse, including the "false memory" controversies, helps to keep things this way.

Doubt.   The single most common error concerning actual severe child abuse made by the mental health field during the past century has been the failure to see, study, and/or acknowledge it (Ross, 1997). Of no small significance in the analysis of professional denial is the fact that the "battered child syndrome" was discovered not by mental health and child care workers but by radiologists (Rascovsky, 1995), spotting the evidence of violence and brutality against children on X rays of broken bones. Also of note, many abusers, before being apprehended or convicted, already had abuse reports on record (Salter, 1995)—reports made by other children, who were disbelieved.

Why are children so often disbelieved and discredited? What is the price of our disbelief? Who has the greater reason to lie, rationalize, and distort (and who has the greater capacity to do so): children or adult perpetrators? Actual methodologically strong studies of false allegations of child sexual abuse (Benedek and Schetky, 1987a; 1987b; Corwin et al., 1987; Everson and Boat, 1989; Jones and McGraw, 1987) show that such allegations are relatively rare and that a false allegation arising solely from a child is even rarer.[14] The fact that false allegations occur at all, however, emphasizes the need for investigators to learn to detect them (Yuille, Tymofievich, and Marxsen, 1995); moreover, the poor interviewing that may produce false allegations may also lead to abuses' being ignored.[15]

Negative biases about young children's testimony—especially regarding suggestibility, memory capacity, inability to distinguish between reality and fantasy, tendencies to lie or to falsify reports with coaching—make it one of the arenas of greatest doubt (Melton et al., 1995). There continues to be ongoing debate about the conditions under which children may lie or may be suggestible (Ceci and Bruck, 1993), not to mention the concern about retractions and recantations[16] (Summit, 1983; De Young, 1986; Faller, 1984).

Solnit (1994) reminds clinicians of the problems inherent in questioning children about possible abuse. They may not be able to distinguish between what adults refer to as good and bad touching. They may not be able to answer direct questions about sexual arousal because of cognitive limitations. They may try to reduce anxiety or fear produced by the questioning by coming up with answers regardless of whether or not they understand what is going on. They may try to guess what the interviewer wants to hear in order to please him/her and diminish the threat. (The situation may be exacerbated when children are caught in divorce and custody battles, and may hope a "right" answer will prevent further separations and magically even lead to reconciliation.)

Rationalization, Disavowal, and Dissociation.   Cultural dissociation in response to reports of child abuse actually resembles the types of dissociative processes—denial, disavowal, and the sealing off of memories—that child-abuse victims use to protect themselves from the knowledge of their own psychological trauma (Herman, 1992; Olafson, Corwin, and Summit, 1993). Sullivan's (1953) important concept of *not-me* self-states, while originally applied to the development of the self-system and the regulation of internal anxiety, may also be construed to operate at a collective level. Consider, in this context, extensions of *not-me* dissociative consciousness based on variations of "each man for himself" and "I don't want to know," such as: "It's not happening in my country," "not in my ethnic group," "not on my street," "I don't have to be bothered with understanding that." The same dissociative consciousness that allows disavowal of one's role (passive and/or active) in the perpetuation of traumatic events, or intrapsychic disavowal and the rationalization of one's actions or their meaning and effects in the case of perpetrators, permits most of us to disavow the human capacity for destructive aggression, greed, and the marginalization of the unfortunate. Political rhetoric, religious dogma, and media-sponsored mystification of aggression make way for the alteration of meanings to suit individual or group purposes of anxiety reduction or power-brokering.

Eliminating personal ownership frees us of responsibility—"It's not my rainforest . . . not my country . . . not my child"—for people and events. Distancing the dangerous and the dreadful as "other" is like a form of manic denial; it magically supports grandiose and omnipotent fantasies of avoiding disaster. Disengaging may reflect our individual and collective wishes to not know about our own potential for violence against children (Solnit, 1994); disavowing our own collaboration in their traumas or focusing on their dishonesty and entitlement reinforces our defensive splitting and lets us off the hook.

Not-Me Configurations in the Mental Health Field.   *Not-me/not-us* thinking patterns also prevail in the mental health field, influencing views on sadistic abuse, forgotten trauma, and the dissociative structuralization of the traumatized psyche—phenomena existing outside the preferred paradigms and therefore *not-us* constructs. In this case, *not-me* consciousness has evolved into a proliferation of attitudes that have been further elaborated into derision and contempt for victims diagnosed as dissociative, and finally into derision and contempt for clinicians who treat severe childhood trauma and MPD/DID.

The disaffiliation between contemporary psychoanalytic theorists and the trauma/dissociation group that preceded them in speaking out against child abuse has been one of the more subtle operations of *not-me* consciousness in the field. In the young, emerging MPD world of the early to mid-1980s, overly directive and overly concrete techniques and practices favored overreliance on hypnosis as the ultimate approach; it failed to integrate such postclassical psychoanalytic developments as acknowledgment of the patient's sensitivities to clinician influence and awareness of coconstruction and conarrational processes in psychotherapy. And while psychoanalytic practitioners may be more likely than other professionals to have worked with people who over time reveal their multiplicity, and to have taken such revelations seriously, they have also inherited the orthodox tendency to emphasize fantasy over trauma and have accounted for the alterations in consciousness of dissociative individuals by diagnosing them as borderline or schizophrenic (McWilliams, 1994). At times, all of the mental health professions seem "to border on a relativism that is bankrupt with regard to real evil" (Grand, 2000, p. 43).

It is not hard to understand that the trauma/dissociation/MPD faction sought to differentiate itself from the constraints of analytic theory and technique, which had practically institutionalized the misrecognition of trauma and dissociative disorders for the better part of a century. It is not hard to understand either how the psychoanalytic community became troubled by some of the early trauma rhetoric that overlooked a century of wisdom about the vicissitudes of transference and demanded that clinicians invest heavily in the use of hypnosis, generally ignoring the dialectic between intrapsychic fantasy and interpersonal and cultural processes in favor of exclusive emphasis on exogenous trauma. Given the lack of dialogue, cross-fertilization, and mutual respect between the two groups in times when therapists treating trauma are under siege by the media and by legal threats, it is vital that the clinical community undertake rapprochement and strive for synthesis; otherwise, who we are and how we can conduct treatment will be defined from without.

Relational psychoanalytic theory, with its emphasis on intersubjectivity, mutuality, interaction, enactment, authenticity, and a sophisticated appreciation for the complexities of transference and countertransference dynamics, can balance the bias evident in much of the trauma and MPD/DID literature toward cognitive, concretized, and managerial approaches. Likewise, the wisdom of two decades of specialized research and practice in trauma/dissociation, the extensive mapping of the terrain of trauma and DID and their intrapsychic and interpersonal manifestations, the understanding of the cognitive errors and distortions characteristic of this population, and familiarity with the experiences of victims of multiple perpetrator and offender group situations, can enrich and enlarge the clinical perspectives of the psychoanalytic community.

Not-Me Configurations, Culture, and Child Abuse

If I had to name one quality as the genius of the patriarchy, it would be compartmentalization, the capacity for institutionalizing disconnection. Intellect severed from emotion. Thought separated from action. Science split from art. The earth itself divided; national borders. Human beings categorized by sex, age, race, ethnicity, sexual preference, height, weight, class, religion, physical ability ad nauseam. The personal isolated from the political. Sex divorced from love. The material ruptured from the spiritual. The past parted from the present and disjoined from the future. Law detached from justice. Vision dissociated from reality.

—Robin Morgan (The Demon Lover)

Individual and collective *not-me* dissociation facilitates perseveration of destructive patterns of selfishness, greed, and unmodulated aggression. Through failure to recognize, and emotional disconnection from, the operative causes, effects, and implications of behavior, we collude with the destruction going on around us, intervening only when disaster strikes at our own doors. The same *not-me* consciousness that allows for toxic wastes to be dumped somewhere "else" or for poverty and starvation to be tolerated in certain (other) places among certain (other) peoples is what makes room for the unspeakable abuses of children without consciousness of our interdependence and shared responsibilities.

Within the network of multiple personalities created by DID individuals, there is a compelling fantasy of having disposed of or eradicated toxic psychic material, just as the perpetrator and society have done through the combination of abuse, denial, and neglect. The MPD/DID patient intrapsychically splits off overwhelming traumatic affects and meanings into container self-states, often child states, which are continually silenced and (intrapsychically) dominated by protector- and perpetrator-identified parts of the self. An absence of critical thinking about the implications of this fantasized extermination coexists with a haunting and looming fear of some inevitable psychic backlash; it takes the form of terror (usually on the part of the host or outer functional personalities) that if the dissociative barriers are allowed to be lowered even the slightest bit, the person will be absolutely overcome and his/her life shut down completely.

As a society we are acting like a desperate DID patient doing everything s/he can to ward off the flood of traumatic affects and meanings. "Fostering a fantasy world that creates an absolute split between good and evil . . . prevents us from entertaining any but the most simplistic solutions to our problems and . . . increases the likelihood that we will perpetrate violence against the most defenseless humans among us" (Milburn and Conrad, 1996, p. 249). DID patients live by the same rules that society teaches the rest of us—ignore bad things, pretend they are not real, create amnesia, call them by another name and they will go away; pretend something never happened and it didn't. This strategy is taught directly or indirectly by the perpetrators, cultivated to survive the abuse, and reinforced by the cultural models of disavowal and minimization.

These strategies of exclusivity and marginalization within mind or within society are dissociative solutions par excellence because they are founded on trance-logic and the omnipotent fantasy of timelessness, "power-over," separation consciousness, and defiance of the laws of causality. The set of derivative forces that most radically contradicts the possibility of ecological harmony is the cluster of narcissism, consumerism, and objectification that together promote the illusion of omnipotence. As Cushman (1994) has described, our culture is configured in such a way that it thwarts social connectedness, common purpose, and group solidarity. Cushman believes that our society has difficulty solving its problems because we do not experience our selves as political beings in a meaningful or devotional relationship with the world around us.

AN ALTERNATIVE PARADIGM: INTEGRATION CONSCIOUSNESS

A feminist perspective on trauma requires us to move out of our comfortable positions—as those who study trauma, or treat its effects, or categorize its types—to a position of identification and action. . . . By insisting that the personal is political, a holy truth of the feminist vision, it is impossible to remove myself and my experiences from my understanding of the etiology, meaning, and treatment of psychic trauma. (Laura Brown, 1995, pp. 108–109)

Ecological, open-system models are alternatives to the *not-me* and dissociative/disavowal paradigm. Postulating mutual, circular influence among all parts of a system and between systems at various levels (Altman, 1995), they hold central the idea that a fragmentary worldview is harmful and dangerous. What is split off and disowned comes back to haunt us in a much more destructive way than if the separation and the disavowal of dualistic thinking had never taken place to begin with (Wilber, 1995, p. 4). In other words, the dissociation of individuals and society does not eliminate pain and suffering, it only anaesthetizes it, perverts it, and leaves it out of relationship and unavailable for transformative change.

Reconnecting the Personal and the Political.   When treating survivors of trauma, particularly hidden and isolating traumas like sadistic sexual abuse, clinicians must be aware of their patients' separation from context and community as children. Recognizing that their healing and integration require realignment with the wider social and historical perspective relative to their suffering is not tantamount, as some critics have alleged, to turning them into whining, entitled, demanding, and permanently infantilized adults who will take no responsibility for themselves. The creation of linkages is part of the process of reassociation after disavowal and dissociation.

Reassociation and recontextualization do not just happen automatically on the intrapsychic level. Movement from ahistorical dissociative awareness through narrativity and testimony does not mean that a DID patient or trauma survivor will cling enduringly to the new identity of (historical) victim; one has to have a history, however, before one can transcend that history toward a more mature identity not solely defined by it. The backlash against recovered memory, psychotherapy, trauma survivors, and the MPD/DID diagnosis, with all of its sincere, insightful, and corrupt variations, has collectively turned back the clock and reversed progress in the recognition and treatment of psychological disorders rooted in child-abuse trauma.

Part Two

Restoration of the Traumatized, Dissociative Self

CHAPTER 4

Major Trends in Relational Psychoanalytic Thought: Implications for Treatment of Trauma and Dissociation

Only in relationship can you know yourself, not in abstraction and certainly not in isolation.

—J. Krishnamurti

In keeping with the goal of building new bridges as well as strengthening those already developed between trauma/dissociation theory and the philosophical and clinical traditions of contemporary psychoanalysis, this chapter reviews major relational theory trends with particular emphasis on those aspects of theory and clinical practice that can enhance our understanding and treatment of severely dissociative trauma survivors.

Multiple mind maps are vying for prominence in psychoanalysis today, where an acute interest in the "social determination of mind" (Wilson, 1995, p. 9) has begun to eclipse the extended emphasis on mind as an isolated object of study. Relational theories tend to draw upon diverse theoretical perspectives from outside of psychology and psychoanalysis such as feminism and postmodern philosophy, where the role of language and power dynamics in human relationships and in the quest for psychological knowledge are factored into theories of psychopathology and advances in clinical practice (Aron, 1996).

RELATIONAL PERSPECTIVES

In general, relational approaches privilege human relationships, intrapersonal and interpersonal alike, over biological drives in the development of the self. Stolorow, Atwood, and Brandchaft (1994) cite the following as key contributions to relationally focused psychoanalytic theory: relational-model theorizing (Mitchell, 1988); dyadic systems perspective (Beebe et al., 1992); social constructivism (Hoffman, 1991); and intersubjectivity (Stolorow et al., 1987).

Some relationally oriented analysts veer sharply away from classical and early postclassical psychoanalytic thought in their views of the role of the therapist, the use of countertransference, the meaning of resistance, and the validity of some theoretical "givens" (Rabin, 1995); contentious misrepresentations notwithstanding, however, they are not so much disavowing as modifying drive theory, the importance of fantasy and instinctual life, and insight as a clinical tool.

Relational theorists posit a view in which both reality and fantasy, both outer world and inner world, play significant and interactive roles in human life (Ghent, 1992a). The intrapsychic and the interpersonal are seen as complementary and interactive processes (Benjamin, 1990); however, the intrapsychic is viewed as constituted primarily by the internalization of interpersonal experience, which is itself mediated by the constraints imposed by biologically organized templates (Ghent, 1989). Conflict is central to a relational analysis of psychological development, but is conceptualized as occurring between opposing relational configurations, between various points and identifications with early significant others, rather than between drive and defense (Warshaw, 1992). Mitchell (1988) reframes the central dynamic struggle of life as occurring between the powerful need to establish, protect, and maintain intimate bonds with others, and various strivings to escape the pains and dangers of these attachments. He describes the contents of psychological life as metaphors for expressing and playing out relational patterns: discovery, penetration, domination, surrender, control, longing, evasion, revelation, envelopment, merger, differentiation, and so on.

The focus of relational psychoanalytic treatment is on understanding and transforming the pathological aspects of relatedness, derived from the patient's internalized models of prior relationships. Consistent with this notion, intersubjectivists focus on helping the patient organize and reorganize experience in less painful and more creative ways so that new and more flexible organizing principles can emerge; with a greater capacity for reflectivity, the patient's experiential repertoire can then become enlarged, enriched, and more complex (Orange et al., 1997). In essence, the intersubjective field created by the emotional availability of the therapist offers a developmental second chance for the patient (Orange, 1995).

Stolorow and Atwood's (1992) intersubjective vision depends on the continual flow of reciprocal mutual influence between the individual's world of inner experience and interpersonal relationships. When this notion of reciprocity (Aron, 1996) is taken seriously, the meanings of clinical material and the therapy relationship itself are subject to continual revision from multiple perspectives; no preexisting theoretical construct is allowed to dominate the discourse—the therapist's perceptions are not intrinsically more true than the patient's. Such a progressive clinical stance, whereby patient and therapist codetermine the course of the therapy process, can arouse high anxiety among practitioners who rely on traditional authoritarian arrangements and classical notions of analytic neutrality. "In order to dispense with the defensive invincibility and omniscience of the neutral stance, analysts must be prepared to bear . . . profound feelings of vulnerability and anxious uncertainty . . . [and to let] go of metapsychological and epistemological absolutes" (Orange et al., 1997, p. 42).

The theoretical underpinnings of the term "relational" reflects the constructivist, perspectivist influence of postmodern philosophy, science, and hermeneutics—namely, the "embeddedness" (Mitchell, 1995) whereby all observations and understandings are regarded as contextual, based on the interpreter's values, assumptions, and constructions of experience. In the absence of any a priori ideology, clinicians are encouraged to stay very close to the patient's subjective experience (Rabin, 1995); by extension, they relinquish the presumption that they have superior knowledge of the patient's psychodynamics (Aron, 1996), thus making way for the patient to act as coconstructor of interpretations and of the process itself. This theoretical position creates a new context for the negotiation of power dynamics and conflicts in the therapy relationship without peremptorily construing the patient's disagreements or protests as pathological or subversive of the treatment; moreover, it leaves room for surprise, for ambiguity, for not knowing. The implications of this theoretical posture for the respectful and productive treatment of traumatized and dissociative patients cannot be underestimated.

As psychoanalytic theory continues to mature, analytic humility and an appreciation for ambiguity and paradox may gradually replace what will eventually be understood as the combined fallacies of objectivity and neutrality. The nature and texture of the psychotherapy relationship and psychoanalytic process change profoundly when the clinician defines him/herself as a "collaborator in developing a personal narrative rather than as a scientist uncovering facts" (Mitchell, 1993, p. 74). Prominent relational theorists like Benjamin (1988; 1990; 1995), Mitchell (1988; 1993), Aron (1996), and Spezzano (1993a; 1993b; 1995) are clear that focusing on a new notion of "neutrality," and the value of interpersonal processes does not exclude the therapist's commitment to the importance of interpretation, insight, and the role of unconscious and fantasy life. The goal is to create the particular interpersonal conditions—developing a therapeutic ambience—where meanings can be constructed and explored, where absolute concern with "objective" truth and consensual reality is suspended.

Ghent (1995) describes the shift from a classical toward a relational paradigm as representing a movement from therapy viewed as informative, insightful, and interpretative to therapy regarded as transformative. For Fosshage (1992), the single most disruptive influence of the shift to relational theorizing is that the modern analyst/therapist has been "dethroned from the position of objective observer and becomes a co-participant" (p. 23). For Mitchell (1993), the healing power of psychoanalysis and the hope it inspires is grounded in the personal and unique meanings generated by individuals rather than in rational consensus: classical analysts may have prided themselves on "knowing and being brave enough to know," while the "current generation . . . tends increasingly to stress the value of not knowing and the courage that requires" (p. 42). For Spezzano (1993a), there is "always more to be said. The point, as a matter of fact, is to keep talking" (p. 179); truth emerges out of therapeutic conversations and confrontations.

According to Spezzano and other relationalists, the objective of therapy is the establishment of an interpretive dialogue that can regulate and contain the affects being defended against by the patient. This simple reformulation places greater responsibility for the quality and freedom of therapeutic discourse on the therapist's emotional availability, creativity, and cognitive flexibility, and less emphasis for positive outcome on the patient's overt compliance and communication skills. Therapy patients want to be known and are always trying to communicate something. Specifically, Spezzano believes that they want their disturbing affects and representations placed "first in a mind that can manage them" (1995, p. 24). In such a view, the success of treatment depends on the ability of the therapist to create an atmosphere where all of the patient's material and enactments can be welcomed, held, tolerated, and examined. Subtle domination by means of unquestioned authority or knowledge as power can be harmful to the therapy; spontaneity, creativity, and malleability are all essential to a productive outcome.

THE SELF AND PSYCHOPATHOLOGY

In relational models (Hirsch, 1994; Mitchell, 1993; Stolorow et al., 1987), the basic units of personality are the "structures of experience," distinctive configurations of self and other that shape and organize the individual's subjective world (Stolorow and Atwood, 1994). Such psychological structures are not mere internalizations or mental replicas of interpersonal events; they are organizing principles through which an individual's experiences of self and other assume their characteristic meanings. This perspective invites consideration of how the effects of power and gender arrangements and trauma can create barriers to actualizing personal agency or memory and to developing self-cohesion and continuity.

The relational view of self is a matrix of intersubjective polarities (e.g., unity-multiplicity, separateness-relatedness) in various states of tension. (According to Seligman and Shanok [1995], identity consists in the capacity to sustain and experience the simultaneity of both separateness and relatedness.) Some aspects of psychopathology can be viewed as imbalances in the tension between multiplicity and integrity/unity. For example, too much of a sense of discontinuity can lead to the fragmentation, splitting, and dissolution most commonly associated with psychotic states (Sullivan, 1956)—the signature of dissociative identity disorder (DID), whether apparent or camouflaged. A reverse imbalance, in the direction of continuity, can lead to the paralysis and stagnation of, say, obsessive-compulsive disorder, often prevalent in the rigid, self-protecting constructions of the severely dissociative patient's internal system. If optimal psychological structuralization means maintaining a balance between organization and an openness to new forms of experience (Stolorow and Atwood, 1994), then psychopathology signals developmental failures either in structuralizing the subjective world or in

consolidating restrictions on one's own subjective field. The dissociative alter personalities in DID are extreme examples of both phenomena operating
interactively.

Through the processes of recognition and conflict within the psychotherapy relationship, the severely dissociative individual discovers a self (or a
set of part-selves) in relation to another subject—the therapist—who is willing to engage to form attachment bonds with, sometimes even to fight, the
disparate, often personified and sequestered, aspects of self-experience. In
cases of trauma, dissociation, and, in particular, DID, unity, integrity, and cohesion—as structural possibilities and healthy fantasies—develop through
being affectively contacted, challenged, and intellectually recognized by another, nondominating subject. The accumulating evidence that both patient
and therapist can survive the interplay of their unique subjectivities is what
stabilizes and strengthens these experiences of evolving wholeness.

TRANSFERENCE AND COUNTERTRANSFERENCE

Relational theorists see transference and countertransference as a reciprocally influential intersubjective system. Stolorow and colleagues (1987) recognize the roles in generating transference phenomena of both the patient's
unconscious *self-object* longings—for the therapist to make up for missed developmental experiences by providing substitutes—and the patient's fears
(the *repeated dimension* of the transference), which are rooted in developmental failures and thwarted strivings. The therapist's psychological structures
and organizing activity have decisive roles in codetermining the transference (Stolorow, 1994). Fosshage (1995) notes that the therapist's experience
of the patient ranges from involvement with repetitive pathological dynamics (e.g., domination/submission) to engagement in developmentally progressive connections, affirmation, and reparation.

Stern (1994) considers transference to be the dialectic of "needed and repeated" relationships; the therapist's countertransference is impacted by the
repetitive and reparative aspects of the patient's needs and transferences.
The therapist's affective responsiveness is most critical clinically because
mutative interactions have the capacity to transform the inevitability of destructive relational paradigms. Success is contingent on the therapist's "surviving" the unfolding transference/countertransference matrix, which in
turn mandates not only maintenance of nonwithdrawing, nonretaliatory

stances (Winnicott, 1969), but also tolerance for traumatic patterns of relatedness and for revelations of extreme human malevolence; "surviving" also mandates the therapist's ability to use language to break through confusion and stalemates when the power of traumatic reenactments has eclipsed reflectivity altogether.

Relational theorists continue to offer innovative ways to conceptualize and use the countertransference experience (Maroda, 1991; 1999; Ehrenberg, 1992), urging the therapist to rely on authenticity, immediacy, and emotional involvement, and to work within the reenactment process rather than to pathologize it, to "translate" or interpret it through the lens of a priori assumptions, or to discount its existence and multiple meanings.

Maroda (1991), like most relational theorists, believes strongly in the importance of the therapist's owning his/her side of the emotional interaction to provide a clear experience of mutuality as an alternative to the domination paradigm so often characteristic of the patient's family of origin and to model a responsible self-observational stance that promotes inquiry and risk taking.

In Benjamin's (1995) terms, relational perspectives make the therapist's countertransference central, not just as a source of information, but also as an instrument that reveals the effect the patient can have on others; such effects must be processed by the therapist and returned to the patient in a usable form.

Mitchell (1995) feels that, by owning and expressing his/her side of the interaction, the therapist is creating something new and important for the patient; a relational therapeutic posture invites the patient to reflect on his/her own involvement in therapy interactions in a more collaborative and potentially less defensive atmosphere.

For Ehrenberg (1992) what is essential is the therapist's willingness to take some kind of emotional risk to reach the patient. Relationalists differ when it comes to how much or how little, when and where and what specifically to share (and not share) with patients, but they all seek to establish mutuality, therapeutic presence, and authenticity.

In Eigen's (1996) view, the therapist's processing of the patient's impact on him/her (either reflectively and/or expressively) gives the patient a sense of being taken seriously. More important, through this interaction, the patient experiences the possibility that someone (at first the therapist, or the dyad, and eventually the patient him/herself) could process previously undigestible and unmetabolizable psychic material.

ENACTMENT/REENACTMENT

The concept of enactment that has become popularized in recent psychoanalytic literature may be one that can bridge the interactional space between concepts of transference and countertransference. Any unconscious interpersonal communication in which gestures, body language, and nonverbal communication play significant roles (Jacobs, 1986) is considered to be an enactment. Like *acting out* and *projective identification*, enactment denotes some form of repeating and representing through behavior rather than by remembering or verbalizing core conflicts or resistances. The term *reenactment*, sometimes used synonymously, refers to enactment of elements of the original trauma in posttraumatic symptoms, behaviors, and/or interpersonal patterns of relating—all characteristic of trauma survivors' functioning (Miller, 1984). Reflecting patients' internal working models of interactions derived from abusive relationships that govern their expectations and behaviors, reenactments become the narrative schemes by which severely traumatized patients understand their engagements with all others, including the therapist (Davies and Frawley, 1994; Fast, 1998). Spontaneous activation of these dissociated beliefs, expectations, identifications, and interactional patterns often takes place quite unexpectedly during treatment, offering at times graphic and immediate access to the patient's internal world and history (and, sometimes, to the therapist's as well). When reenactments do not lead to endless stalemates or unbridled acting out on the part of either patient or therapist (or both), and with sufficient time and space for mutual reflection, these unnerving therapeutic events can lead to magnificent breakthroughs.

In enactments, the therapist inadvertently and inevitably plays out a given role in the patient's psychic life before either patient or therapist becomes aware of the process or its meaning. The parts that are being played are not only elements of the patient's psyche but elements of the therapist's psyche as well. From this egalitarian perspective, therapists and patients are always doing things to one another—and the dyadic reciprocating field of interaction must always be kept in mind in appreciating the meaning and clinical utility of enactments and reenactments (Aron, 1996). The parts being played often relate to culturally defined self-constitutional factors: racial, ethnic, or gender roles or more subtle forms of culturally prescribed behaviors involving authority, aggression, and sexuality.

The process of enactment allows the patient to use the therapist to relive parts of his/her earlier life (Frayn, 1996). Or, it allows patient and therapist both to exist within each other's internal worlds (Bollas, 1987). From this perspective, patients are constantly oscillating between an introspective reporting mode and behavior-discharging communication. It is important to keep in mind here Aron's (1996) essential point that we must recognize enactments and projective identification as continual processes rather than as discrete events, especially in treating survivors of early complex traumas who create multiple simultaneous enactments and reenactments in order to become known to themselves and the other. The actual transformative therapeutic potential that relational theorists believe can emerge from work with enactments is not primarily based on intellectual insight alone. Rather, progress evolves directly out of increased mutual observation, creative verbal and nonverbal exchanges, and the play of (new) interaction. For the severely dissociative patient whose life has been permeated with the abuse of authority, domination, and betrayal-paradigms of relatedness, the experience with an authority figure who is humane, benevolent, nonretaliatory, open to feedback, and willing to change can, in and of itself, be profoundly disarming and reparative.

Far more important than any interpretation of an enactment is the therapist's response (Bloom, 1997). We clinicians must first change something within ourselves, in our internal relationship to the patient; only then can we change our responses to the patient. What is called for on our part to resolve the kinds of complex and painful enactments we cocreate with severely dissociative trauma survivors is a singular combination of emotional availability, integrity, honesty, and willingness to be completely misunderstood and unappreciated.

SURVIVING DESTRUCTION

A relational theory of treatment for dissociative disorders must address both the patient's and the therapist's survival—of destruction by the complexities, pains, and challenges of working within a traumatic transference/countertransference matrix where reenactments of torture, betrayal, and danger not previously understood or described in the clinical literature are taking place. Clinicians must recognize the damage done to severely traumatized, dissociative patients by their perpetrators/caretakers and validate their pain and stress; however, because such individuals are extremely wounded, they can be extremely wounding to those who share intimate psychological space with them. Since unmetabolized trauma and betrayal often lead to more enactments of trauma and betrayal, therapist and patient can get caught in re-living aspects of the past that destroyed the patient's core sense of self. Similarly, the therapist may unconsciously deploy defenses used to survive his/her own early traumas and catastrophic disappointments.

Winnicott (1969) emphasizes that the holding functions of the therapy relationship and the patient's use of the therapist as a transitional object create a critical healing opportunity: the patient can test the limits of his/her omnipotence and destructiveness. Discovering that the therapist can survive that destructiveness is the fundamentally integrative experience of treatment for an individual who was exposed to utter brutality and predation throughout childhood; indeed, experiencing the therapist's survival is the heart of what is transformative about psychotherapy for patients with DID and other severe posttraumatic conditions.

Severely dissociative patients have unique capacities and needs to test and push the survival capabilities of their therapists to the limit. They need to play with and play out many of their fears and fantasies of omnipotent destructiveness in order to discover their own boundaries and their appropriate relationships to, even the actual existence of, themselves and other people. Severely dissociative patients need to discover the possibility of benevolent and nontraumatically mutative interaction. They need to revisit the quintessential assaults on the core self and identity that were emblematic of their childhood experiences. This is frequently accomplished through placing the therapist in the positions of the child-victim, perpetrator, and collaborator in unconscious reenactments that can potentially reveal traumatic relationship dynamics of the past (Davies and Frawley, 1994)—or blow the therapy container apart altogether.

Surviving the therapy process is a formidable challenge; the process of treating a dissociative trauma survivor inevitably means experiencing some of the patient's fear, pain, rage, hatred, disillusionment, and despair. Most contemporary psychoanalytic clinicians believe that part of the healing power of a therapy process comes from the capacity to respond from an experience-near vantage point (Kohut, 1971; Stolorow et al., 1987), to get inside the inner world of the patient. The relational therapist's responses to all parts or self-states of the patient (e.g., the young and vulnerable, the seducers, the killers, the drones, the collaborators, and the self-betrayers) will facilitate the emergence of powerful transferences and become the basis of mutative interaction that s/he can eventually internalize and use to develop more expansive, less compartmentalized solutions to intrapsychic and interpersonal problems. Along the way, however, the therapist will be tested and strained to the breaking point.

How the therapist tolerates painful affect-states and remains in contact with both the patient and him/herself will be fundamental to the patient's internalization of new object experience. In this struggle between domination and mutuality paradigms of relationship the therapist's defenses may be completely assaulted. Rivera (1996), contending that a commitment to scrupulous personal honesty is the best insurance that therapists will neither burn out nor act out on their tortured and terrorized patients, identifies the need for in-depth treatment of clinicians whose defenses "have never been tampered with [lest they] crumble" and for the periodic return to treatment by the rest "to ensure that they remain a relatively clear and clean vessel for the use of their trauma survivor clients" (p. 187).

In patients with DID the ante of the traumatic relational paradigms is upped compared to other traumatized patients. The dynamics of reversals, captivity, isolation, sacrifice, blackmail, appeasement, condemnation, the assaults on hope, faith, and trust, and the attack on reality testing must all be considered. Hence, the early phases of treating the most severely dissociative patients often involve many urgent approaches to the precipice of self- and other-destruction followed by last-minute saves. The middle and later phases of treatment have their own challenges to survival, organized primarily around affect tolerance, deepening of trust, and learning to "surrender" (Ghent, 1990). When mutual survival is successfully negotiated, the patient's internalized patterns of domination, submission, avoidance, and coercion give way to conscious and voluntary surrender to the mourning and grieving process. Some identifications have to be relinquished, others must be renegotiated, and most attachments and identifications will be reconfigured in some ways. Both therapist and patient alike have to rework identity and worldviews in terms of their mutual impact. The clinical challenges of this work are enormous. There is no way to shortcut or bypass painful mergers with the patient's trauma and the split-off aspects of the patient's self.

Part of therapy is helping the traumatized patient experience and understand nonexploitative, mature, loving relationships. Inevitably, for the therapist, this will involve assaults and abuse of the attachment bond s/he has developed with the patient. Without this strain and searing pain the therapist cannot know an essential part of the patient's experience. An individual who has been severely traumatized and has developed a complex dissociative world to simultaneously contain and lose him/herself in has based that world on layers of self-deception, omnipotent reorganizations of interpersonal and intrapsychic realities, and the steadfast avoidance of contact with painful reminders of the agonies and betrayals of childhood. Such an individual will not relinquish a massive, meticulously constructed empire of defenses in the presence of a therapist who cannot tolerate pain, confusion, ambiguity, complexity, and the impact of traumatic relational dynamics.

In a welcoming ambience where confusion and ambiguity are tolerated and protest responses and confrontation are valued, the patient's increasing experience of his/her own and the therapist's aggression and survival leads to what Bromberg (1991; 1996a) refers to as the patient's developing confidence in his/her ability to move from dissociation and alienation to negotiation of intrapsychic conflict and authentic human relationship. In this realm the coexistence of more than one thought/feeling/identification/alter personality, more than one person/belief, can be tolerated and worked with at the same time. Such a developmental shift toward the use of reflection and toleration of ambiguity, intrapsychic conflict, and pain is central to the recovery process for all severely traumatized patients. The process is grounded in the new object experience that occurs in and through the reciprocal transference/countertransference entanglements and the mutuality whereby patient and therapist work their way out of the tangles together (Aron, 1996).

CONTEMPORARY (RELATIONAL) PSYCHOANALYTIC PERSPECTIVES ON DISSOCIATION

Recent advances in psychoanalytic thinking have emphasized *nonlinear dynamics, states of consciousness, self-organization,* and *dissociation,* thereby changing theoretical views of psychological structure and psychological growth (Bromberg, 1994) and bridging the unnecessarily wide gap between psychoanalysis and trauma/dissociation theory. For Bromberg, dissociation is not inherently pathological: the process can be considered basic to human mental functioning and central to the stability and growth of personality. For Goldberg (1995), dissociation plays a part in normal development and normal living, a key role in productive and creative work, and a significant role in survival in both ordinary and extraordinary situations. And for Davies (1996a), multiplicity need not be construed as solely trauma related; indeed normal multiplicity can be viewed as endemic to the progression of ego development, consistent with the poststructuralist vision of multiple self-states and with recent developments in cognitive psychology.[1]

Echoing the work of major dissociation/DID theorists (Putnam, 1988; 1989; 1992; Ross, 1989; Kluft, 1987a; 1995; Kluft and Fine, 1993) Bromberg (1994) projects dissociation as "intrinsically an adaptational talent that represents the very nature of what we call consciousness" (p. 521). He conceptualizes the human mind as a system of discontinuous and shifting states of consciousness from birth to death: "the psyche does not start as an integrated whole, but begins and continues as a multiplicity of self-states that maturationally attain a feeling of coherence which overrides the awareness of discontinuity" (Bromberg, 1993, p. 162). If "feeling of coherence" is nothing more than an adaptive illusion—an important and perhaps developmentally complex illusion—whose form and content are in large measure culturally and interpersonally determined, then the study of the dissociative disorders becomes the comparative study of adaptive and maladaptive illusions and trance states that actually protect and variously cultivate and compromise the self.

Integrated or organized multiplicity operating under the adaptive illusion of unity where conflict and paradox are tolerated and welcomed may in fact reflect maturation—"a distributed self" (Pizer, 1996a, p. 503) with the capacity to contain and sustain conscious relationship with the contradictory multitudes of self-experience. The dissociative self, in contrast is overburdened by shocking discrepant relational juxtapositions—"strained toward the traumatic breaking point" (p. 504)—and unable to negotiate contradiction in such a way as to avoid fragmentation by experiences of domination, nullification, and defeat.

In normal development, and with appropriate responsiveness from caregivers, transitions across states of consciousness are smoothed out of awareness; healthy illusions of unity and integration facilitate maturational achievements (Stern, 1985). Under conditions of chronic traumatic impingement, neglect, or violence and sexual exploitation, however, these state-changes are unmediated and the illusions of unity of self never quite realized. Paradoxically in such cases, as dissociation attends frequent and disruptive state-transitions and amplified illusions of internal separateness, it actually permits psychological survival (and sometimes even incredible developmental achievements in spite of staggering emotional devastation). Dissociation thus emerges as both a form of fragmentation and a defense against fragmentation.

Bromberg (1994) suggests that dissociation is not itself fragmentation, citing Ferenczi's (1930) brilliant insight that fragmentation may not be a consequence of trauma as much as it is an adaptation to it. In dissociating to cope with trauma, the psyche may be enlisting its inherent adaptational capacity to compartmentalize, freeze, and disconnect. Instead of remaining a passive, helpless victim to a fragmentation experience, the protective wisdom of the dissociative capacity of mind absolutely reclaims the fragmentation—orchestrating it, personifying it, and camouflaging it. Then, forever dancing on the edge of annihilation, the dissociatively organized individual creates and deploys a kind of controlled fragmentation while in fantasy avoiding, and in some corner of the mind perpetually reliving, the horrendous visitations to the psychological sites of the original traumatically disintegrating experiences. Anticipating disaster, sustaining a life that is itself a disaster zone, and ultimately remaining a psychological disaster in some ways wards off the ultimate disaster—loss of the attachments to perpetrators and loss of "self-as-disaster," the only self there is. This is a mirror dance because it takes place intrapsychically and interpersonally and these two dimensions potentiate one another until life itself becomes kaleidoscopic or cubist to the stationary observer.

Dissociation splits affect and cognition, observer and experiencer, mind and body, self and self into parts, leading to fantastic permutations and schisms in ownership/disownership, knowing/not knowing, responsibility/irresponsibility, and victim/perpetrator dynamics within the psyche and in relationships. Stern (1996) suggests, in cases of unremembered childhood sexual abuse, that dissociation is "the appropriate model for motivated not-knowing in much of our clinical work . . . [and] that in the coming years, dissociation will come to be at least as important in psychoanalytic thought as repression is" (p. 255). Bromberg (1995a), in fact, suggests a role for dissociation in the conceptualization of all of the personality disorders; and indeed compartmentalization of mind and dissociative knowledge/affect-isolation do appear all across the personality disorder continuum.

For a child—who probably doesn't have the requisite language, abstraction, or symbolization skills to integrate the traumatic experience in the first place—dissociation under stress, particularly the stress of potential loss of (security with) attachment figures, may come more easily than it does for an adult. As Stern (1996) points out, all that the child might know is that something very horrible has happened, that something feels wrong, and/or that something is confusing: sexual abuse might be encoded as something bad that has to do with touching but might not be internalized as anything sexual per se. Since the confusing, disorganized events are disruptive and challenging to the smooth flow of self- and other-representations, the experience can then be split off (Horowitz, 1986); without a narrative context, fragments not encoded or sequentially linked and ordered may or may not result in a viable memory (Stern, 1996).[2] Unlike repression, according to Stern, such dissociative experience is not ejected from consciousness. "Rather, the experience never enters consciousness at all. It is dissociated, never known, at least not in any clear and emotionally salient way. In most conscious respects, it is as if the experience never really happened" (p. 258).

For some relational theorists (e.g., Hirsch, 1994), dissociation occurs across a continuum of problems and represents split-off, internalized interpersonal configurations and the affects associated with them. For others, dissociation as a defense, as a social process, as a significant "arranger" of traumatic human experience, is the container and deflector, the divider and conqueror, the protector and destroyer of self, other, and terror within the internalized psychic landscape of trauma. According to Stern (1996), dissociation is *both* a means of coping and a significant resource for constructing views of the self and the world. It is not (p. 259), "necessarily limited to the absolute prevention of experience; it often merely drains experience of the feeling and the potential for narrative vigor that even the most terrible memory must have to be real." As Stern points out, when personalities are built around this sort of absence, the possibilities for articulating experiences of abuse become increasingly remote; adult victims who have dissociated abuse experiences may remember only "unformulated shards of something that there may not even be any words for, because there were none at the time" (p.258).

Under conditions of trauma, the acquired, developmentally adaptive illusion of unified mental functioning becomes impossible and is useless in coping with overwhelming threat. In Bromberg's (1996b) view, the traumatized mind resorts to the primitive but effective device of dissociation. The foremost goal is to absolutely avoid the repetition of trauma. Of course, the dissociative defense creates only the illusion of invulnerability—it cannot guarantee any real protection from pain and danger. What is actually avoided are the memories, feelings, and meanings of the trauma. The tragic irony about dissociatively organized experience is that it sets up the individual using it for what Kluft (1990) calls the "sitting duck syndrome," where revictimization is almost inevitable.[3] The individual dissociates the very knowledge needed to protect him/herself and prevent repetitions of traumatic relational experiences (Van der Kolk, 1989); the pressures of unintegrated relational experience toward manifestation in reenactment are intense.

Thus, paradoxically, dissociative experience, while out of awareness is continually replayed in relationships. Dissociation gathers strength as an organizing/disorganizing architect within psyche, social system, and culture, in the fertile medium of chronic, uninterrupted, and unrecognized trauma. Dissociation is the tricksterlike process of human self-protection/self-deception that can sever and recombine, sequester and nullify, neutralize and reorganize, experience, over time (i.e., destroying time), at unconscious prompting, and, sometimes, at will.

Goldberg's (1995) discussion of the "sensory cocoon" of the dissociative patient's life experience and self-construction, along with his emphasis on the requisite deceptive practices, exquisitely captures one of the primary characteristics of dissociation—a kind of autism, along with an exile from both the interpersonal world and the tumultuous and passionate internal world of the psyche. It forecloses, however, the dialectical nature of dissociative process, which involves more of an interplay of permeability and impermeability, authenticity and inauthenticity, hiding and seeking, and "hope and dread," to use Mitchell's (1993) apt description.

Winnicott's (1965) formulations of the true and false self are more useful in their acknowledgment of the struggles of neglected and assaulted individuals who must creatively resolve the dilemmas of survival and attachment, live long enough and develop enough psychologically to have the opportunity to experience transformative relationships. Eigen's (1996) essential elaboration on Winnicott's formulation describes the false self as protecting the true self, or acting as a substitute or counterfeit. In this view, the false self capitalizes on the weakness, shame, and grief of the true self; the false self converts the true self's hatred of its corruptibility to hatred of weakness as such, and gloats over the true self's shame, provoking it to hide, disappear, or seek the false self's protection.

On the other hand, such dichotomies as true/false, real/unreal, authentic/inauthentic do not reflect the subjective experience of the dissociative patient, whose mind embraces multiple and always shifting positions to cope with dissociated vulnerability and dissociated terror and pain. Further, the dissociating patient is always simultaneously galvanizing and destroying hope in an effort to leave the door open for transformative contact while also insisting on preserving his/her readiness for the return of past trauma (Bromberg, 1995a). By sustaining an ongoing traumatic internal reality, played out and reinforced through enactments, in which potential pain and exploitation are always just around the next corner, the dissociating patient paradoxically creates his/her own position of safety from which to negotiate change and new object experience.

Bromberg's theory is grounded in his sensitivity to the dissociative patient's paradoxical need for insularity and contact, to be permeable and impermeable, to simultaneously reveal and conceal, and most of all, to "preserve the dissociative structure while surrendering it" (p. 521).[4] The patient's duplicity, dissimulation, and confabulation—frustrating as they might be for the clinician—must be contextualized in their full paradoxicality through their relationship to survival, self-destruction, and, most of all, hope. Otherwise, as clinicians and theorists we run the risk of blaming the victim for his/her pathology, or wasting our energies decontextualizing the psychopathology from its origins in the helplessness of trauma (and efforts to avoid retraumatization). This is an extremely seductive and appealing possibility since the strains of working with these patients—the effects of being at the mercy of dissociative strategies—can lead to countertransference enactments of all kinds including the intellectualization of theories that are themselves based in a collapse of paradoxical thinking and on camouflaged sadism, despair, and hatred of the patient.

Bromberg's invaluable contributions to psychoanalytic dissociation theory serve as the most essential theoretical backbone of this book precisely because he has systematically integrated awareness of the "experience-near" description of the dissociative process and its underlying motivations with a great respect for the patient's struggle and an informed awareness of the dangers and pitfalls of treating dissociative patients.

> Because the anticipation of misfortune is the principal way a traumatized person protects himself from future trauma, the promise of cure (which is always implied by a therapist, even if not explicitly stated) makes the process of attempting to free a traumatized patient from the expectation of misfortune probably the most complex treatment issue a psychoanalyst faces. (1996a, p. 64)

Bromberg's thoroughgoing appreciation of the paradoxes inherent in the treatment of dissociative disorders paves the way for transcending some of the divisiveness that has existed in the professional discourse about disso-ciation. In order for a traumatized individual to allow his/her self-truth to be revealed, and then altered by the impact of the therapist and the therapy relationship, the therapist must join with the patient's system, and yet si-multaneously stay separate from it. That is, the therapist must maintain his/her own self-observation and sensitivity to the symbolic and metaphoric significance of the patient's experience, while at the same time entering deeply into and joining with the patient's experience, psychic ma-terial, history, and personified self-organization. Finally, the therapist must view psychological health as "the ability to stand in the spaces between realities without losing any of them—the capacity to feel like one self while being many" (Bromberg, 1993, p. 166).

When the arrogance of isolation is replaced with the appreciation of rela-tionship and affective connection, tension-states that promote integration are sustained rather than bypassed. In Bromberg's terms (1996b) such de-velopmental shifts facilitate the development of the capacity for "genuine repression" including activation of self-reflection and the interpretive and collaborative restructuring of identity. This idea of "genuine repression" is not just semantic: it emphasizes the fact that many individuals can be pri-marily organized by dissociation, that repression is in fact a developmental advance that has been underestimated as an actual achievement, and that it takes a capacity for conflict tolerance and a workable, healthy illusion of a unitary self to make repression possible.

Dissociation is a method of conflict avoidance. Repression implies con-sciousness of conflict and a self with enough continuity and capacity to ex-perience conflict. Hence, repression is a developmental achievement that evolves out of a negotiation process of previously unlinked self-states. The presence of intrapsychic conflict, which stands in contrast to dissociative en-actments and evasion, is what fuels developmental progress and the hu-manizing process of psychotherapy. Ultimately, this negotiation process leads to a capacity for authenticity in the present, and, as Bromberg says, "ownership of an authentic past." This means having a self, with feeling, continuity, reflectivity, responsibility, and presence—not necessarily an ab-sence of multiplicity. In trauma-theory terms (Van der Kolk, 1996) this de-velopmental shift is tantamount to creating the capacity for the patient to be mindful of current experience while creating symbolic representations of past experience, with the goals of taming traumatic terror and desomatizing memories.

MERGING EPISTEMOLOGIES OF RELATIONAL AND DISSOCIATION THEORIES

Relational positions try to respect the dialectical tensions between the intrapsychic and the interpersonal domains of psychological experience, to move beyond either/or dichotomous thinking and to appreciate the power of interpersonal trauma and malevolent social and interpersonal contexts in shaping affects and self- and object-representations. Relational approaches, deeply indebted to feminist critiques, move beyond simplistic notions of neutrality, resistance, or the unitary self; in the case of trauma survivors, they integrate knowledge of the damage done with the strengths and healthy resistances to domination buried and camouflaged beneath the maze of symptoms and traumatic reenactments. In this view, severe dissociation and pathological multiplicity (definable as the internalization of malevolent power dynamics leading to hierarchical structuring of subjectivity, and not as some inherent defect in or manipulation by the individual) can be seen simultaneously as problem and solution, as a method of re-creating and transcending personal and social history. Both relational and feminist theories privilege the multiplicity of human consciousness, describing the various ways in which the individual's normal multiplicity is feared, suppressed, and manipulated in the service of survival and developmental challenge (Mitchell, 1993; Flax, 1993; Bromberg, 1993; Rivera, 1996).

Current psychoanalytic understanding of the decentered nature of self acknowledges the discontinuous and shifting states of consciousness and the healthy illusion of unitary selfhood in a dialectical relationship (Bromberg, 1996b). Since the processes of subjectivity are overdetermined and contextual, the human mind is not homogeneous, unitary, lawful, or internally consistent (Flax, 1993). For Flax, the concept of a unitary self is unnecessary, impossible, and a potentially dangerous illusion: "unity is an effect of domination, repression, and the temporary success of particular rhetorical strategies" (p. 50). The self consists of multiple self-states, an interplay of co-creating systems, which are neither spatially situated nor temporally fixed at some endpoint of stratified, archaeologically accrued development (Bromberg, 1993; Mitchell, 1993). The previous notion of a unified self gives way in relational thought to a view of the self as an "amalgamation of many fragments, narrative threads and voices" (Kennedy, 1996, p. 95; see also Mitchell, 1993); coherence, permeability, and integration of these many voices are regarded as the central issues in evaluating mental health and maturity.

Recent contributions from the trauma/dissociation and feminist literature are consistent with this emerging paradigm of multiple self-states. Feminist perspectives highlight the role of dominant cultural and political ideologies in the conceptualization of the self. bell hooks (1995), for example, claims that "psychoanalytically, it is clear that the unitary self is sustained only by acts of coercive control and repression" (p. 249). For hooks, the focus on unitary identity oppresses minority groups by rendering invisible the complex and multiple subjectivity of individuals. Consistent with this is Flax's (1993) view that the unitary self is only sustained by splitting off or repressing other parts of its own or others' subjectivities.

In discussing the nature of subjectivity, Flax (1993) reminds us that temporary coherence into apparently solid characteristics or structures is only one of the many possible expressions of human subjectivity and personality. Flax's view, which embodies a prescription for the treatment of severely dissociative individuals, emphasizes fluidity over solidity, process rather than topographical perspectives, and contextual rather than universal outlooks in conceptualizing self-development. In this framework no singular form of the self is the regulative ideal or the absolute definition or objective of human evolution and maturity.

Colin Ross's (1991) view of multiplicity as a normal organizational principle of the human psyche is in harmony with these conceptualizations, although it emphasizes psychological, spiritual, and anthropological implications. According to Ross, in Western industrialized culture natural multiplicity has been suppressed by a "cultural dissociation barrier" that separates out the executive self or dissociated ego from the mind's other part-selves. Ross compares this system of executive ego domination to a kind of "internal apartheid." As Goodwin (1993a) also points out, in our society many of us pretend that our everyday, pragmatic executive personas are the only selves we have—and we forget that not everyone shares this assumption. She, like Ross, reminds us that older cultures often provide ritualized arenas for state-changes in individual consciousness (grief states, ecstasies, regressions, and displays of anger and revenge, etc.). In psychotherapy with trauma survivors who have anything but a unitary worldview, mood state, or philosophical stance, the therapist may feel overwhelmed, disoriented, or manipulated not only by the content of the patient's state-changes but also by the suddenness of their onset.

As a disorder based on caretakers' misuse of power (domination, betrayal, sadism, neglect), DID is the ultimate paradigm of the collapse of the transitional, the dialectical, and the paradoxical in intrapsychic and interpersonal life. Contrary to most public misrepresentations of the disorder, diversity is dangerous to, and the illusion of unity highly valued by, the DID individual. What is reflected in MPD/DID symptomatology is the quintessential paradigm of hierarchy and authoritarian power imbalances—the one dominating and negating the many and the many either silenced, begging for recognition, or complicitous with the power of the one or the few. From Ross's (1991) and hooks's (1995) perspective, these forms of internalized domination and polarization reflect and are reinforced by the patterns of power enactments in the dominant culture, but also the domination and coercion of child-abuse scenarios synergistically reinforce and reify dissociative practices and support the feigning of a unitary self commonly found in severely dissociative patients. The social arrangements and intrapsychic phenomena rooted in hierarchical relationships of oppression can only lead to reification of dissociative barriers where denigration and disempowerment are internalized and where paradox, inclusivity, and ambiguity are occluded by hypervigilance and dichotomous thinking.

RELATIONAL PERSPECTIVES ON TREATMENT

Relational models offer particularly useful perspectives in approaching chronic-trauma-syndrome patients whose subjective worlds are complex survivalist constructions, whose core developmental processes have been assaulted and derailed throughout childhood, and whose patterns of relatedness are organized around domination and abuse. The emphasis of relational theories on internal structuralization of human experience and concomitant, recurrent patterns of behavior and fantasy (Stolorow et al., 1987) encourages articulation of the patient's intricately woven subjective organization, its traumatic origins, and the relational processes that maintain it. Moreover, the philosophical premises underlying most relational theories insist on the development of the therapist's alertness to the dangers of imposing his/her theory or perspectives upon the patient's subjective experience. This sensitivity can minimize further psychological violations of already chronically traumatized individuals.

It is not only therapists, however, who may contribute to the obfuscation of severely dissociative patients' internal experience. Some voices of consciousness are purposely lost, forgotten, and forced underground by perpetrator/victim relationship dynamics and complicitous cultural contexts. In such cases, coercive dissociative conditions and the barriers to locating, experiencing, and believing the internal voices are developed into personified part-selves whose function is to feign unity of consciousness, block reflection, and interfere with remembering trauma or experiencing traumatic affects—to delegitimize the multiplicity of internalized voices and block evidence for a dissociative diagnosis. Hence the early work of therapeutic encounter and dialogue is to access the multiplicity of voices and the barriers (cloaking devices, hostile alter personalities, addictions, distractions, dissimulation, lying, cover stories) to experiencing these "forgotten" voices and parts of the self, and to create an arena where the voices can interact and perhaps confront one another for the first time in the presence of a *protective witness*.

Sometimes these opportunities are created by the therapist's wedging him/herself (or accidentally stumbling) into the spaces between the patient's fragmented states and experiences with a question, an empathic commentary, a confrontation, or a statement about his/her own experience in the moment of the transaction. Sometimes the most helpful thing to do is to draw the patient's attentions to gaps, inconsistencies, and subtle shifts in behavior and relatedness in an effort toward mutual reflection. As Levenson (1996) explains from an interpersonal perspective, the self-system is a conglomeration of defenses operating to maintain self-equilibrium and minimize the emergence of situations that threaten to evoke anxiety. These defenses may include inattention, avoidance, disavowal, and, most relevant to severely dissociative individuals, a series of interpersonal maneuvers designed to distract, deflect, and in general, to contain anxiety. Therapeutic inquiry, according to Levenson, is more about *deconstructing stories and locating omissions*. Investigating omissions is a search for the absences or black holes in the patient's narrative that represent the repository of anxiety and issues or experiences being excluded from awareness.

In the severe dissociative disorders, transforming the relationship with the past means what Winnicott (1965) called turning "ghosts into ancestors." It involves overthrowing the yoke of psychic slavery, organized and sustained by terrorizing, possessive/possessing imperial part-selves (i.e., malevolent introjects, personified identifications with the perpetrator), and establishing an intrapsychic democracy where neither ghosts nor tyrannical ancestors have any dominion. This revolution can impact positively on the capacities for hope, for symbolizing, for deploying restorative fantasy (Smith, 1989; Reis, 1993; Pizer, 1998; Schwartz, 1994). Through the systematic repairing of memory and imagination (Pye, 1995), the dissociative-disorder patient moves from being a victim of his/her mind (and of control by the perverse mind of the perpetrator) to authentic ownership of that mind and body and spirit.

The term "relational" implies a focus on relationship not only with other people and things but also with internal personifications and representations (Ghent, 1992a). That focus in treatment is essential to facilitate the shift from dissociation to negotiation of meanings, conflicts, and identifications (Bromberg, 1993; 1994; Pizer, 1992; 1996; Schwartz, 1994). Addressing individual subnarratives, each in its own terms, and enabling negotiation to take place between them is the essence of structural personality growth (Bromberg, 1991). But negotiation can take place only when there are intersections—crossroads of emotional contact—instead of dissociative sleight-of-hand, camouflage, and the internal reenactment of forgetting and suppressing voices of pain or protest. Successful recognition among dissociated self-states leads to what Rivera (1989) calls the capacity to identify (with) different points of view and divergent voices as "I" rather than singling out any one as the whole story, and what Bromberg (1993, p. 166) calls "the ability to stand in the spaces between realities without losing any of them." The presence, distortions, and absence of relationship are critical avenues of therapeutic inquiry leading to engagement with all aspects of the patient's self/selves. The dissociative patient's elaborate matrices of exclusion and avoidance of anxiety (often posttraumatic anxiety) must become the focus for a renegotiation of non-trauma-based identity to take place.

Proponents of self psychology (Kohut, 1971), intersubjectivity theory (Stolorow, et al., 1987; Orange et al., 1997), and relational psychoanalysis (Mitchell, 1988; 1993; Aron, 1996) all agree that rigid application of theory must be transcended in order to encounter and then interpret from affective and empathic proximity the patient's inner experience. Emphasizing the uniqueness and integrity of the individual and his or her way of representing the world, they mandate that the therapist enter and comment on the patient's experience from the patient's frame of reference (Kohut, 1959; Stolorow et al., 1987), rather than impose a priori assumptions about who the patient is or what s/he needs. This stance is crucial to the treatment of individuals who have survived chronic violent impingement by figuring out what others expect from them. Prior to therapy, no one has engaged these objectified and dehumanized individuals in authentic dialogue. Even well-intended therapists who impose a predetermined set of meanings on the patient's life experiences can fall into the trap of replicating their domination by the caretakers of their lost childhood worlds. Intersubjective and relational perspectives are inherently inimical to power dynamics and their potential for derailing treatment; those dynamics are defused when confronted explicitly as part of the therapeutic discourse rather than tacitly legitimized and made subject to enactment.

A QUESTION OF BALANCE: PARADOX, TRAUMA, AND SEVERE DISSOCIATIVE DISORDERS

Because dissociative experience is fundamentally paradoxical (me/not me, real/not real, past/not past, present/not present, them/not them), internality and externality are collapsed in the psyches of patients with severe post-traumatic conditions. Their reversals of ownership and responsibility, real and false identifications with victim and perpetrator positions, and motivated forgetting of complicity and collaboration epitomize the posttraumatic fluctuations in their psychic states. Many severely dissociative patients have trouble knowing what they are actually responsible for: they may assign themselves excessive responsibility for everything that has happened to them, for forcing their caretakers to be abusive or for enjoying the abuse, that is, for events/conditions objectively beyond their control. Yet at other times they feel they are innocent victims—although often of the therapist, rather than the abusers—and they have difficulty accepting responsibility for frustrating the caring responses of people around them (therapists included).

It has been difficult for the mental health professions and the media to understand the essential paradoxical, biphasic feature of trauma, PTSD, and the dissociative disorders whereby DID patients describe, then deny negative views of their caretakers/abusers; remember, then (from moment to moment or month to month) recant abuse memories; and alternate between believing and doubting virtually everything they themselves say about their histories, identities, and most of all their victimizers. Baffled by the complexity and reversibility of the psyches of these patients, clinicians can be hard-pressed to come up with reasonable and responsible attitudes toward them. "One does not want to minimize the pathogenicity of external trauma, but one does not want to place such trauma on a pedestal, from where it can crowd out the internal amplifications that are likewise pathogenic" (Wilson, 1995, p. 18).

Psychic trauma involves the forced recognition of realities that most people have not yet begun to face. It often manifests as history that has no place: it does not belong in the past, where the trauma was not fully experienced; and it does not belong in the present, where its precise images and reenactments either are not fully understood or are totally denied, minimized, or reformulated (by listeners, helpers, and society as a whole) into more palatable representations.[5]

The clinical use of the concept of paradox has been a major contribution to the psychoanalytic literature. It came first from Winnicott (1969; 1971), and has been elaborated by various relational theorists (Benjamin, 1990; Modell, 1990; Ghent, 1992a, 1992b; Eigen, 1981; Pizer, 1992; 1996; 1998). Paradox includes the realm of the *transitional* where reality and fantasy can become wonderfully indistinguishable, where there is no point in determining whether a psychic element is reality- or fantasy-based. Even mutually exclusive elements can coexist in a mind that can successfully negotiate the paradox of, say, the father as the man who sadistically rapes the patient as a child in the basement when no one is looking, and as also the one who saves him/her from abuse or neglect by the mother, or as the only one in the family or the world who doesn't ignore him/her or who treats him/her specially.

The developmental perspectives of relational psychoanalytic theory have placed particular value on the individual's capacities for tolerance of both conflict and paradox leading to integration and maturation of the personality. Winnicott (1971) regards the failure to perceive and tolerate a paradoxical reality as a defensive operation of the ego. Indeed, he asks therapists to tolerate and respect paradoxes, and to try not to resolve them prematurely. Ghent (1992b) states that paradoxes must be acknowledged also without attempted resolution yet at the same time be viewed as directional signals pointing to a new level of comprehension. Pizer (1992) conceives the negotiation of paradox as the essential vehicle of the therapeutic action of psychoanalysis. Within the preservation and sustained experience of paradox lie the capacities for play, creativity, and flexibility in the development of the self and relational worlds.

The mind of the severely dissociative patient cannot bridge contradictions, however, as a result of its overload of discords and incongruities. Instead of functioning as a plastic container for mutually inconsistent representations, identifications, or memories, it operates out of fear of disintegration or retraumatization. Instead of using intrapsychic conflict to develop increasingly sophisticated resolutions, it avoids mental conflict altogether in order to sustain an illusion of unity and normalcy, and to conserve the psychic energy necessary to minimize painful states and sustain necessary attachments. There is great utility in incorporating paradox into our understanding of the nature and treatment of dissociative conditions, where intrapsychic conflict is somaticized or reenacted interpersonally but never felt, and ambivalence is a distant and dangerous possibility.

PARADOX AND THE DID DIAGNOSIS

Colin Ross (1995a; 1996), viewing DID as inherently paradoxical, says it is both real and not real. It is not real because no one can possibly have more than one actual person living inside—the alters or self-states in MPD/DID are not real persons or personalities; they are dissociative symptoms. On the other hand, the disorder is quite real because those very symptoms (alter personalities or split-off self-states) are subjectively compelling to the patient, and often to the therapist. Whereas skeptics get fixated on only one part of the paradox, that of one body/one person, the therapist must work inside the whole paradox to maintain viable connections inside and outside the patient's internal world. The therapist's mandate is to neither dismiss nor become overly engrossed in the virtual reality of multiple selves, to work *within* the patient's dissociative frame of reference instead of debating with the patient about its existence.

In other words, multiplicity is both a "useful heuristic" (Beahrs, 1994), not to be taken completely literally, and a legitimate complex posttraumatic stress disorder to be treated on its own (structural) terms—one whose real phenomenology reflects rigidification, concretization, and in some sense perversion, of normal processes or aspects of selfhood and self-development. We must acknowledge the existence of multiple internal realities and their potential for dissociation and personification in the alterity phenomenon of MPD/DID, and we must also focus on the intrapsychic and relational meanings behind the organizational and representational decisions and movements of the dissociative process as it takes place during the therapy hours. The structural and transferential elements of DID must be considered dialectically and simultaneously.

Yet another paradoxical aspect of DID is that it is both a complex character-disorder syndrome and a complex, multilayered posttraumatic stress disorder. Chronic child-abuse trauma leads to specific character problems including disturbances in relationship patterns, intimacy, and sexuality, manipulativeness, chronic defensiveness, avoidance, and so on. (Briere, 1992b), and the character pathology can in turn lead to a vulnerability to revictimization experiences (Van der Kolk, 1989; Herman, 1992). That dialectic can become a reciprocally reinforcing spiral that keeps the patient in a state of continuous traumatic reliving—actual and symbolic. Therapy must address both sides of the dynamic while remaining sensitive to the need for homeostasis in the individual's self-system, the objective being creation of the right relational conditions to maintain continuity and negotiate change simultaneously (Bromberg, 1993; 1994).

The pathway to accessing hidden meanings and hidden aspects of the self, and to articulating traumatic relational paradigms reenacted between therapist and patient is a microanalytic focus on the moment-to-moment shifts in the patient, in the therapist, and in the interactional process. Overemphasis on the intrapsychic content and structural manifestations of severe dissociative disorders may lead to reifying the symptoms of survival, but overemphasis on the process and transference alone, to the exclusion of the dissociatively organized and shifting subjectivity of the patient, may lead to an abstract, distancing approach to treatment that misses the mark of direct contact with dissociatively sequestered self-experience.

Only *direct contact* with dissociative self-states with their alterations in perception has the capacity to change the cognitive realities, transform the rigid internal worlds, and challenge the belief systems of severe trauma survivors. Direct contact with the affective and perceptual substrate of dissociative part-selves allows the therapist to penetrate the trance logic or rigidified belief system contained in that part-self, to ascertain some of the historical events, perpetrator messages, and fantasies that consolidated the cognitions and motivations of that part-self, and to gently disrupt that system. This process culminates in facilitating the patient's experience of new thoughts, revealing old and experiencing new feelings, and in the strengthening of an observing ego. Ultimately such contact, and disruption of the dissociative construction of self followed by reintegration, leads to the patient's reclaiming of his/her own mind and life.

Entry to the perceptual substrate (memories, somatic sensations, fantasies, beliefs, etc.) walled off in dissociative chambers is often catalyzed when the therapist notices subtle changes in his/her own experience, in the patient's behavior or communication style, or in their interaction. Empathic inquiry about, or mention of, the change in sensory, affective, or thought process can lead to drawing out of self-states or alter personalities not previously engaged in treatment. By paradoxically accepting and disrupting the ideologies of individual self-states, their mutual exclusion and domination, the therapist can establish a foundation for dialogue in and among part-selves whose relationship was previously defined by impermeability and control.

For example, helping a desexualized host personality understand and accept that her highly sexualized alter personalities—trained to initiate sex with adults in the contexts of child prostitution and pornography—are also victims, also vulnerable, and also deserving of respect assisted the patient in moving through some of her shame and disavowal of her past traumas and resulting dissociative identifications; simultaneously assisting her seductive alters in recognizing that their need for attention had been purposefully sexualized by her perpetrators liberated them to experience a level of vulnerability previously segregated to the host and traumatized child-states. Likewise, supporting the capacity of a patient victimized by his father as part of a man-boy pedophile group to accept and dialogue with the parts of himself that believed he *chose* to kill small animals as well as the parts that believed he was "blackmailed" into doing so when the group threatened to tell his mother about his sexual "compliance" rendered the dissociative barriers between his self-states more permeable and gave him more access to grief, rage, and sorrow. This integrative process interferes with the pathological agency and relative defensive autonomy of part-selves that have dissociated from the current environment and from information that is not consistent with what has already been accepted as "real." Eventually, the patient's lifestyle of dissociation can be converted into a lifestyle of differentiation.

PARADOX IN THEORY AND PRACTICE

The compulsive, dangerous, and often repetitive reenactments of the past that define so much of a trauma survivor's life experience cannot be viewed simply as testimony to the traumatic event(s) themselves (Caruth, 1995b). Paradoxically these reenactments bear witness to a past that was never fully experienced as it occurred. Traumatic symptoms register the force of an experience not yet owned or known. In the space of unconsconsciousness the event is preserved in its literality; it is fully exposed only in connection, and only through relationship, with another place in another time.

This book proposes paradox, along with recognition and mutuality, as a central principle of therapy with severely dissociative patients. Paradox changes that which is in its orbit; dissociation keeps things as they are, frozen in time, space, and character. The intersubjective processes of recognition and mutuality lead toward the paradoxical awareness that can be transformative: "paradox stretches us and invites us to transcend the familiar, it expands the purview of awareness and poses a mystery" (Ghent, 1992b, pp. 136–137).

Ehrenberg (1992) counsels psychotherapists to sensitize traumatized patients to the real tragedies they have suffered at the hands of others and to the ongoing tragedies they perpetuate against themselves. Bromberg (1996a) advises the therapist also to be clear that his/her goal is not to cure patients of something that was done to them in the past, but to cure them of what they still do to themselves (and to others) to cope with what was done in the past.

According to many relational theorists following in the spirit of Winnicott (1971), effective therapy consists of a containing space in which illusions can flourish and in which multiple realities can collide and intersect. When the DID patient can experience the contrast between his/her archaic objects, internalized traumatic relational paradigms, or posttraumatic belief systems and the therapist's reality against a backdrop permissive of doubt, suspicion, and incredulity, then the rigidified dissociative self-system will slowly begin to tolerate increasing conflict and ambiguity. The patient will, in turn, substitute less rigid defenses and come to establish an identity based on a more complex, multidimensional view of self and others.

ALICE

DID patients' memories are stored in layers. The emergence of new material from the underlayers—previously unthought and as yet unintegrated—is typically accompanied or interrupted by some kind of reenactment. This case is no exception.

Alice had been making progress in her professional and interpersonal life. By the early middle phase of treatment, she was acting out less and spontaneously remembering more. She had just started going beyond her sexual abuse by her stepfather and grandfather, which she had originally romanticized as signaling specialness and love—notions elaborated in her imagination to make the physical and emotional pain of her victimization more bearable—to discover material suggesting that she had also been subjected to violent, sadistic abuse.

Those recollections, totally at odds with the beliefs she had constructed to sustain her attachment to her perpetrators, inundated Alice and triggered a sudden change in her posture, some apparent confusion, rapid eye movements, and several minutes of nonresponsiveness to my gentle questioning—whereupon a somewhat sexualized child-alter surfaced, who said she was scared and asked if I would let her sit on my lap.

Trying to contain my own discomfort, I asked about the connection between her fears and her need for physical contact. Alice, seeming a mixture of conscious and unconscious alters fronted by a childlike state, replied that my holding her would make her feel safe enough to talk; later she added that it would make the bad feelings go away. All efforts to invite her to talk about her experience without physical contact were met with either stubborn silence or a sorrowful look.

When I tried to articulate the double bind we were in together ("I need words to understand what you're feeling, what you're afraid of, and why you're insisting on physical touch as the only solution—and you need me to hold you so that you can tell me"), because that strategy is usually effective with DID patients, Alice said only that maybe she shouldn't have come today. When then I reminded her that other personalities in the system claimed that when her stepfather "invited" her to sit on his lap he would fondle her genitals as a prelude to escalating sexual involvement, Alice said that her stepfather had told her he loved her and that touching was an expression of love.

I suggested that sex and affection were all mixed up in her life, that she has been willing to pay a big price for love but that real love doesn't have a price tag, and that her other part-selves too seem confused about self-protection and self-sacrifice. She asked the meaning of the word "sacrifice"—and I referred her to her other parts for the answer because I didn't want to completely support this child-alter's delusion of complete separateness (such that, unlike other alters, she either didn't know or pretended she didn't know she wasn't the size of a child), but also because I was frustrated by the lack of participation by her other parts and wanted her to listen to their voices in her head (especially about subjects that have already been discussed several times in treatment with different alters).

In a quiet moment, the other parts did explain sacrifice to her; her anxiety increased noticeably, then shifted to what I perceived as a stance correlated to anxiety-reduction and control when Alice iterated her conviction that I was rejecting her by refusing her the oasis of my lap. I speculated aloud that doing otherwise—symbolically adopting her, in keeping with another of her requests, as yet another sexualizing father—would not be helping her come to terms with what really happened but would be helping to keep her away from the pain. I want to hear about the pain, I tell her, so we can understand her feelings and her needs around sex and affection. (Alice had a history of dangerous promiscuity, including an almost complete inability to say no to anyone initiating sexual contact with her, and also a history of sexual compulsivity for managing painful states of mind.)

When, after considering my comments silently for a time, Alice's child-alter again declared that my refusal to hold her proved that she was unlovable, I remarked that her pressuring me was similar to her stepfather's pressuring her. I expanded (in slightly less complex language than I used with Alice's adult alters) on the reenactment that might be going on.

Now she reverted to bargaining about hugs instead of lap-sitting until I asserted that I was not comfortable with that kind of physical contact, that it felt forced, and that I believed that—even if it remained nonsexual as she claimed she trusted it would—it would be bewildering to someone whose life has been freighted with so much confusion about sex and affection. I added that I could see how not getting the kind of validation she was used to could itself be upsetting and bewildering, but I reminded her that I was here to discuss just those feelings.

Trying to link in other elements of Alice's dissociative system, I also reminded her that many of her other parts didn't like or trust me (some hating to be touched at all), and accordingly would not be supportive of the intimacy she is after. I was assuming, as always, that despite some amnestic barriers, I was addressing the whole patient, and I spoke (as I usually do) as if the whole patient (i.e., including adult parts) was listening, bringing up natural love feelings toward parents, sexualized attachment, desires to avoid pain, and some episodes from

Alice's history, as well as the ongoing reenactment of seduction, sacrifice, and rejection.

Finally, a break: as Alice again lamented that no one loved her or ever would, I observed how deep her shame—the feeling of unlovability—was, and I wondered if other parts counted on her to hold or resolve through physical contact that feeling for them; I commented on the pressure of her wish to be held and wondered what that might be about. Unable to sustain the child position with intensifying affect, Alice shifted to a more adultlike presentation to tell me how people would just use her, so she would take whatever she can get from them and then feel even worse.

I fixed on her shifts between feeling special and protected and feeling unlovable and worthless, and on how long she has been managing them by switching from vulnerability to control and seduction. Her needs could be met without her selling herself out, I repeated, and without her trying to get me to do the same by crossing a professional boundary or doing something that didn't feel right. "We can work hand in hand without touching," I said—and Alice and her child alter, shifting back and forth, at last seemed connected to feelings and began to talk about her mother's complicity in giving her to her stepfather the first time. Something had broken through the stalemate.

The adult (host/functional) alter, who had been moderately coconscious for most of the session, interjected her impression that I seemed overly interested in the abuse experience she had started out describing. "One voice in my head said you were getting turned on by it, another said it would make you angry, and the other said no, you just wanted to help me find a way to talk about it as you always do."

"So you had three different, strong reactions to my encouraging you to talk and you became overwhelmed and you switched. In response to the perception that I found it sexually gratifying to hear the details, you went into a child state to manage the possible sexual interaction—just as you've said you used to do with your stepfather." I hypothesized that it seemed safer to replay a familiar abuse scenario to ward off the more dangerous awareness that was emerging, and Alice agreed, answering that the choice was automatic.

Then she asked me an uncharacteristically direct question, which I acknowledged as a promisingly authentic communication showing her ability to hang in with her anxiety instead of dodging it and taking dissociative flight as she had throughout her life. "Were you aroused and stimulated by what I was saying?"

I reflected a moment and said no, that I had actually been feeling some revulsion and that I was trying to contain that feeling without making her feel that she, rather than what she was beginning to tell me, was revolting . . . and also that I was listening real hard since she seemed to be bringing up an entirely new level of trauma. Alice said she picked up on the revulsion but did think it was about her. "Arousal and revulsion are all mixed up in me." Alice was able to make use of these comments to begin sorting out some of her own past and present confusion about sex, affection, and free will and to increase her self-observational skills regarding her dissociative system.

Toward the end of the session, pressing the intimacy further and perhaps seeking (or testing) further safety, Alice asked me if I would acknowledge sexual arousal when asked about it if indeed I ever did experience such feelings when she or other patients talked about traumatic material. Because there was little time left and the question was so potentially loaded and complicated, I told Alice that I would give her a brief answer for now but that further discussion was essential. After briefly exploring what she felt her own needs would be in this context (and she admitted she was not sure she would ever even want to know), I explained that many feelings I experienced during sessions would remain part of my private reflections on our clinical process and only some would seem appropriate for sharing. How, when, where, and with whom to share them were decisions I had to make on a case-by-case, moment-by-moment basis. I also explained that honesty, intimacy, and authenticity were not necessarily equivalent to revealing all feelings.

In our ensuing dialogues about what had just taken place, I told Alice how hard it is to know what and when patients and therapists should share, but added that I felt it important that she stay with her own traumatic material and feelings about the therapy relationship and explore whatever was coming up. Alice expressed relief at being treated with (unaccustomed) respect "like a real person" and pleasure at hearing what was going on for me. She also, however, commented that such treatment made her feel pressured to "show up" more completely (i.e., to be direct and vulnerable and self-aware simultaneously)—which was something that would take some getting used to.[6]

The work in this session seemed to create the space in Alice to re-member more of the sadistic abuse and to tolerate holding contradic-tory feelings about her perpetrators. She began to realize how her requests for physical contact correlated with strategies she had used as a child to bargain for less painful treatment. And she recalled how, when her relationship with her perpetrators changed from one of se-duction to one of terrorization, she had feebly attempted to restore the milder sexual exploitation.

As a rule, any increase in intimacy can trigger immediate fears of re-traumatization in treatment of severely dissociative trauma survivor patients. Alice had never come to terms with the facts that her omnipo-tent approaches to controlling her abusers had not worked and that re-capitulating them in her adult life only brought her trouble. Now these connections were becoming directly accessible, through affect and memory, and were not just abstractions.

It was not yet time for Alice to completely relinquish using dissocia-tion to manage her here-and-now interpersonal challenges; it was clear that she had to be allowed to play with moving back and forth among her alter-states as a way of negotiating changes in her identity and sense of history without feeling that she would have to give anything up be-fore she was ready. I needed to respect her dissociative defenses—to honor her need to change and stay the same without imposing my im-patience, expectations, or agendas.

Later in our work I was able to share my frustration in the face of her dissociative flight and her ways of projecting rejection onto others: she had cultivated a talent for leaving the relational field while pretending to be engaged. Alice was increasingly open to feedback about her inter-personal style, and became a partner in a sturdy therapeutic alliance.

Beyond Survival: Humanization, Negotiation, Reparation

In a relational psychoanalytic model of therapy, the truth emerges from a process of inquiry, discovery, argument, and agreement involving two peo-ple in psychological community (Spezzano, 1993). Through intersubjective discourse, dissociative strategies are replaced by pathways of free associa-tion, dialogue, and negotiation. Rigid identities based on false power and false helplessness can be renegotiated to create more fluidity among parts of the self previously compartmentalized and disowned, and a real sense of agency and a realistic appraisal of danger and limitations can begin to develop. Negotiation is directed at achieving some shared reality based on respect for the subjectivity of the other; it stands in marked contrast to communication processes such as indoctrination, forced compliance, submission, and unequal participation (Goldberg, 1988; Pizer, 1992).

Psychotherapy provides a container, a holding environment (Winnicott, 1969), a cohesive temporal-relational context (Bromberg, 1996a), an anchor of tenderness, where the past, present, and future can be reliably addressed by way of the enacted and observed interpersonal experience occurring between therapist and patient. In this process, there should be an effort to welcome and communicate with the patient's multiple voices, personifications, multiple subnarratives, and multiple (historical) perspectives. When such diverse self-representations are described, symbolized, and reenacted with a receptive and emotionally available therapist who has an informed awareness about the nature of trauma, including the subtleties of dissociative adaptation and identifications with perpetration and complicity, there is never a silencing of unwelcome or unacceptable voices (Rivera, 1989; Bromberg, 1993, 1994; Schwartz, 1994). Through the therapist's efforts to build a multidimensional relationship with the patient's fragmented self, the patient's voices are brought into contact and dialogue with each other, into a capacity for conflict and collision and eventually for mutuality and harmony.

The task of approaching traumatically sequestered aspects of self is a daunting one. Even when therapy is conducted in a thoughtful way by a skilled clinician, severely dissociative patients will experience aspects of the therapy process as similar to his or her abuse, leading perhaps to forms of unconscious opposition resembling what was felt toward the perpetrator during the original trauma. Bromberg (1991) posed the question of how psychotherapy can enable someone who has fought all his or her life to keep traumatic aspects of self-experience from being thought or exposed to find a voice and enter dialogue. How can a patient who has learned to maintain a sense of being in the face of chronic catastrophic anxieties learn to experience disorganization and chaos as generative and healing?

"Finally every conflict has to be fought out in the sphere of transference" (Freud, 1912, p. 104). The transference/countertransference matrix is the medium for healing. Enactments represent the forms and transformations of experience within it. This medium makes it possible for severe trauma survivors to revisit and make conscious the full house of malevolent object relations and activates a healing configuration where benign maternal and paternal images and playful, creative aggression replace self-defeating patterns and abusive identifications.

Through effective navigation of the transference/countertransference matrix, the therapist facilitates the transfer of *the unthought known* into thought (Bollas, 1987). The patient comes to experience elements of his or her being that have not been knowable before. This new form of knowing is enabled precisely because the therapist's position of stewarding "potential" and "transitional" space helps the patient to tolerate the experience of not knowing, in Ogden's (1989) sense, as well as other tension-states from where more authentic affective and relational experience emerge. The essential developmental experience of restitution following disruption (Kohut, 1977) is internalized by the severely dissociative patient who develops a confident expectation of humanizing responses from the internal and interpersonal worlds.

As the dissociative patient internalizes the therapist's inclusive, observational, and empathic stances, and the mutuality-based patterns of interaction and power negotiation, the patient begins to treat him/herself with compassion, creativity, and respect. From this there is a continual and gradual erosion of dissociative defenses that have distanced the patient from his/her own suffering. The nonredeemable suffering of unbridled reenactments, revictimization scenarios, and fear of grieving is replaced by "redemptive suffering," whereby the patient stays affectively connected and fully aware of him/herself during periods of taking reownership of the previously disavowed and disparaged victim-self. Eventually suffering itself becomes associated with shared humanizing contact and a deepening capacity for joy and creativity rather than an unending abyss of isolation and misery. As the dissociative patient makes room for deep grief and suffering within him/herself, the integration process is well underway. The patient no longer is afraid of him/herself. Knowing what to be afraid of and what not to be afraid of, the recovering dissociative patient can actually begin to protect him/herself in complex interpersonal situations without dissociating or leaving the relational field.

The severely traumatized patient is not simply in need of reliving traumatic experience, of magical and concretized reparation rituals, or of gaining insight to moderate impaired reality testing. The dissociative survivor of chronic childhood holocausts requires a mutually transforming relationship with another human being who can help him/her find a voice to express the unspeakable and reconstruct a self that can create, hope, and love without denying his or her tormented past. The ultimate goal of *integration* is the establishment of an identity based on inclusion and recognition instead of repudiation and disavowal, with a developed sector of self for transitional experiencing where meanings, identifications, and historicity can be created, destroyed, and reconstructed joyfully without adherence to totalistic rules and ideologies of submission (Schwartz, 1994). A psychotherapy initially fraught with confusing, dominating reenactments and chronic displays of autistic, dissociative self-remedies can evolve into what Atwood and Stolorow (1984) refer to as a dialogue between two personal universes.

CHAPTER 5

From Inclusion to Integration: Basic Concepts in Psychotherapy with Severely Dissociative Trauma Survivors

The extremes of emotional excess and explosion that we call psychopathology are based on normal and otherwise healthy psychological mechanisms that have been called into play to handle situations for which they did not evolve.

—Donald Nathanson

Psychoanalysis has long understood that these primitive defenses . . . (splitting, projective identification, idealization or diabolization, psychic numbing, etc.) . . . both characterize *severe psychopathology and also (once in place)* cause *it. But rarely in our contemporary literature do these defenses "get any credit," so to speak, for having accomplished anything in the preservation of life for the person whose heart is broken by trauma.*

—Donald Kalsched

Childhood-trauma refugees are streaming in record numbers into clinics, mental health centers, and private practice settings. Their accounts cover a spectrum from intrafamilial incest and torture to well-organized sadistic and criminal perpetrator groups involving sophisticated mind-control techniques and the commoditization of child abuse. The patients themselves are educating their therapists in the treatment of severely dissociative trauma survivors—with their wisdom, their informing reenactments, their symptoms' disturbing challenges to theoretical orthodoxy, their suffering, their brilliant avoidance of grief, mourning, and remembering, and their astonishing capacities for reactivating developmental strivings in the face of histories of massive interpersonal violence, betrayal, and neglect. As often-isolated clinicians grope through the landscape of psychological trauma in an environment marked by the risk of imminent breakdown, the psychotherapy relationship can be suddenly turned upside down. A momentary catastrophe can become the root of a transformational process. Or a moment of promise can dissolve into agonizing misunderstandings, chaos, or tragedy—boundary violations by the therapist, premature termination by the patient, an urgent need for hospitalization, a suicidal gesture, a malicious lawsuit, the stalking and harassment of the therapist and his/her family.

VARIATIONS ON A THEME

Clinicians can now read about treatment of posttraumatic stress and dissociative disorders from just about every conceivable theoretical perspective, ranging from the immediacy of cognitive, hypnotic, and behavioral techniques to the immersion in transference and countertransference phenomena from classical and contemporary psychoanalytic points of view. Most strive for a middle ground. Trauma authorities differ on the utility of hypnosis, the value of integrating psychodynamic perspectives, the purpose and structuring of memory work, the use of countertransference, the role of hospitalization and medication, and so on. And the psychoanalytic schools are divided with respect to the fantasy/reality aspects of trauma and dissociation, the nature of neutrality, the impact of interpretation, insight, and enactment, the feasibility of reparation, the merits of confrontation, self-disclosure, and empathy in treatment.

Some clinicians discourage the patient's expression of dissociative pathology; such "benign neglect" posing as treatment is actually on the rise as a result of the growing role of managed care in mental health services. Steadfast avoidance of dissociative states or their underlying trauma history leads to little structural change in the patient's personality, however, so that "neglect" is closer to clinical abandonment. Those who equate willingness to confront dissociated aspects of a self—an essential process for trauma theorists or relational psychoanalysts—with the unprofessional relinquishing of neutrality also endorse potentially retraumatizing ideologies of suppression; they contend, in fact, that recognizing alterity is tantamount to cocreating it.[1]

The clinician who refuses to address dissociative identity disorder (DID) may provoke patients "either to dissociate, further sequestering that for which they will receive no help, or to create even more dramatic proofs that the condition [exists]" (Kluft, 1995, p. 360). Such a misadventure can pressure the patient to shield the therapist and the therapy from the alter personalities: the clinician will see fewer traces of personified dissociation and feel convinced that the policy of "nonreinforcement" is actually healing the disorder—whereas the patient is merely learning how to be more compliant, and, worse, is unconsciously reenacting the submissive identity reconstruction consistent with the original trauma dynamics. The therapist is shown exactly what s/he wants to see, or what the patient perceives s/he can handle—an increasingly well-shaped host alter personality (or set of persona-restoring self-states) who mirrors the clinician's need for a successful (nondissociative) case by becoming one, at least, temporarily. The disbelief in multiplicity and alter states or the refusal to engage with them because of a priori beliefs is emblematic of the old idea of naïve patient and all-knowing therapist, which contemporary relationally oriented theorists have come to consider as totally mythological and collusive (Aron, 1996; Renik, 1995).

The therapist should be someone with whom the patient can reexperience trauma within a new context and thereby experience for the first time what has been absent in the past (Modell, 1990). Such a stance emphasizes that the essence of psychoanalytic treatment is not in making the unconscious conscious or increasing the capacities and strength of the ego, but is rather in providing a setting in which healing can occur because connections between previously split-off and lost aspects of the self can be reestablished (Rycroft, 1985). Elaborating the psychoanalytic approach to DID, Barach and Comstock (1996) identify the need for the therapist to help the patient tolerate affect, form a cohesive sense of self, develop coherent object- and self-representations, differentiate fact from fantasy, and resolve the negative effects of compulsive reliance on dissociative defenses.

Now, some two decades after the rediscovery of DID, it appears that the interface between psychoanalysis and the trauma and dissociative disorders field will advance new forms of strategic integrationism (Kluft, 1988a) and facilitate constructive dialogue among traumatologists, cognitive psychologists, and psychoanalysts. All clinicians should be able to draw on different methodologies, including perhaps especially those that do not fit with their preferred styles. And different patients (or the same patient at different times) may respond to different modalities—for example, supportive work, medications, hospitalization, and containment at some points, and exploratory work, confrontation, and direct use of countertransference experience at others.

In discussing variations in treatment approach, it is important to remember that retraumatization can take place in *any* therapy situation. For patients with dissociated injuries, confused histories, and tangled or fragmented memories, the trap of collusion with a therapist's misrecognition, domination, or narcissistic needs is a definite possibility. When a therapeutic posture or underlying belief system permits repetition of traumatic nonrecognition experiences, for example (itself a form of clinical abandonment according to Bromberg, 1995b), that posture will reinforce the patient's conviction that others do not want to know who s/he really is; ironically, since most trauma survivors are ambivalent about being known because of the pain of the challenge to their identities, bonds, and belief systems, the therapist's misrecognition may be felt as a relief—for a while. At a deeper level, however, the failure it signals drives a wedge of despair into an already despondent and cynical psyche, confirming the abandonment and lack of concern on the part of the adult world that made possible the traumatic childhood experiences in the first place.

Our patients are not naïve and oblivious to the tensions therapists have to confront and/or the biases and theories clinicians rely on to make sense out of these tensions. Severely dissociative patients who have witnessed countless adults abuse children and skillfully manipulate them and others to avoid detection have keen observation skills. One thing they most certainly understand is power. The refusal to work with dissociative states recommended by conservative critics of traumatology assumes that patients can be fooled by pseudo-objectivity, when it is precisely the persuasive power of the therapist that fosters the patient's collusion to suppress and inhibit his/her own complex subjectivity—collusion that echoes the collusion of a lifetime. Anyone who is aware of the damage done by perpetrators of child abuse in the misuse of authority, specifically in undermining the victim's perceptions and reality testing, will see the dangers of revictimization inherent in sidestepping the multiple subjectivities of the patient.

DIVERSITY IN APPROACH

Not only the wide variety of clinical orientations, but also the wide spectrum of needs, resources, and abilities of the dissociative patient population must be taken into account when designing and implementing treatment. Patients differ in terms of accessibility to and capacity for therapy, prior history (constructive, neglectful, or destructive) with the mental health system, extent and complexity of abuse and number of perpetrators involved (and their past and current connection), capacity for and commitment to self-care, capacity for attachment and interest in relationships, capacity for symbolization, the presence of other psychiatric or medical disorders or of sociopathic traits or other particularly destructive comorbid characterological patterns, motivation for treatment, and overall physical health. Some dissociative patients can do character restructuring, memory work, and intensive mutual reflective work within the transference/countertransference while others may only be able to make use of competent supportive psychotherapy.[2] Some dissociative patients need to explore or express aspects of their spirituality and/or creativity in the therapy process; for others, such explorations or expressions only trigger useless enactments or are otherwise disruptive. It should always be remembered, however, that the subjectivity of every traumatized patient has been debased, defiled, and shattered by a fellow human being or group of fellow human beings. The patient's exposure to interpersonal savagery and his/her dissociative reactions to it must be gradually replaced by prolonged exposure to nonviolent, nonexploitative, and nondominating respectful relationship experiences.

There is tremendous range in character, temperament, and disposition among psychotherapists as well. Some will be most comfortable with more directed, less ambiguous approaches to healing, and for them relationship factors will not be primary; to diminish relationship factors for others would be to betray what they believe are the chief agents of human development and transformation. Some clinicians use formal hypnosis as an essential adjunct to treatment (Kluft, 1995; Fine, 1994); others find it unnecessary, problematic, or retraumatizing (Briere, 1992b; Enns et al., 1995; Lindsay and Read, 1994).[3] There are those for whom even the mention of spiritual matters or the inclusion of sand-tray work or stuffed animals might never happen—and there are those who espouse the introduction of all of them. Certain therapists find the concretized "mapping" of a patient's personality system, like that of a family therapy diagram, useful, while others prefer what

Marmer (1996) calls "acquainting yourself with the overall architecture of the person" (p. 202)—more like walking through a building slowly side by side with the patient than like asking him/her to generate a blueprint so the therapist can find his/her way alone. Feminist and social constructivist approaches facilitate discussions about the politics of abuse, complicity, and gender oppression in family and cultural systems, and about how the traumatized patient can find a place in a world based on such politics; many clinicians who are not so inclined and/or informed would see those conversations as detours from the central tasks of helping patients better understand their psyches and personal histories and learn more effective and appropriate coping skills.

Interpersonal and relationally oriented therapists reverse the figure-ground arrangement advanced by mainstream MPD/DID theorists: cognitive changes are secondary to emotional working-through. The therapeutic action is where the reenactment is, where the retraumatization is, where the trauma drama unfolds to be met, recognized, struggled with; enactments/reenactments are the royal roads to restored affectivity. Patient and therapist fumble together, guide one another, and come to respect one another's authority over time; the therapist consistently affirms the ascendancy of their mutuality. In contrast to traditional psychoanalysts, who may focus on the experience of the self as unitary to the point of refusing to talk to alter personalities for fear of reifying dissociative tendencies, relational psychoanalysts emphasize the dialectic between unity and multiplicity while helping a patient develop observing ego functions and resolution of omnipotent defenses.

According to relational perspectives on treatment, no intervention is an isolated event; each is mediated by the therapist's belief system, reactions, and interpretations—and they, in turn, influence what the patient thinks, feels, and eventually presents (Miller, 1996; Aron, 1996). According to Miller, therapists control for their influence on patients by "understanding that their conscious and unconscious behavior are the proximal stimuli that evoke, maintain, or transform the schemas that the patient uses to organize and interpret their interaction" (p. 395). Therapists can also balance power and control for their influence by welcoming criticism, exploring patients' reactions to the clinical methods in use, and persistently invoking patients' own inner authority. The subject of influence thus becomes part of the therapy dialogues, not ancillary to or subversive of them.[4]

Distinctions Among Psychoanalytic Influences in the Treatment of Dissociative Disorders

Although the literature on DID has always recommended incorporating psychodynamic perspectives (e.g., Ross, 1989; Putnam, 1989; Kluft, 1991a), explicit psychoanalytic conceptualizations—classical (Brenner, 1994; 1996; Barach and Comstock, 1996; Marmer, 1996), post-classical (Smith, 1989; Ferguson, 1990; Schwartz, 1994) and feminist (Rivera, 1996; Waites, 1993; Davies and Frawley, 1994)—have only recently begun to appear as the trauma/dissociation communities have welcomed integration and cross-fertilization as reprieves from their isolation and marginalization within the mental health field; their emergence also attests to the maturation of the field.

Relational perspectives are more sensitive to the ways an individual's construction of his/her subjectivity reflects prevailing social conditions, power arrangements, and language practices. Relational and feminist perspectives combined (cf. Mitchell, 1993; Bromberg, 1994; Flax, 1993; Rivera, 1996) tend to be concerned more with meaning than with truth, more with the complexities of identity politics than with ego-defense analysis, more with exploring multiplicity and the decentered self as a valuable resource for the patient than as something only to be worked through or resolved.

If we think about DID as a trauma/neglect-driven disorder (i.e., trauma-structured subjectivity) rooted foremost in sadistic abuse, torture, neglect, and exploitation of children, and embedded in the historical, economic, political, and cultural contexts where the inequities of capitalist patriarchy are institutionalized, then it is only secondarily a disorder of defense and identity (viz., Marmer, 1996). A primary focus on defense and identity fails to recognize that the nondisordered self is also multiple, and that the key to severe dissociative conditions is the lack of sufficient and intact linkages among self-states—not alter construction, personification, or multiplicity per se. Correspondingly, that focus fails to contextualize the patient's experience, thus unintentionally exacerbating existing splits between etiology and symptomatology, between recognition of violence and confrontation with its effects, between individual and social responsibility, and ultimately between public and private realities.

Construing DID as a trauma disorder (of extreme stress) is not meant to privilege one form of psychological pain over another, alleviate severely dissociative patients' personal responsibility for their behaviors, or reinforce pathological entitlement and victim stances. But to decontextualize any aspect of a trauma survivor's complex adaptations to malevolent social and familial systems is to "dissociate" a diagnosable disorder of defense and identity from the circumstances that give rise to disordered defenses and a fragmented identity in the first place. To sustain the important link between individual psychopathology and the cultural conditions that generate or cultivate it, we must make room for a human rights and social justice perspective in the process of assessment and treatment.

Applying Relational Perspectives

> Our patients bring to us not only their suffering but their creative attempts to heal themselves. As blind as they are at times to their own issues, they are often keen sighted about their therapists and other patients. The idea of the healthy well adjusted therapist curing the patient is a myth. The therapist must be candid enough and human enough to treat the patient, as a fellow traveler in life, not all that different from the therapist. (Chefetz, 1997, p. 264)

Adult survivors of severe childhood abuse need many things in treatment but first they need the emotional presence and psychological availability of the therapist. Second, they need a therapist who is informed about both the dynamics of chronic interpersonal psychological trauma—including the dissociative and characterological adaptations and the dynamics of perpetration, victimization, and complicity—and the archetypal by-products of dissociative disintegration as they appear in dreams and in the personifications of the MPD/DID individual's internal world. Third, these patients need a treatment environment that promotes explorations and inquiry, not an environment that seals over the past and addresses only adaptation without also disentangling and de-enmeshing the patient from abusive power dynamics and traumatic relational patterns; the therapist should not echo the pressure of familial and cultural backlash to conform, comply, and adjust. Finally, they need a tolerant witness, one who explicitly states and implicitly demonstrates that s/he is prepared to hear and discuss anything and everything the patient feels and believes (however bizarre or unusual), anything the patient remembers (entirely or partially, regardless of whether the memories are real), anything the patient has done or believes s/he has done (no matter how awful or gruesome or shameful), and anything and everything the patient has to say about the therapist and the therapeutic process. The therapist must make clear that while there are some actions that will not be permitted in the therapy relationship—sex, violence, emotional abuse, property damage—there are no words s/he will be unwilling to listen to.

The therapist's pledge to help the patient make sense out of his/her experiences—no matter how baffling, to be amenable to witnessing and *feeling with*, and to remain open to the possibility of traumatic realities to which the therapist personally may not have been exposed creates the kind of ambience where extreme dissociative defenses can be relaxed and where suppressed voices can emerge. This contract does not produce a false memory free-for-all. It does, however, anchor compassion and ensure acceptance for someone who is brutalized, alienated, and bereft. The therapist must never forget that compliance and protection of the (powerful, needed) other at one's own expense is central to the programming of all child-abuse victims, so without a repeatedly tested and proven belief that the therapist can tolerate exposure to horrific material about the treatment of children, the adult survivor will not venture to bare his/her multiple subjectivities and traumatic memories.

A relational approach to treating trauma and dissociation emphasizes knowing the patient through direct relatedness, direct experience, direct emotional contact (Bromberg, 1991; 1998; Davies and Frawley, 1994; Ehrenberg, 1992; Maroda, 1999). From these perspectives, which are influenced by intersubjective theory, feminism, and interpersonal psychoanalysis, the therapist does not relate to the patient as if s/he were only a resister and distorter of reality. Therapists working in the transference/countertransference matrix believe that what cannot be remembered or narrated can often be discovered through reenactment, making the very "distortions" and "resistances" believed by other clinicians to be in need of their subtle authoritarian modifications the medium for learning about the patient (Marmer, 1996). Through the immersion in that matrix, therapists inevitably become part of the problem on their way to cocreating solutions with patients (Mitchell, 1988). This means that both parties must accept the loss of their bearings during the interactional process, and must trust—subsuming distrust and presupposing the temporary disappearance of hope and faith—that insight will emerge after the enactment and confusion about who is doing what to whom have run their course.

DISSOCIATIVE DISORDERS, DEVELOPMENTAL FAILURES, AND DEVELOPMENTAL PERSPECTIVES ON TREATMENT

Because chronic violent trauma throughout childhood freezes, deregulates, and deforms almost all developmental processes, DID (and most other severe dissociative conditions) is, above all, a disorder of development, development gone awry. The cohesive and continuous self-experience of normal development is replaced by a patchwork of state-dependent organizations each operating under its own rules, which may or may not be relevant to, or even in any form of dialogue with, one another. Confabulation and self-deception supplant self-knowledge and self-observation, distraction and numbing stand in for affectivity; precocity and intellectual skill mask developmental deficits; compulsive delinking and the actual inability to make connections take over for natural continuity, curiosity, and the bridging functions of the well-developed psyche. Core beliefs in safety, benevolent authority, and personal goodness are shattered (Ulman and Brothers, 1988), memory and cognitive abilities are disrupted, and the capacities to trust, attach, and self-regulate are all fractured in significant ways. Dissociation replaces intrapsychic conflict. And because chronic trauma socializes the individual to accept authoritarian modes of relating and institutionalizes the belief that the self is damaged, worthless, or inherently bad, it restricts the effective use of fantasy, aggression, and critical thinking in the service of development. Domination/submission (and its eroticization) is deeply internalized in the intrapsychic realm as the only solution to the challenges of human relations and becomes the only adaptive paradigm in the individual's repertoire.

The adult dissociative survivor can feel deeply tormented, defective, and sick on the inside while passing in the mainstream culture as a compliant model citizen. The multiple levels of developmental failure lead to seriously impaired volition, as defined by both subjective experience and objective assessment. Of course, certain self-states can be inhibited while others are dramatically willful; self-agency may be limited to whatever functions are performed effectively by the dissociated self-state that has access to the mind at any given point in time (Bromberg, 1996a).

Like all psychoanalytic psychotherapies, relational treatment of severe dissociative disorders is a developmental process, oriented around sequences or stages reflecting retrieval, recognition, and activation of previously derailed development (Stolorow et al., 1987). Relational treatment is also conducted within the essential dialectic of "knowing" and "not knowing" (Ogden, 1989, p. 3)—of denial and intrusion, in the terminology of post-traumatic stress disorder. In trauma-oriented therapies, the need to be known and "found" alternates with the need for absolute camouflage and protection from revictimization; human contact—every human relationship, including one with a therapist—is simultaneously dangerous and longed for.

The establishment of deeply integrated psychological functioning in a DID patient must involve the resolution of the developmental deficits that have resulted from chronic trauma and neglect (Barach and Comstock, 1996). However, maturation, developmental stages, and concepts of unity and multiplicity must not themselves be concretized and reified or understood as simple cumulative or linear processes. Broader concepts of personality development are required to link treatment of problems as complex as severe dissociative disorders to psychoanalytic developmental concepts. In traditional approaches to developmental psychology, one stage is seen as leading to another—oral stage to phallic to genital; paranoid-schizoid position preceding depressive position. But what is more important is the relationship among stages, phases, and aspects of self.[5]

A relational vision of personality development does not deny that dissociative strategies for self-protection and self-construction are dysfunctional phenomena that create imbalances and rigidities in what would otherwise be freely interpenetrating, dialectical realms of experience. However, this perspective insists on contextualizing the patient's limitations and adaptations in the interpersonal and cultural matrices of childhood, and on acknowledging the survival value and, at times archetypal brilliance, of dissociative solutions to chronic violence and neglect. Therefore, developmental maturation in the context of treating dissociative disorders needs to be conceived of in dialectical terms where stages and modes of experience evolve in and of themselves and in fluid relational interchanges with other modes.

Child alter personalities, the most common alter states in DID patients (Ross, 1997), exemplify the simplest application of these dialectical concepts of development. At the end of a successful treatment one may hope to see the erosion of dissociative barriers so that child alters no longer appear in split-off form and the adult no longer has to manage his/her vulnerability by disconnecting aggression, mature functionality, and memory from need-states. Simultaneously, however, one hopes to see the patient able to move in and out of adult and childlike self-states, feelings, and identifications without losing awareness or a sense of self-ownership. Moreover, the rigid, impermeable protective barriers the patient will have mostly worked through in treatment may continue to be useful at certain times and under certain circumstances. A fluid or "distributed" (Pizer, 1996) multiple self and a unified or integrated self are not mutually exclusive.

In Leowald's (1960) terms, the developmental perspective on treatment means that the therapist always relates to the patient from the "standpoint of potential growth" (p. 20) rather than from a position of encouraging insight or analyzing defenses. Treatment involves the participation of two essential aspects of the traumatized patient: an adult who struggles to succeed, form relationships, feel accepted, and—most important—to forget; and a child who strives to remember and find a voice to scream, to tell, and to rage (Davies and Frawley, 1991).[6] The therapist's internal, inclusive vision of the patient's wholeness and integrity facilitates the truly mutative ongoing interactions that foster the patient's self-deconstruction and self-actualization. The fact that treatment for dissociative trauma survivors moves through developmental phases mirrors the fundamental reality of childhood trauma survivors.

Grand (2000) cautions against naïve optimism and the therapist's subtle betrayal of the patient through unrealistic reparation fantasies. Viewing recovery as a linear or "progressive movement from the nonlinguistic to the linguistic, from fragmentation to cohesion, and from solitude to mutuality is to suffer from an excess of hope. Such hope imagines that the traumatized self can finally locate the other who should have been there, and in that meeting, death itself will be defeated" (p. 37). Psychotherapy may be a powerful vehicle for the reestablishment of developmental processes and personality transformation, yet, as Grand poignantly expresses, psychotherapy is "not larger than death, and it is not larger than the solitude of survival" (p. 37).

COMMON STAGES[7] AND PASSAGES IN TREATMENT

In an effective treatment, the patient's initial reliance on the therapist as bridge between self-states and container of affects, tensions, and history is gradually replaced by the patient's developing observing ego, capacity to codirect the healing process, and abilities to activate aggression in the service of self-protection and tolerate complexity and ambiguity. These accomplishments do not signify that the patient has attained conscious control over all dissociative processes. They do mean, however, that reactions that were previously automatic become optional and volitional and can be reflected upon: the driving motivational system initially fueled by pain avoidance, aggression against the self, and attachment to perpetrators is now propelled by self-respect and a healthy sense of entitlement. One patient aptly described this middle stage of therapy as the point when everything "seems to be coming together and falling apart at the same time."

The first treatment goal in therapy with a severely traumatized patient after establishing an initial working alliance (trust, safety, informed consent) and stabilizing his/her hyperarousal and numbing symptomatology to maintain functionality is recognizing the dissociative disorder, which may be buried beneath years of unsuccessful (or partially successful) treatment. This diagnostic mandate is best realized when the therapist engages the patient in shared inquiry and observation of recurrent patterns of relatedness, omissions, and absences; it need not happen in a dogmatic, formulaic way.

Because addictions seem to be the glue that holds dissociation in place, the patient's relinquishing of compulsive patterns is often a prerequisite to the discovery of dissociative ones. Most severely dissociative patients do not openly present their dissociative symptoms until they recover from their addictive behaviors or relationships—to, for example, self-mutilation, food, work, sex, drugs, alcohol, shopping, computer games, abusive others, and so on. Detailed explorations of their subjective experience of addictive behavior often reveals the alterations in consciousness, trance logic, internal dialogues, and power struggles that typify extreme dissociative disorders.

For example, one patient whose initial complaint was compulsive sexual promiscuity reported the behavior without feeling and in general, stereotypical ways that obscured the subtle shifts and state-changes it involved. When he was asked to identify the moment-by-moment experiences of moving from not feeling sexually aroused to having sexual thoughts to struggling with impulses to act out to playing out the mental arguments to inducing a kind of trance to finding himself in dangerous sexual scenes that he didn't remember getting into, the dissociative process that underlay the whole sequence began to be revealed. Later on in therapy, after he started to recall traumatic moments in his past and could resist the initial momentum and not act out sexually, the remembering, and the revealing instead of sequestering, disrupted the fixity of his traumatic reenactment patterns. This process of bypassing addictive cycles is the beginning of the dissolution of some of the more rigid dissociative defenses.

When the patient/therapist dyad addresses the anxiety that inevitably floods the patient's personality system without resorting to either dissociation or rescue, a deeper and more emotionally accessible relatedness to self and others can arise from the experience of tolerating the affect. If trust breaks down, or if patient or therapist (or both) sidestep the temporary disorganization, the infusion of anxiety may remobilize the original dissociative defenses. But when addiction patterns are contained and well analyzed and the severely dissociative patient can consistently appreciate the phenomenology of his/her own dissociation, s/he can finally engage in a continuous mutual reflection process without interruption by every new wave of posttraumatic affect, without avoidance due to another crisis, and without distraction by relapses of addictive behavior.

The revelation and recognition of the structures of dissociation is anything but a smooth or continuous process. Not surprisingly, the most difficult dissociation-supporting addictions to detect and change are the ones reinforced in the "normal" social world (like workaholism and perfectionism, both particularly common in higher-functioning DID patients). While the process of recognition varies from patient to patient there is always a bargaining for the trauma and dissociation to be less serious than it is, and few patients move into awareness of their dissociative processes without a good fight (and sometimes flight). This "fight" has often been misconstrued by critics as reaction to the foisting of an inappropriate diagnosis onto the patient. But what is really going on in most instances is that once the patient's dissociative organization (including cloaking devices, distractions, and cover stories) is exposed, his/her defensive and camouflage functions flip into overdrive; they deny or minimize the revealed multiplicity to prevent retraumatization even when one or more alter personalities are simultaneously appreciating the therapist's recognition and breathing perhaps the first sigh of relief in a lifetime.

One patient experienced this biphasia in concrete and paradoxical ways: a level of deep relief alleviated a chronic suicidality in one aspect of his psyche, while threats and images of knives (suggesting that he cut himself) emanated from another aspect of his psyche. After first denying that these fleeting images of knives and impulses to cut had ever surfaced before, he remembered that they had, once, many years ago, the only other time he had been in psychotherapy and had tried to talk about the possibility of sexual-abuse trauma. For this man, like so many severely dissociative patients—especially those with histories of organized child abuse—recognition of the dissociative process is a terribly mixed blessing. Following provisional acknowledgment of dissociative disorders, patients can go back and forth a hundred times in accepting and denying the evidence of systematized dissociation. Often it is only late in treatment that they begin to fully grasp the overwhelming role that dissociation has played in their lives.

The unfolding of pathological multiplicity in treatment requires a willingness on the part of the therapist to empathically enter the patient's fragmented subjective world and to notice and inquire about the patient's shifts in consciousness, omissions, and inconsistencies in behavior or memory or self-representation. For clinicians wary of managerial methods, empathic inquiry and resonance, participation in enactments, confrontation from within the transference/countertransference matrix, and mirroring processes may be powerful enough to work through dissociative defenses without resorting to hypnosis or behavioral or cognitive treatment techniques, especially with higher-functioning patients. Regardless, the recognition of dissociation and pathological multiplicity—like other aspects of working in "potential space"—requires ongoing humility and negotiation to bridge reality, illusions, and disparate self-states because our "knowing" is always approximate and selective.

The diagnosis and treatment of severe dissociative disorders need not become a process of domination and concretization. It can take place dialectically and dialogically. Accordingly, a therapist should not represent his/her interpretation as correct, complete, or definitive. Rather, s/he should offer different options for the patient's consideration and reflection to represent or register some aspects of his/her self-experience. Negotiating the potential diagnosis has more to do with finding new ways of symbolizing and accessing the self than with reifying the self and its experiences.

Following the shared recognition of chronic dissociation between therapist and patient, there is often a dramatic shift in the patient's relationship with him or herself and a changing mixture of relief and terror and of denial and acceptance of the diagnosis. The patient gradually begins to deconstruct an old, and reconstruct a new, identity based on new information from his/her internal world as well as from reflecting on (and, at times, arguing against) the therapist's perspectives. This is the point in treatment when more systematized forms of denial and disavowal deployed by the patients to sustain their dissociative system can be articulated, and when patients begin to show some increasing ability to tolerate anxiety and depressive affect states. Now discussion of traumatic memories can move from focusing on the dynamics of shock, avoidance, doubt, and the quest for validation to developing the psychological functions requisite to disengagement from deeply entrenched sadomasochistic paradigms and advancement beyond helplessness. Severely dissociative trauma survivors switch back and forth between taking on the new challenges and remobilizing dissociative defenses—so progress, too, is nonlinear.

Motivated by reminders of the past trauma to avoid annihilation experiences, hostile protector-parts of the survivor emerge out of the unconscious—sometimes like a flash flood—to seize control of the patient's consciousness and of the therapy at many points along the way. The quality of the therapist's ongoing negotiations (occasionally wrestling matches) with these personified rebel and demon figures is, in large measure, what creates the trust that allows the trauma patient to move past isolationist and survivalist strategies of coping toward authentic engagement and true mutuality. Some patients remain in this coming-to-terms with multiplicity phase for an extended period, often regressing into addictive behavior, and not all have the necessary ego resources to enter the next phase. Some severely dissociative patients may be able to tolerate only long-term supportive therapy focused on managing life crises and preventing posttraumatic decompensation. (And many may not ever have the requisite skills or resources to pursue or complete psychic restructuring.) In any case, the defenses of survivors of extreme trauma should be assessed before proceeding with uncovering/memory work and processing of trauma (McCann and Pearlman, 1990). That destabilizing but ultimately integrative work—accessing memory and fantasy material located within or among alter personalities—also includes building relations between previously disconnected and reciprocally disavowing aspects of the self.

During intensive memory recovery and abreactive work, it is essential that the therapist provide sufficient contact, relational continuity, and support to sustain the patient's functionality and demonstrate that regression is an inevitable part of progress. This means working especially hard to keep patients out of the hospital, in their jobs or school, out of disability and welfare programs, and away from the seductions of short-term solutions that may provide immediate stagnant gratification but militate against restoring the dialectic between progression and regression in the patient's life. For example, because many severely dissociative patients have chronic unmet dependency needs, their yearnings for direct reparenting at critical junctures in the treatment, if enacted, could eclipse the essential balance between breaking down and building up that is the basis of most depth therapy.

ABREACTION

Integrating the developmental needs represented by the elements of denial and intrusion that alternate in severe posttraumatic stress dissociative syndromes is a balancing act. The therapist must at once avoid discouraging disclosure, consciously or unconsciously, and reinforcing the trauma by clinically inappropriate pacing that causes emotional flooding in the patient (Courtois, 1992; Chu, 1992b); compulsive, unexamined reenactments and malignant abreactions repeat the sadomasochistic dynamics of the original trauma.

Abreaction usually refers to the experiencing of intense feelings when recalling a disturbing past event in response to some trigger. According to Ross (1997), however, abreaction exists on a spectrum with purely informational recall of trauma on one end, and full-tilt abreaction with behavioral reenactments and dramatic behaviors on the other end. Abreaction connotes discharge but—in contrast to the overlapping construct of enactment, which begins unconsciously—abreaction most often implies a consciously and/or volitionally mediated reexperiencing.[8] And it is best when facilitated; during abreactions, one person guides another through what, in enactments, the two of them become temporarily lost in reliving. Both have their place in effective treatment; in fact, depending on the efficacy of the therapuetic process, enactment and its analysis may lead to either spontaneous, or well-guided and appropriately paced, abreaction. Both may be conceptualized as the only means by which traumatized patients' unconscious strivings to be known can become manifest and articulated. Both are ways for old and new object experience to be brought into consciousness and ultimately into dialogue.

During abreaction, a patient may experience a cathartic moment or a peak of painful emotions, somatic and/or psychological, which can represent elements of the original dissociated childhood traumatic events or elements of any trauma from any age (Sachs and Peterson, 1996). It is important to affirm that the facilitating of abreactions does not per se cause patients to become dysfunctional or to remain in regressed states;[9] indeed, abreactions are not regressions at all, but regression-*like* and transient (Sachs and Peterson, 1996). However, noting the potential for mismanaged or unmodulated abreactions—especially full-tilt abreactions with behavioral reenactments and dramatic behaviors—to lead to malignant and lasting regressions, Ross (1997) emphatically states that those are fundamentally retraumatizing to patients, and not at all essential for healing. Stressing the importance of the therapist and patient's modulating and controlling the reexperiencing of traumatic material, and reminding clinicians that emotional discharge is not in itself a therapeutic intervention, Van der Hart and Steele (2000) also emphasize that without integrative mentation abreactions may be destructive and disrupt the patient's healing.

While abreaction is a central feature of all stages of psychotherapy of severe dissociative disorders, its form and frequency change as the patient's degree of reliance on dissociative defenses shifts. Abreactive material seldom reveals a chronological map of the patient's childhood traumas (Barach and Comstock, 1996); in fact, it can relate simultaneously to the patient's traumatic past, the patient's experience of the therapeutic and extratherapeutic present, and the patient's fantasies. Early in treatment there is a greater likelihood that spontaneous and potentially destructive abreactions will take place, because the therapy relationship harbors unknown psychic landmines and because surfacing memories (be they fragments, somatic sensations, and/or nightmares) are apt to trigger transitory shock or psychic overload.

Some patients experience the therapist as torturing them from the minute they come into treatment (Marmer, 1996). For survivors of childhood torture and organized sadistic abuse, this is understandable. The rearrangement of a piece of office furniture, a change in the therapist's appearance, an illness or vacation, even a neutral expression, can sometimes set off uncontrollable reactions in a severely traumatized patient. Because the stories of survivors of organized perpetrator groups reveal that their abusers imbued everyday situations with posttraumatic triggering valences that kept the victims spinning endlessly in unconscious reenactments and flashbacks[10] and prevented them from escaping or exposing the perpetrating system, the therapist may be faced with a situation where no stimulus is a neutral one.

Revisiting the affective, sensory, and cognitive experience of traumatic events cannot be bypassed if the treatment goal is to restructure the traumatized psyche. But abreactive work is difficult because it causes somatic pain, behavioral reenactments, and hallucinations analogous to the original traumatic experience (Ross, 1989), or amalgamations of traumatic experience and fantasized elaborations. There are moments when the patient literally must leave the relational field to retrieve fragments of experience—and there are also aspects of traumatic memories that can only be retrieved through mutual examination of and reflection upon the enactments taking place between patient and therapist. Although abreaction and the integration process do not always involve significant loss of control, some relational disruption is usually inevitable when highly dissociated material appears on the horizon of consciousness—especially for the first time. That disruption itself, however, can be used as a key to enter a deeper level of association to new material, or as a rehearsal for the next abreaction of a newly accessed memory fragment.

To be effective, abreactions must occur within a trusting, well-boundaried therapy relationship (Steele, 1989).[11] From a relational perspective, the patient is not simply benefiting from affect discharge, cognitive interpretation, or integration of dissociative events, or merely internalizing a new object experience (the therapist) who relates differently from abusers. The patient is developing new self or ego capacities by virtue of internalizing healthy (i.e., respectful, nondominating, and nonauthoritarian) interactional processes (Leowald, 1960).

Abreaction helps the patient move unarticulated, unformulated, and unwitnessed experience into the potentially transformative space of the therapy relationship. Whether the decontextualized fragments of personal history being reexperienced are memories of receiving electric shocks or feelings of having been betrayed or lied to, the process allows the patient to acknowledge viscerally that the trauma occurred (as opposed to dissociating it), and to relegate it to the past (instead of continuously reliving and reenacting it) so that the trauma takes on symbolic rather than predominantly sensorimotor or behavioral properties (Van der Hart, Steele, Boon, and Brown, 1993). Clinical experience confirms that the patient can now attempt new techniques—restorative fantasy, for example[12]—to master it. What might actually have happened in the trauma, what one wished had happened, and what one was told happened or didn't happen will emerge simultaneously and/or intermittently during successful abreactions and later in free associations.

Many survivors of severe child-abuse trauma will eventually be able to recall or want to reveal fragments of their abuse history that will be excruciatingly difficult for the therapist to witness and tolerate without barging into the patient's narrative offering empathy or interpretations, or withdrawing, or becoming incredulous, before the patient has adequately felt and represented the experience. Yet, allowing the disturbing abreaction to go on too long may make the patient feel too much like s/he is replicating the original trauma. Finding the proper balance between commenting, containing, and silently witnessing is one of the most difficult challenges of doing therapy—and abreactive work in particular—with survivors of severe trauma.

Listening to a person's memories of sadistic traumas can revolt or paralyze the therapist (or stir him/her to tears) as much as it can the patient, and sometimes the only appropriate response is the natural one—shock—or silence, followed by an emphatic protest on behalf of the patient (who may be quite unable to think or feel this on his/her own). Though it is fashionable nowadays in light of the false memory movement and the recent aggressive critiques of psychotherapy to champion the value of therapeutic objectivity and the skepticism about the accuracy of patients' memories, it is not always easy or even ethical to remain emotionally indifferent. Indifference may also be clinically ineffective: it is possible that not responding empathically to material the patient is experiencing as real may do more damage than good—although such authors as Barach and Comstock (1996) believe that a neutral therapeutic stance can give the patient room to explore anxieties as he/she works to create a cohesiveness of his/her own history. The desirability and utility—and possibility—of clinical neutrality is an issue that divides the clinical professions, especially those of us who lean in the direction of believing in the authority and validity of many of our patients' reported experiences from those of us who are mindful of the limitations of memory or fearful of reinforcing so-called false memories.

Many DID patients locked into the trance logic of traumatic thinking or hypnotized by the messages their perpetrators gave them can only begin to disrupt the fixity of these frozen states and register another emotional reaction by sensing the therapist's response. With some patients, of course, any comments, empathic or otherwise, on the part of the therapist can interfere with the patient's spontaneous reflections or the emergence of traumatic memory and affects.

ELENA

Elena, a female DID patient in her early forties in the late middle phase of treatment and who has already recovered a large amount of traumatic memory remembers an abusive incident in her childhood when a group of men after raping her, forced her to crawl around the floor naked and act like a dog while they laughed at her and called her a fat, ugly worthless dog whose only value was to lick their shoes.

It was only after experiencing the impact this narrative had on me that Elena, who was almost frozen in the belief that what the perpetrators had said was the absolute truth, could arrive at her own discovery of degradation and humiliation, and only after she acknowledged her heartbreaking feelings that she and I were able to speculate on the probable intentions of her abusers. Shifting her focus from her extreme and paralyzing shame to the intentions of her abusers—and recontextualizing the episode with what came before and after it, including how they engineered her "forgetting" it, and so on—ultimately revealed Elena's lifelong pattern of feeling degraded and behaving in a subjugated way in all her relationships. Using accrued information to point out to the patient that her perpetrators were probably training her for future abuse as well as using her for momentary sexual gratification helped to contextualize the incident in terms of the particular sex-ring in which Elena was held captive. Among other things, the memory work freed up some aggression necessary for Elena to become (for the first time) thoroughly angry at the perpetrators.

Victims of prolonged and repeated traumas may need to reevaluate virtually every assumption underlying their thinking habits in order to continue to process new memory material and in order to disengage from the social trance and derealization processes that have held them hostage intrapsychically. When the patient's entire assumptive world begins to change, then his/her dissociative self-system is likely to be radically altered in many internal locations at once; that may feel to the patient like a loss of moorings, even if the new meanings contain the possibility of redemption, benevolence, and solidarity.

Following some catharsis—dramatic or otherwise—and the reactivation of observing-ego functions, dissociative experience can shift into a permeable relational mode where self-generated and flexible applications of meanings and new identifications replace traumatically induced cognitive fixity. In this phase, all of the messages, beliefs, and cognitive distortions internalized from (or implanted by) the perpetrator(s) must be reviewed and systematically deconstructed. Traditional trauma theorists like Van der Hart et al. (1993) and others (Ross, 1989; Fine, 1996) call this aspect or phase of treatment cognitive restructuring and the correction of cognitive distortions. Both existential issues and the psychological roles of different alters within the patient's personality system can be illuminated so that the patient develops a greater breadth of understanding for his/her own survival strategies, and a greater appreciation for the more extreme alter personalities that have been rejected or marginalized because of the difficulty of their mandates in the traumatic environment.

In a relational psychoanalytic approach—which is not necessarily incompatible with the cognitive approach despite certain stylistic and philosophical differences—this integration of abreactive experience comes about in part by the therapist's creating an environment where enactments are understood to be inevitable. Transformative elements in this tradition are an emphasis on the patient's experience of his or her impact on the therapist, the therapist's observation/participation, and the cocreation of the traumatic dynamics and conarration of the meaning-making process. According to Bromberg (1993), the model of the therapist knowing the patient through direct experience can lead to the patient's creative and imaginative use of his or her own (previously split-off, or rigidly held) experience and ultimately to the pleasurable, consensual construction of a more inclusive reality; that, in turn, allows for narrative meaning-making not previously available within the patient's closed dissociative system.

> Elena's initial memory of the humiliating incident was triggered by her strange resistance when I offered to be flexible about her appointment time in order to accommodate her upcoming surgery. Her rebuffing of what I felt to be generosity and her chronic inability to accept anything good from me stirred my frustration and anger: I felt disregarded and blocked from offering protection and assistance. Our wondering about this dynamic between us seemed to shake something loose in her psyche. As she associated to profound and unalterable worthlessness and disgust with herself, another in a series of complex and bizarre memories emerged about her involvement in a highly sadistic multiple perpetrator group, encompassing training for prostitution and participation in sadistic acts against others.

It is often the case that the patient's experience of his/her impact on the therapist and/or the therapist's self-disclosure during both the revelation/remembering and reenactment phases may make way for insight and reparative relationship experiences that fundamentally disrupt the fixity of posttraumatic patterns.

To manage abreactions and reenactments cooperatively is for the patient as well as the therapist a direct experience of mutuality. As Ghent (1990, p. 108) points out, the act of "surrender" in the presence of a facilitating, trustworthy other is itself healing. Such an experience stands in stark contrast to both the patient's masochistic submission in the original trauma and to unconscious reenactments that may be contained and managed by the therapist but never felt or worked with directly. In surrender, the patient experiences the wish to be found and recognized, to move beyond false self-constructions, and to become authentic and emotionally present.

Cooperative abreaction is also an example of paradox in relational therapy. The dread and annihilation anxieties that accompany abreaction can be reexperienced and reintegrated in a firm holding environment where restitution reliably follows disruption (Kohut, 1971); the restructuring process liberates hope and attachment strivings frozen by chronic despair, shame, and rage. In addition, effective abreaction may clarify relational configurations and subjective organizing principles of childhood, fostering development of the capacity for continuity, narrativity, and historicity, revitalizing the dissociative survivor's relationship with his/her self. Finally, the experience of having one's testimony witnessed and accepted is a fundamentally healing experience especially for survivors of extreme childhood torture and victims of organized abuse groups who were convinced that they would never be believed by outsiders and were terrorized into silence about their perpetrators' secrets. The willingness of the therapist to listen empathically to the patient, and the survival of the therapist and the patient following these revelations, releases a burden of terror the patient has been carrying (usually for decades) and this mutual survival almost always allows opportunities for other traumatic material to surface.

From Fragmented Objects to Multiple Subjectivities

Once the preponderance of reenactments in early treatment has subsided and explorations of the patient's past are conducted in a more mutually orchestrated way, the next transition involves encouraging a shift from obsessive concern with controlling defenses to relating to and being curious about the internal world. This transition parallels what relational theorists (Benjamin, 1988; Ghent, 1992b; Winnicott, 1969) call the developmental shift from object relating, a relatively primitive mode of human connection based on projection, identification, and limited intersubjectivity, to object use, where the external other—and, in the case of severely dissociative patients, aspects of the self—can be encountered and used for growth and expansion. For the therapist to become fully useful, s/he must become "real in the sense of being part of shared reality and not just a bundle of projections" (Winnicott, 1969, p. 712). S/he becomes real through the patient's testing the limits of his/her tolerance, patience, and availability, for example, through collisions between their worldviews, through the patient's experiencing his/her passionate commitment to the work and observing his/her struggle with difficult conflicts and painful emotions.

The therapist must initially function as a relational bridge over which different parts of the patient's self can come to learn of each others' existence, history, and functions once dissociation has been recognized. In this role, the therapist must attempt to acknowledge empathically all of the patient's conflicting developmental and defensive needs. During this period, in order to establish communication across the range of the patient's dissociative system, the therapist may often have to confront quite aggressively the domination of some alters by others or expose duplicitous manipulations aimed at obscuring minority intrapsychic positions. Sometimes conflicts over trust, control, and power have to be hammered out directly with different alters; at other times the therapist has to return such issues back to the patient's system, where struggling with conflicting feelings can replace reliance upon dissociation and reenactments of trauma.

There are situations when a patient's criticism of the therapist is not just an effort to protest, offer feedback, reenact sadism, and so on, but also a conscious effort to deflect the panoply of inner voices that would confirm the diagnosis of DID or threaten the attachment bond with a perpetrator. And there are situations when the therapist must become a player in the patient's internal world so that the patient will have an alternate perspective from which to observe his/her divergent attitudes, affects, and behaviors. If a hostile, intimidating alter is bullying the patient's child alters, for instance, the therapist may have to go beyond simply understanding its protective function or its reasons for being angry and abusive: s/he may actually have to debate and negotiate with the hostile alter in order to disrupt the pattern of reenactment of early traumas—a pattern that interferes with memory and affect integration and the development of healthy forms of self-protection.

As integration begins to evolve, and as the amnestic barriers between self-states begin to decrease, the patient becomes more and more able to manage continuity of consciousness, preparing for deeper transference work on core characterological patterns of self-hate, fear of dependency, identification with the aggressor, shame, and sadomasochistic dynamics. Of these, dependency conflicts seem to be among the most difficult for severely dissociative patients to reconcile. They often move back and forth among sexualization of attachment, adamant and defensive claims of autonomy, and forms of entitled ownership of the therapist, or between clinging, and crisis-generating behavior—all of which mask the patient's fundamental vulnerability and uncontrolled dependency needs (*I hate myself for needing you and I hate you for being the one I need; I've always been able to do it on my own and now I know I can't—being with you reminds me that I can't and I hate that*).

The Observing Ego and Inclusivity

Beyond stabilization, one of the most important goals in treating trauma-induced dissociation is helping the patient develop sufficient observing-ego functions, including the capacity to tolerate conflicting affects and identities as well as the disturbing meanings embedded in traumatic memories. At the outset this process overwhelms and repeatedly retraumatizes the fragile self held together and managed by dissociative devices, because development of observing ego functions in severely dissociative patients cannot avoid encountering the multiplicities that classical psychoanalytic theory, hypothesizing a unitary base of personality functioning, essentially bypasses. Where psychic life is predominantly organized by dissociation, observing ego entails reflection by one aspect of the self on other, formerly dissociated alters or parts (Bromberg, 1996b). Accepting the existence of loathsome, offensive, pitiful, or worthless part-selves is a preliminary phase in the development of observing ego capacities; cultivated during psychotherapy, they become capable of making links between personal pain and trauma, self-organization, and the power arrangements within the family and dominant society.

In Altman's (1995) wide-angle model of self-observation, a socially embedded self develops expanded observing ego capacity, such that therapy can concern itself with the invisible and unconscious ways in which traumatic patterns of domination and oppression have been built into the life and psyche of the patient. The wide-angle model stands in contrast to the automatic-shutdown, self-soothing behavior that typically follows hyper-arousal once traumatic material has entered consciousness (Van der Kolk, 1987).

A Posture of Inclusion

The effective therapist encourages differentiation and integration processes to foster synthesis of object- and self-experiences that contain positive and negative affective tones. Dichotomous perceptions/representations can then be joined into a single central consciousness as opposite experiences are shifted from polarized trance states into spontaneous dialogue. Dialogue with some part-selves may be characterized by hate, terror, and intimidation at first, but it may be the only place to start. The goal is to keep the dialogue moving and prevent its collapse into a reenactment of silencing, polarization, or violation. The therapist has to support the struggle among aspects of the self so they do not fold into reconfirming original beliefs/positions in the internal world, and/or reinstating dissociative defenses. That support helps the severely traumatized patient to shift from dissociation to building the capacity to sustain the tensions inherent in intrapsychic conflict (Bromberg, 1993), which requires confrontation with not only dissociative habits but also fears about surrendering them. Such fears may emerge in concretized form as the constant anticipation of danger from the therapist or as the clamor of different alters for time with the therapist, unaware that each part benefits from the time spent with any other part. Or, the fears may be expressed more subtly, as workaholism, missed sessions, chronic attempts to distract the therapist or steer the dialogue toward superficiality, confusion of internal and external cues, or other dissociation-reinforcing behavior. The patient misinterprets his/her burgeoning anxiety as heralding revictimization. When the therapist can persuade the patient to allow the old way of life to fall apart to make way for a new one, and to tolerate the transitional anxiety, the process of integration can begin.

Healthy development involves equal opportunity for all facets of a personality to be recognized and to evolve. Unless the therapist can embody a posture of inclusiveness, s/he will replicate the central cognitive-relational errors of multiple personality disorder itself—exclusion, overgeneralization, domination, polarization, and sacrifice. The approach to the psyche that respects the balance of unity and multiplicity in psychological life celebrates intrapsychic diversity and the tensions between the literal and the metaphorical. In contrast to some of the other psychoanalytic paradigms proposed for severe dissociative disorders where conflicts are worked through and progress is expected to unfold in a linear fashion, relational models emphasize not the elimination of tensions, conflicts, and internal diversity, but the increasing ability to function comfortably and creatively in the context of tension, and, in some cases, to leave things unresolved.

Therapeutic pluralism (Kluft, 1988a), embodying the vision of paradoxical awareness, respects diversity and approaches the reconciliation of internal differences and intrapsychic opposites without losing sight of the validity of each element and without imposing false synthesis. Treatment addresses not individual psychic elements and states but the relationships among elements, and the relations between relations. Such a counterhierarchical and necessarily dialogical posture particularly suits disorders of pathological dividedness and victims of interpersonal violence, because—even though their need for alters and radical dissociation may be significantly diminished through therapy—the complexity of their internal experience dictates a continual collision of needs, desires, and beliefs. Therapists can help patients care about, and also confront and set limits on, all parts of the self, and cooperate internally instead of complying externally and reenacting self-destructively.

The negotiation of a cohesive sense of identity can only take place when there is creative participation of all of the patient's selves as well as participation of the therapist in the entirety of the patient's dissociative self-system (Bromberg, 1993; 1994). Multiple self-states must be listened to and negotiated with (Bromberg, 1993; 1994; Pizer, 1992; 1996; Schwartz, 1994) and brought into relationship with one another and the patient's here-and-now reality (Putnam, 1989; Ross, 1989) through the therapist's inclusive, dialogical connection with all the permutations of the traumatized self's organization, and through the therapist's awareness of traumatic reenactment dynamics and his/her own shifting self-states and countertransference (Davies and Frawley, 1994; Bromberg, 1993, 1994). Most experts in the treatment of multiple personality disorder (Putnam, 1989; Ross, 1989; Kluft, 1987a; 1995; Chu, 1998), and trauma (Herman, 1992; Briere, 1992b; Courtois, 1992; van der Kolk, McFarlane, and Weisaeith, 1996) advocate for the same underlying philosophical approach, variations in clinical methodology and ideological stance notwithstanding.

It is essential to treat each emerging alter personality or self-state with curiosity and respect, in an ambience where each can find its central theme and voice and can enter into a conscious, observing, and felt relationship to the others without being prematurely forced into merging with the whole because the clinician needs an integrated presentation. Neither incredulity nor fascination is appropriate; neither neglect nor reinforcement of delusions of separateness will work. There is evolving consensus across clinical subspecialties to the effect that recognition and direct, inclusive contact with dissociative self-states (including the affects, meanings, memories, fantasies, and identifications they represent), is fundamental, along with symptom stabilization and creation of an environment of safety.

The main problem with dissociation is that it fuels forms of psychic terrorism and sabotage; neglected and disowned aspects of personality, in an effort to seek recognition, tend to find abnormal, usually destructive ways of expressing themselves. Pluralist developmental perspectives welcome both unity and multiplicity in psychic life and weight them equally; unfortunately, many treatments of dissociative conditions fail because of the inability of patient and/or therapist to maintain the tension between those opposite poles. Simultaneous alliances must be forged with the patient as a whole and with his/her individual alters or less personified self-states.

Therapeutic inclusivity entails receptivity to surprises in the intersubjective dialogue, and a corresponding willingness not to silence or disavow any of the patient's voices. Arousing a new capacity for self-reflection in the patient, with or without anxiety, is important because severely traumatized, dissociative individuals have survived by avoiding introspection, focusing on externality, and exercising hypervigilance (Briere, 1992b). Some therapists are unable, too fearful, or philosophically unwilling to contact or refer to alter personalities. Others, hypnotized by the phenomenology of the disorder, become so engrossed in interacting with part-selves that they lose track of the whole-person construct (Chu, 1988; Greaves, 1988; Ross, 1989).

Unreflective treatments can collude with the patient's defensive efforts either to block access to split-off parts or to encourage a kind of elaboration of part-selves that cements the delusion of separateness or produces secondary gains. Overemphasis on unity as a result of the therapist's existential or theoretical agenda may be experienced by the patient as yet another way the person with power wants to control him/her. Relational and trauma theorists alike endorse working back and forth simultaneously between the individual as a whole, his/her parts, and the relationships among them, with the therapist in a transitional space where reality and fantasy do not always have to be immediately discriminated.

The therapist's sustained interest in the whole person, including recognition of all the separate and coconscious dissociated elements, contrasts favorably with the divide-and-conquer manipulations of the perpetrator and has a cumulative countervailing impact on the patient's internal bondage and entrapment in silence. (This impact can be especially powerful when the therapist is willing to look for and speak empathically to the invisible victim and villains in the patient's world.) The therapist's soothing and containing presence and the disarming effects of a consistently nondominating style help metabolize the tremendous anxiety released when the patient's dissociative barriers begin to come down. Often, corfronting the patient's cognitive distortions empathically (Chu, 1992a), or challenging them with play, metaphor, and humor communicates the important message that the whole person is greater than the sum of his or her parts. The development of respect, rapport, and mutuality with each aspect of the patient's dissociated experience and identity, however, is an organic part of the integrative process.

PAUL

Paul brought a macho, military-identified alter in the picture after several years of therapy. Disowned or ignored until then, the Vet was linked as some kind of witness/protector to the severe traumatic memories that were sealed off in the "fog" Paul was on the verge of penetrating. He so threatened Paul's compliant, adaptive part-selves, however, that we devoted several weeks expressly to negotiating the development of cooperation, empathy, and loyalty between him and them.

Constructing that internal bridge meant first convincing the others to allow the Vet to speak at all, helping them tolerate the intrapsychic tension arising from his dystonically rude questioning of my competence and authority, and confronting the entrenched beliefs of all the part-selves about the unreality, dangerousness, or uselessness of all the rest.

It next meant establishing trust between the Vet and me. Our first bonds were rooted in my working respectfully with his anger, distrust, and defensive autonomy—by both honoring his positions within the system and challenging some of his more extreme beliefs, prejudices, and trance logic.

Toward fostering the internal alliance, I suggested that the Vet treat the other alters as comrades in the trenches rather than as useless, weak, and shallow young men, and that he ask their assistance in his quest to secure time in therapy and begin to face whatever was contained in the fog. The Vet deflected my suggestion but proposed one of his own: he was willing to consider the others as younger brothers whom he had not seen in a long time, and who had not been exposed to military training and were therefore vulnerable and needing his protection and guidance. From that perspective only he was initially willing to communicate directly with the other parts about his needs.

By considering my input but coming up with his own metaphors and setting his own limits, the Vet was beginning to finesse his emerging dependency needs while sustaining defensive autonomy. He soon began, however, to experience anxiety and share his fears of incompetence and cowardice associated with facing the terrors contained in the "fog." We spent considerable time redefining the terms weakness and strength to ensure that the feeling of vulnerability would not by itself propel the Vet out of the relational field to redissociate (or be redissociated by the others).

Eventually, he was able to move back and forth between grateful relief that I would be accompanying him on his forays into the "fog" and fears that depending on me meant that he was not as strong as he had previously believed. In order to move forward the Vet had to tolerate being vulnerable to my betraying and abandoning him, and being annihilated by the unprocessed traumatic material in the "fog." He also fluctuated between welcoming this new model of masculinity and fearing the loss of control implied by its internalization.

Not surprisingly, Paul's high-functioning, adaptive alter personalities responded with alarm when they recognized that the Vet was developing depth, complexity, and texture in the course of the therapy dialogues and becoming a personality to reckon with. The Vet's transformation and integration would make his long-avoided and excruciatingly painful traumatic memories inescapable by the others.

Following this acknowledgment, the Vet was able to recognize that he had distanced himself from the collective history of intrafamilial multiple perpetrator abuse—isolating the other part-selves' stories and memories as "pulp fiction." The Vet was responsible for more complex extrafamilial torture and organized child abuse, and by attempting to separate the two, Paul's system had perfected dissociative strategies that facilitated functionality, self-protection, and complex amnesia all around.

With the recognition of the history of negation on both sides, some of the affective and empathic walls that sustained Paul's pathological multiplicity came tumbling down. In the wake of this preliminary communion, some of Paul's deepest grieving for his lost innocence took place. Ultimately, all aspects of Paul came to confront not only their delusions of separateness, but the ways in which one set of part-selves perpetuated the others' fantasies of omnipotence. Integration was well underway when all were able to (simultaneously) reflect on their own (and the others') strengths and vulnerabilities, competencies and limitations, integrity and arrogance.

Paul's midtreatment movement toward integration was marked by a particular revelation by the functional adaptive alters (who had previously given many hours to denying and debating their multiplicity and the veracity of the memories that had emerged from other alters to that point). Paul reported that for the first time these parts of himself that had always imagined they were Paul had recognized—following more waves of deep sadness and grief—that they were only parts in a complex person and not the whole story.

EXPANDING THE CONCEPT OF SELF-HELPERS

From a relational perspective, alter personalities are regarded as self-helpers created to resist or rescue at least parts of the individual from the shattering experience of trauma. Though varying in function, responsibility, history, and maturational level, every alter must be considered of equal value— there are no "good" and "bad" personalities even if both patient and therapist are tempted to so label them. An abused child organizes his or her internal world for at least partial psychological survival by focusing on separation, idealizing, and merger fantasies to ward off disintegration anxieties (Kohut, 1977). Elaborated dissociative states like alter personalities can bind anxiety and chronic narcissistic rage and redirect them into their own "faulty selves" instead of onto the predatory perpetrators and failing caretakers.

The despised, worthless little girl alter (who holds the abuse because she believes she "deserves it") encapsulates fear, pain, abandonment, and dread, and protects the rest of the system from these disruptive affect states, while the quivering but lovable, compliant girl alter with no memory for violation or betrayal (who imagines she can please the perpetrator and everyone else) sustains hope for nurturance and reparative relationships; together they make it possible for the functional adult, persona-restoring alters to evolve, and for prostitute alter(s) to develop—mutating the child's experience of helplessness into (both fantasied and real) power and mastery, by eroticizing needs for attention and affection, tolerating objectification of the body, and ultimately liberating her to work. Since all effective plantation systems need overseers, this constellation of alter personalities allows the development of a defensive protector (through partial identification with the aggressor's power and control) to keep them all in line, to keep disturbing affect at bay, and to ensure that the dissociative barriers remain in place (a double agent, of sorts). However, if there is increasing pressure from chronic torture and degradation, this already working combination will allow a demon (or two, or three) alter to develop who minimizes (real and imagined) pain to the whole personality by becoming completely callused (encapsulating intense shame and humiliation), turning hatred and rage (away from the perpetrator) onto the inner children's needs and vulnerability, denigrating (and setting-up for harm) the prostitutes who "asked for it and deserve whatever they get," and deflecting and isolating intense physical and emotional pain from sadistic abuse through extreme identification with the perpetrator's omnipotence, contempt, and lack of guilt. All these splits and personifications allow the child-victim's body to do what s/he is told by her perpetrator and prevents the perpetrator's retaliatory rages and punishments from being further unleashed on the child-victim.

This dissociative virtuosity (Herman, 1992), among many things, allows the child-victim to encapsulate (and to some extent, neutralize) the worst aspects of the perpetrator's malevolence; s/he can minimize the risk of perpetrating against others (when not coerced into doing so by the perpetrator) and thus retain (albeit, dissociatively) some of his/her original innocence, and most importantly, some of his/her dignity and integrity. Unfortunately, this type of psychological organization leaves the victim vulnerable to many forms of interpersonal betrayal and exploitation experiences in adulthood (including vulnerability to involvement with abusive partners, sociopaths, predators, pimps, etc.). Upon encountering such an elaborate, personified dissociative system, the therapist has to (eventually) find creative ways to remind the individual part-selves of their inherent interdependence. This news is not welcomed, understood, or accepted—at least not initially—least of all by those "in charge." With the persistent, sometimes playful repetition of the liberating and dangerous knowledge that mutual interdependence once saved "their" lives and that mutual empathy and recognition can now be integrative and healing, the impenetrable system of extremely personified dissociation can become (internally and interpersonally) porous.

The dissociative patient eventually continues to rediscover the interdependence among the part-selves on his/her own. For example, a gentle alter who managed to imagine wrapping him/herself up so as not to feel the full force of the violent penetrations of savage sexual assault comes to understand that the malevolent internal counterparts who "cooperated" with the perpetrators were thereby protecting other aspects of the self. Each has been misunderstood by the others, each sacrificed a great deal, and each still operates in a limited, self-reinforcing trance state until the point of contact and conflict with the therapist and the other parts of the dissociative self-system.

Severely dissociative individuals find it almost impossible to believe that their various fragments (including the most infantile, dependent, and sadistic) can be brought into wholeness or into accepting, honest relationships. Their functional personae (their Nancy Reagans, according to one patient, their Donna Reeds, according to another), desperate to pass for normal and craving the lifestyles promised on television and in magazines, can undermine treatment in the most socially sanctioned of ways; in males, for instance, they might be reactionary military types deferential to any higher authority and entirely lacking in empathy. Many therapists are, unfortunately, prone to reward such functional alters while overtly or subtly pathologizing or rejecting a patient's defensive, defiant, and regressive aspects. Cultural pressures to deny child abuse, valorize the capacity for "resilience," and sanction authoritarian child-rearing practices all contribute to alleviating the collective sense of guilt about crimes against children and to tempting clinicians to favor compliant personalities.

Some therapists elevate to the status of cotherapists the "internal self-helper" personalities (Adams, 1989, p. 138; Allison, 1980)—highly centering, unifying, and protective and also informed about the individual's life history and dynamics—completely ignoring their limitations. Like excessive play therapy with child alters and the banishment of self-destroyers, such reification of the internal self-helper phenomenon not only endorses hierarchy in the patient's system but also reinforces the cultural value of compliance over protest and actually constricts the notion of constructive service to the self. Allying too closely with any one aspect of self may intensify the dissociation, pseudomaturity, and defensive precocity generated by the original traumas. Accordingly, the therapist must balance validation of all part-selves with reminders of their limitations, fostering the patient's working through barriers to valuing all parts of his/her intrasubjective world.

A SIMULTANEOUS RELATIONSHIP WITH
THE WHOLE PERSON AND ALL OF ITS PARTS

An empathic relational field fostering establishment of basic trust with a therapist who apprehends the patient's struggle to know and to avoid knowing can begin to serve as a wedge between the old trauma-domination paradigms holding the survivor hostage—intrapsychically in the dissociative theater of the mind, and interpersonally in reenactments—and a new emergent self with hope for another way of life. The therapist's dilemma is to take into account contemporaneous, often hidden, and sometimes competing subjectivities residing in one individual (Sands, 1990).

An alter personality is the most highly coherent and personified form of a dissociative state. It usually coalesces around a particular affect, set of functions, and sense of self (body image, ideology, set of meanings) and exhibits only a limited repertoire of behavior, with access to only a limited number of (often state-dependent) memories (Putnam, 1989). Actually, alter personalities can be quite complex, clustered in groups and overlapping, so that what have been traditionally construed as alters may in some cases be subsystems of identities of the larger whole working in tandem.

Most organized and personified part-selves (and in some cases subsystems of the self) maintain their position and equilibrium in the internal world through what Kluft (1984) calls a narcissistic investment in a sense of separateness, which manifests as claims by one part-self or ego-state that it doesn't inhabit the patient's body, has different parents or relatives, or is not of the same race or gender. Ruptures in this delusion (or pseudo-delusion as Kluft refers to it) of separateness often produce overwhelming anxiety and will almost certainly be followed by desperate attempts—state-changes, attacks on the therapist, motor discharge, abruptly ending the session, threats, dissimulation, and so on—to reestablish the protective dissociative barriers that had effectively contained the overpowering affect states and the disturbing meanings they generate.

The advantage that this narcissistic investment in separateness holds for the patient is that it allows for significant development of functional achievements despite massive early traumatization. (One patient described the process as similar to the launching of the Space Shuttle, where one part of a rocket is jettisoned so that another, more important part can reach its destination.) The investment in separateness also shields the patient from access to authentic human relatedness, however, and from observing ego abilities and the shaping and transformative experiences produced by contact with internal states and helpful others. When perpetrators threaten child-victims about the consequences of revealing their abuse and tell them that what happened didn't really happen (it was a dream or it was imagined, the victims deserved or asked for it), they are counting on the children's submission and dissociative capacity to encapsulate sexual-abuse trauma and keep it away from healing or revealing experience.

All aspects of the patient's subjective experience must be invited into the therapy relationship—respecting, of course, the needs for safety, agency and autonomy, proper pacing, and sustained trust. (This is in contradistinction to the discriminatory directive strategies undertaken by practitioners who may feel out of control in the complex, volatile, and readily polarized relational field between themselves and dissociative trauma survivors: their efforts to "manage" such patients can precipitate combinations of defiant and submissive antics that form an ineluctably regressive spiral.) Dissociative experience—isolated, silenced, and well-camouflaged—continues to exert influence, but because it is often unmediated by thought or language, having been encoded in somatosensory or iconic levels of memory (Van der Kolk and Van der Hart, 1989), the results of its reactivation (via flashbacks, nightmares, body memories, behavioral enactments, etc.) are not easy to understand or integrate with other aspects of the patient's personality.[13]

Enhancing the dissociative patient's sense of subjective responsibility (especially to him/her self) and agency is crucial to any therapy. The helplessness clearly involved in the defense of dissociation should not be equated with automatic release from moral, ethical, and legal accountability when enactments cross criminal lines (viz., Braude, 1995, and Radden, 1996). Clinicians generally get better therapeutic results when they combine empathic sensitivity toward the subjective experience of helplessness with a firm expectation that the patient is fully responsible for his/her actions and decisions, incomplete control notwithstanding. The capacity to hold this paradox internally leads to more integrative behavior and enhanced observing ego capabilities.

Ultimately, the severely dissociative patient desires to repudiate different parts of the self (and to seduce the therapist into doing the same) for that is how psychological survival was ensured and how the pathological multiplicity evolved in the first place. In DID, alter personalities organized around functionality usually wish to destroy or suppress those that interfere with daily living, including traumatic-memory-holding child-parts. Similarly, defiant alters containing traumatic affects and virulent identifications with perpetrators (historically unwelcome except by the abusers in moments of privilege), may denigrate the compliant passivity of the functioning alters and attempt to do away with them in a variety of actual and fantasied enactments.

All alters fear destruction because they have been created, in some measure, to ward off and contain annihilation anxieties; many alters also fantasize that the therapist is out to destroy them. Some hostile alters, stuck in their original trance states and playing them out in the transference, begin to talk with the therapist about the worst aspects of the trauma including the phenomena associated with liking and willingly participating in the abuse; and, having learned from their sadistic perpetrators to use physical pain to distract themselves from painful emotional states and disturbing meanings, they may beg to be hurt or raped in order that their dissociative defenses can reorganize.

One such alter of a patient who has been involved in gruesome underworld child pornography, murder, and cult abuse pleaded to be hit and humiliated so that he could "flatten himself out and become two-dimensional once again." His request came when the level of emotional vulnerability became unbearable following his (the alter's) revelations of participation in organized sex-death rituals. Other alters surfaced during the next session, terrified that the perpetrator group somehow knew that their secrets were getting out; childlike, they pleaded for a promise of no physical harm to the patient and a pledge that he would never be returned to the perpetrator group.

Such incidents constitute the unconscious tests, reenactments, and double binds that challenge the progress of therapy; whether or not some of the events patients describe have actually happened is often beside the point. Double binds in particular must be articulated, as they usually contain themes of prior abuse. Unfortunately, therapists may easily fall into the polarizing trap of participating in acting out double binds, thereby replicating (instead of deconstructing) the psychological essence of the original trauma. In the name of psychotherapy, they may unconsciously repeat parental patterns of domination, neglect, complicity, and dissociation, failing to recognize the unconscious meaning of the tests and failing to offer new object experience to facilitate mastery of the original traumatic relationships. As already noted, the most useful new object experiences that can be internalized are those cocreated by the patient and therapist in an interactional process—that is, ones that are diametrically opposed to the traumatic relational paradigms of the survivor's childhood.

CONTINUITY AND CONSISTENCY

One of the greatest difficulties for dissociative patients is giving up unilateral control of treatment direction and allowing the therapist to moderate or disrupt their obsessive, authoritarian, self-denigrating forms of self-protective behavior. Pathological multiplicity has become a way of life for them, and they sometimes try to orchestrate the actions of several helping professionals at once; the result is a distinctly unhelpful mishmash of unintegrated relationships. Given the complexity of treating severely dissociative patients and the traumatic transference pressures, the multiple-therapists solution may be enticing on both sides—but inevitably, unless the clinicians involved are in constant dialogue, they and their patients will be plagued by outrageous splits, confused loyalties, and divergent perceptions of events. A single therapist for treating the problems of pathological multiplicity is almost always, therefore, preferable, and it is essential that s/he arrange and monitor referrals when adjunct services are necessary.

As each part of the dissociative individual must come to see itself in the other dissociated, disavowed aspects of the self, recognizing similarity where difference was once rigidly constellated, so the patient must eventually learn to tolerate differences in (and with) the therapist from whom sameness is often adamantly demanded as a means of controlling putative dangerousness. The therapist advocates for "federation," "distribution" in Pizer's (1996) terms, and "pluralism" in Samuels's (1989) terms, and consistently questions the exclusionary outcome of the polarizing, and domination impulses in his/her interpretations. This therapeutic posture slowly, pervasively, and persistently disrupts dissociation and leads to bridging processes that enable resolution, lack of resolution, and ambiguity to coexist.

INTEGRATION

Integration is the final stage of psychotherapy, but this notion of "stage" is somewhat too reified for what actually takes place in psychotherapy (or for that matter, in human development). Integration is both a process and an outcome. It is ongoing and cannot be precisely measured. It is never solely intrapsychic and cannot take place in isolation from the assignment of individual and collective responsibility in cultural context. Realistic goals for psychotherapy should reflect relative changes in intrapsychic, interpersonal, and life functioning, and should address the patient's capacity for negotiating power dynamics in current (and past) relationships.

> *I finally feel I have a right to exist. I used to get scared when I read the books that talked about integration for MPDs—I didn't want anyone doing me that way. Integration isn't like a cake mix recipe, it's more like a soup where everything naturally becomes a part of everything else but where there are still some pieces left that are familiar from what they were before. How can someone fuse someone else together? It happens only when and if it's ready and then it happens on its own, no one has to do anything to make it happen.*

—Lori (DID patient entering final phases of treatment)

Integration needs to respect the subjectivity of the patient and must be negotiated between each patient and therapist, not dictated by some abstract ideal of what post-dissociative or post-DID mental health looks like. Single-self models of integration (Barach and Comstock, 1996) are useful but may not apply in all cases.[14] In fact, most individuals who have developed complex forms of DID from early childhood will probably continue to use dissociation in some form or other to cope with life stressors even after an enormous amount of working through of the traumatic aspects of their early experience.

Micro-integrations, medial integrations, and macro-integrations occur throughout treatment. Their development is often nonlinear, simultaneous, and supportive of the capacity for productive use of regressive experiences. An instance of micro-integration could be an encounter with a new part-self, or the crossing of an amnestic or dissociative barrier, or the recall of part or all of a new memory that changes a patient's understanding of his/her history and identity, or the working through of a confusion between old and new object experience with the therapist.

A medial integration could be the disappearance from internal and interactive life of certain defensively reified alter-personality constructs (without loss, and perhaps with enhancement of the patient's overall functioning), or the grasping of painful overarching meanings about the intentions of perpetrators and the patient's loss of innocence, or the patient's departure from enmeshments and situations fraught with destruction and betrayal. A medial integration may describe what takes place when therapist and patient share a difficult or moving emotional experience or resolve a complex treatment stalemate that allows for a deeper level of trust or for access to new levels of previously sequestered material.

Macro-integrations may reflect both the satori experiences common to many growth processes and/or the more sweeping and generalizable shifts in awareness that take place in the second half of therapy where the patient becomes increasingly differentiated from the abusive matrix and the cultural collusion, and where clearly assertive, self-protective, and creative solutions to life problems are born. Some macro-integrations occur when spontaneous psycho-spiritual notions arise from deep within the patient about his/her journey through the landscapes of trauma and dissociation, about the greater meaning of his/her life, and about the nature of human experience itself. As simple as it sounds, one major macro-integration is the adult survivor's realization that s/he was a child when subjected to trauma.

For many survivors, certain linchpin beliefs and fantasies or perpetrator teachings hold many levels of dissociation in place at once. Just as in a game of pickup sticks, the movement of a strategically positioned alter personality, fantasy, memory, or belief can lead to the rapid rearrangement or even deflation of dissociative defenses. Integration then involves the patient's tolerance for out-of-control states and transient periods of disorientation while internal reorganization, recategorization, and reconfiguration take place. Ultimately integration mandates the development of healthy (not sociopathic) senses of entitlement and ruthlessness and the refusal to put up with any shred of revictimization or any reversals of blame or responsibility for interpersonal violence and its effects.

Without access to this healthy aggression, survivors cannot disengage from complex circuits of interpersonal enmeshment in perpetrating and complicitous systems. Consequently, integration must replace with a sense of privilege a lifetime of diminishment, a grandiose sense of immunity from harm, resistance to all forms of denigration and exploitation, and confrontation with sociopathic modes of relating. Integration means a survivor recognizes abuse for what it is, doesn't refer to it euphemistically, and has worked through false memories of nonabuse. Integration does not mean that the survivor cannot continue to love his/her parents; it does mean the love involves no measure of self-sacrifice, self-denial, or self-sabotage. (Loving their perpetrators, either up close or from a distance, after redefining relationship to them, can be pivotal to the healing of some survivors. For others, especially those for whom any contact could be dangerous, the goals of integration involve moving on and not looking back.)

From a relational psychotherapeutic stance, integration occurs when two or more previously separated aspects of self, in their own time and of their own volition, recognize each others' existence and experience to the extent that there is a shared memory, grieving, and relinquishment of dissociative controls. A true "witnessing" of the internal other, a capacity to see the self in the other, and a grieving for the loss of omnipotent fantasies, defenses, and the illusions they protected must take place. This does not necessarily mean agreement, blending, and absence of conflict, but it does mean mutual recognition. Recognition involves conscious cooperation and a decentering process (Crossley, 1996), whereby dominating monologues become transformed into empathic dialogues.

In actual practice, integration is a subtle ongoing process where new experiences of contact and mutuality restructure a personality previously organized around disavowal, hierarchy, and separateness. Whatever form it takes, integration is a by-product of the pivotal treatment goals of mutual recognition, internal empathy, self-love, self-forgiveness, and cooperation. These processes, which lead ultimately to an increased capacity to tolerate paradox and conflict apply to a long-term, psychoanalytically informed psychotherapy, but they have particular significance for severe dissociative conditions—disorders of internalized domination and dividedness. Effective treatment leads to both intra- and intersubjective rendezvous to supplant the internal vacuum, or war zone, where the severely dissociative patient begins the therapy process. Integration should be unique for each individual and reflect his or her emergent capacities, needs, and "destiny drive" (Bollas, 1989, p. 3); it should not be based on the theoretical orientation of the therapist.

Rivera (1989) combines clinical notions of integration with poststructuralist philosophical challenges toward articulating a relational perspective on how the integration process operates. She addresses an individual's subjective experience vis-à-vis the power relations that structure social practices and identity formation; she considers notions of a unified self or a well-defined individual identity as ideological fictions that may blur awareness of differences within and between human beings. The therapist regards dissociative barriers as interfering with the patient's freedom to construct an identity from a wide range of options; the goal of treatment becomes helping the dissociative individual to hold in a single consciousness different and often contradictory emotional states.

Similarly, Bromberg's (1993, p. 166) description of the patient's evolving ability to "stand in the spaces between realities without losing any of them" and to "feel like one self while being many" speaks to integration via the pathway of recognition. Identity is constructed on the basis of inclusivity, not renunciation, repudiation, or disparagement. Health and integration are also always about being able to consciously choose and reject external realities and circumstances and extricate oneself from anyone or any context that feels abusive, invalidating, or exploitative. Integration-based freedom to circumambulate in the internal world does not however, equate with unconscious free reign in the external world. Although recovery does not mean an ability to handle all situations at all times, a survivor needs to know where s/he can and cannot be and with whom.

INTEGRATION VERSUS ADAPTATION

> Some will get lost, never finding their way to the center, others will collapse beneath the weight of hopelessness and try to paper over the cracks and grimly survive, yet others (perhaps most) will turn away from the rawness of the experience and take refuge in premature knowing, settling for an imitation of themselves, medicating in some way or another the symptoms that are a whisper from the depths, the soft call to interiority and the hunger for truth. (Chassay, 1996, p. 5)

Integration involves developing capacities to tolerate ambiguity, paradox, and conflict. It does not mean, however, complete adaptation. Coherence of self is one thing, conformity is another. Integration must involve the reinstitution of previously derailed and deformed protest responses so that the formerly traumatized and fragmented patient can aggressively respond on his/her own behalf, deconstruct the duplicity and double binds of the familial and social context, and sublimate his/her aggression in the service of self-love and respect for the rights for others.

No integration is underway as long as the patient does not understand the power arrangements that led to his/her victimization during childhood. In integration, critical thinking and self-assertion are no longer avoided: the patient previously limited to dissociative fantasies will now be able to enjoy and discuss fantasies that are not marked by overgeneralization or concretization or constrained by fears of reprisals by perpetrators. When a patient is "integrating," s/he can think or speculate without becoming terrified, and can examine the perpetrator's scripts without becoming entranced by them, and can examine the therapist's suggestions without automatically complying with (or defying) every one of them.

With the invitation to learn how to rely on, challenge, and enjoy the authority of others as equals, integration represents a return of the authority of the patient. It signifies that s/he can know there is tremendous evil in the world, that s/he has been terribly betrayed, and that without using dissociation s/he can discern some meaning and value in living. Integration means the patient has stopped choosing between different parts of him/herself and has moved beyond denial and narcissistic fantasies of separateness as a mode of psychic living. Integration means that the patient no longer avoids his/her suffering but allows it to exist in an internal place from which it can inform other aspects of life. Integration means that intrapsychic experience no longer bypasses the mind, language, symbolization, and relationship on its way to the body. Integration means that the patient knows a lot of what happened to him/her as a child and does not let those violent and violating experiences define his/her essence.

CHAPTER 6

From Domination to Recognition: The Restoration of Intersubjectivity and Paradoxical Awareness

If you want to shrink something, you must first allow it to expand. If you want to get rid of something, you must first allow it to flourish. If you want to take something, you must first allow it to be given.

—Lao Tzu

In the severe dissociative disorders, more "self" is wrapped up in disavowing multiple selves, diverse subnarratives, and alternate realities than in investing in actual self-knowledge or self-reflection; more "self" is wrapped up in holding back traumatic affects and memories than in doing anything else. Briere (1992b; 1995) calls that which is desperately avoided "the resting level of trauma." He conceptualizes this unmetabolized psychic mass as existing in contradistinction to self-capacities that enable the individual trauma survivor to cope with life, to keep the resting level of trauma from flooding and overstimulating the personality system.

How do we begin to reach and effectively communicate with individuals who have virtually closed themselves to all possibilities for vulnerable human relationships in order to seal off internalized trauma and prevent its recurrence? How do we as clinicians build healing relationships with individuals who are buried beneath layers of illusion, self-deception, and fortified avoidance? How do we help trauma survivors develop self-cohesion, agency, and courage sufficient enough to process the enormous amount of pain and anguish locked away in unintegrated, unmetabolized, disconnected self-states? Therapy is a dance between regression and progression, between deconstruction and reconstruction, between mindlessness and mindfulness. This chapter explores the destruction and reconstruction of the severely dissociative patient's subjectivity and capacity for paradoxical awareness.

"ACROSS THE GREAT DIVIDE"

Relational psychoanalytic theories attempt to avoid reductionistic thinking by welcoming the tensions in various pairs of apparently opposing principles—by acknowledging with equal regard the intrapsychic and the interpersonal, the intrasubjective and the intersubjective, the individual and the cultural, reality and fantasy, and autonomy and interdependence (Aron, 1996). The therapeutic postures that correspond to such a dialectical formulation can help offset the propensity for reification inherent in the phenomenology of severe dissociative disorders while respecting and permitting access to the unique subjective experiences of deeply traumatized individuals. In practical terms this means, for example, avoiding prolonged debates with the patient about whether an alter personality is real or manufactured and instead finding a way to relate to the patient simultaneously as a whole and as a part-self.

By sustaining a clinical perspective that appreciates paradox, therapists can integrate all aspects of DID without becoming mired in speculation about the validity of dissociative diagnoses. The two-person (or, perhaps more appropriately, multiple-person) psychology of contemporary psychoanalysis (Mitchell, 1988; Greenberg and Mitchell, 1983; Greenberg, 1991; Stolorow et al., 1987) supplies a progressive theoretical vehicle for understanding the perplexing experience of severely dissociative patients.

Individuals with severe dissociative conditions suffer from emotional swings between states of psychic deadness and unspeakable terror. Between these two extremes, they behave almost nonchalantly, as if nothing particularly disturbing has overtaken them. Under stress, however, their overall internal chaos leads to a psychic "scattering" and to the temporary exile of the managing and observing ego. Even though most patients (and for that matter, many therapists) cannot see it, this confusion and apparent chaos is almost always ordered according to a unique internal organization. As Kluft (1991) has suggested, it is primarily the intrapsychic structure of the alter-personality system more than the behavioral manifestations of dissociative identity disorder (DID) that is the key to understanding and helping patients.

Relationally oriented psychotherapy at its best provides the opportunity for dialogue, empathy, and conflict with the complexities and diversity of the dissociative patient's experience. The processes of negotiation, mutuality, and intersubjective discourse are in a sense revolutionary models for relationship because they access and elicit recognition of previously unavailable aspects of the self, and they systematically undermine internalized and interpersonally enacted forms of domination and authoritarianism.

Sometimes the only way a severely traumatized patient can represent or formulate previously unarticulated traumatic relationships and developmental experiences is through profoundly alarming or otherwise disturbing his/her therapist. Hence, the most productive focus in treatment is on transference/countertransference relationships. This approach echoes Bollas's (1987) advocacy of the therapist's feeling his/her way into the patient's internal object world: the patient not only talks to the therapist about the self; s/he also puts the therapist through intense experience, effectively inviting direct and intimate knowing of his/her self and internal objects.

POWER, INFLUENCE, AND THE RESTORATION OF THE FRAGMENTED SELF

Rivera's (1996) clinical and philosophical perspective on the fragmentation of consciousness typical of severely dissociative individuals emphasizes adaptation over pathology and meaning-making over defense-analysis. DID is rendered "an attempt to create meaning where meaning has been eroded or destroyed . . . to make order out of threatening chaos using the elements of the chaos. . . . [Its] purpose is to create a language to speak about the unspeakable" (p. 65).

Recontextualizing self-construction and self-development by raising patients' awareness of their own subjugated subjectivity mandates an affirmative, ongoing therapist/patient commitment to address the realities of relational reinforcement, institutional legitimization, and inadvertent victim-perpetuation of power imbalances. Both parties must monitor and reflect jointly on the conscious and unconscious ways in which they can be seduced into replicating the dynamics of dominance-submission, sacrifice, betrayal, collusion, subjugation, and exploitation—often in the name of healing, integration, abreaction, support, rescue, or anxiety reduction.

The severely dissociative patient who has been exposed to domination and captivity needs to be encouraged to find and speak his/her own mind and to articulate his/her feelings and beliefs regardless of how outrageous, multiplicitous or inconsistent they may seem, and regardless of how much they collide with the therapist's worldview. Where discord and disagreement were formerly potentially life-threatening for the trauma victim, the survivor in therapy slowly comes to learn that conflict and differences can clarify and deepen the treatment relationship and each one's relationship to him/herself.

Identification with the perpetrator is a primary medium through which the effects of trauma reverberate intrapsychically and interpersonally, and the echoes in the psyches of survivors will be competing with the messages and interpretations of the therapist. Accordingly, identification with the therapist, and by extension with his/her relational style and values, can be pivotal to the disruption of rigid and repetitive patterns of trauma-based relatedness. It is partly through the power of the idealizing transference (Kohut, 1971) that a traumatized patient can even come to imagine or believe that s/he can leave an enslaving internal and interpersonal world.

Identification with the therapist's power (to access feelings, subvert denial and collusion, value differences, etc.) and with the benevolent use of that power, constitutes a central intrapsychic and relational shift that contrasts with the patient's compulsive use of dissociation out of fear. The patient must come to believe that the therapist (and the therapy relationship) could actually be as powerful as the perpetrators, or more so—and that the therapist's power (to confront denial and domination, to tolerate pain and ambiguity, to communicate with passion and authenticity, to mobilize and protect democratic forms of relatedness etc.) is accessible and shareable, not rooted in coercion, self-sacrifice, or subjugation. This conception is a necessary precondition for a patient's relinquishing ties to malevolent introjects and feeling fully empowered him/herself. Clinicians must repeatedly investigate and openly discuss the patient's experience of their use of power and willingness to share it as well as their therapeutic technique, especially in terms of the patient's sense of freedom to differentiate him/herself from biases and influences with which s/he has identified. Treatment is complicated, however, and a patient's access to new interactional experience limited, when s/he absolutely will not tolerate any aspect of the therapist's authority or constantly assaults the therapist's vulnerability, trustworthiness, and goodwill (with, e.g., criticism, boundary violations, relentless demands).

Some severely dissociative trauma survivors must vehemently fight against internalizing the influence of the therapist's relational style and benevolent use of power because it threatens to dismantle fragile self-organizations based on unholy alliances; therefore, they may unconsciously engage in sadomasochistic reenactments of the traumatic past to reinforce their own adhesive and enslaving attachments to perpetrators. Purging the patient's thoughts, applied meanings, and experiences of the therapist's influence is, in Mitchell's (1993) view, anyhow impossible because the therapy dialogue by its very nature entails mutual reflection upon interactional dynamics, including the patient's ways of using, misusing, or avoiding using the therapist's participation.

Mitchell's relational perspectives represent an increasingly refined two-person psychology, an enlightened, reciprocal psychotherapy process, and ultimately a pathway out of the trauma-replicating patterns of ideological totalism and relational domination. Charting a course for integrating the patient's narratives, fantasies, dissociated identities, and historic recollections with the therapist's experience of the patient, they encompass the multiple realities of both participants and maintain open channels for ongoing revision and reconstruction. The very encouragement of direct contact with alter personalities and self-states leads to a more inclusive observing ego, a more reflective intrapsychic and interpersonal morality, and a compassionate democratization of mind.[1] These are developmental achievements of the highest order.

A relational philosophy values democratic forms of integration whereby the therapist does influence but does not dominate the patient both in terms of the meaning of the patient's material and the ultimate goals of treatment. Similarly, the eventual decision about the veracity of memories and associations accessed during the therapy process belongs to the patient, although the therapist clearly has a role to play and will undoubtedly have impact on the outcome. Ghent (1994) captures the paradoxical interplay of real and transference relationships—a benevolent collaboration between patient and therapist—in asserting that the patient always wants simultaneously "to be sure that the analyst 'gets it' the way the patient experienced it, and . . . to have the analyst help him go deeper [so that he can] 'get it' on a level that had previously been inaccessible" (p. 485).

An integral part of psychotherapeutic work is the creation of spaces for marginalized testimony or subverted discourses to be heard, specifically, those that have been excluded from representation by society's dominant (and dominating) master narratives (Price, 1995); it also involves the deconstruction and challenging of pathological stories and identifications, such as "I am worthless," "I am damaged," or "I am evil," to generate more historically accurate, compassionate, and self-affirming alternatives. Making such spaces must include investigating the subtexts and influences of the debates about false memories as well as the influence of perpetrators' thought-reform practices and other unconscious and coercive influences in child-abuse trauma. The cultural forces of denial about and collusion with child abuse, in combination with specific messages and ideologies inherent in abusive family systems and the distorted thinking of abusers, actually determine much of the form of dissociative identity construction in chronic trauma survivors.

The journey toward self-understanding then involves both an internal and external linking process (Bion, 1993) so that disparate aspects of the self can encounter one another and dialogue, and then systematically challenge and eventually dismantle the aggressive unlinking processes of the dissociative mind—the faulty associations that have held the traumatized individual captive to massive denial, the irrational logic of perpetrators, coerced belief systems, or preoperational and concrete operational thought. Clinicians treating trauma and dissociation need to be educated not only about memory and its vicissitudes but also about the dynamics of incestuous families, of perpetrators and perpetrator groups, of coercive thought-reform and its social influences, of complicity, collusion, and collaborationism, about the psychobiology of trauma and dissociation, and about the relationship between the abusive power arrangements in the culture and the internal worlds of severe trauma survivors.

LINKING THE CHARACTEROLOGICAL WITH THE POSTTRAUMATIC

Inclusivity in treatment implies a willingness and an ability to work with both character disorder and posttraumatic aspects of DID and other severe dissociative conditions. In such complex disorders of extreme stress the characterological and posttraumatic features are mutually reinforcing; the interaction between them, as well as an individual's deficits in psychosocial resources and intrinsic psychological capacities, influences the construction and personification of self-states and the development of divisions among them. For example, both borderline and avoidant personality traits (and organization) may be particularly reinforced by the highly dissociative patient's double-binding, violent, and deceitful early environment, lifelong unconscious trauma reenactment patterns, and ongoing biphasic posttraumatic symptomatology (i.e., numbing, hyperarousal, and intrusive symptoms).

During treatment it may be difficult to tease apart the characterological and posttraumatic elements, and as Kluft (1988b) has noted, various therapeutic approaches seem to focus on only one or the other. Unfortunately, treating the character disorder aspects of severe dissociative conditions without acknowledging the underlying traumatic affects and memories can produce a highly intellectualized process with minimal structural change (Putnam, 1989; Kluft, 1987a); it might even deepen the dissociation between the patient's adaptive (functional/compliant) and less adaptive selves, and could reinforce defensive precocity developed in childhood). (A patient may be well analyzed but never quite "reached" [Bromberg, 1991]). On the other hand, trauma-oriented therapies that seek only to access memories and alter personalities, that encourage the patient to abreact, express, and integrate painful material from the past, may result in overt changes in symptomatology but leave intact the untreated narcissistic, personality-disordered aspects of the patient's disturbance.

Individuals with unexamined notions of omnipotence and aggression remain incapable of intimacy and mutuality. Indeed, as Kluft (1988b) observes, failure to work with the problematic character traits of the DID patient very often result in a relapse into dividedness, and Brenner (1996) points out, in support of Kluft's recognition of the importance of the enormous characterological issues in the DID population, that "psychic welding" (p. 156) of alters through hypnosis alone is insufficient treatment and rarely works to hold a supposed integration together. Bliss (1986) concurs with Brenner, acknowledging that, despite the centrality of autohypnotic phenomena, DID requires more sophisticated treatment than hypnotically based alter integration.

Posttraumatic symptoms represent incomplete responses to the original trauma; like other defenses, they must be valued and affirmed for their latent transformative potential. Challenging the pathologizing of victims' responses to trauma, Briere (1996) maintains that the intrusion symptoms of PTSD are an inborn self-healing activity. In this "counterconditioning" view, for example, flashbacks, intrusive thoughts, nightmares, and/or traumatic preoccupation might represent the mind's natural attempt to desensitize and integrate previously overwhelming and unintegratable, affect-laden traumatic material through small, repeated, moderately distressing dosing until the survivor attains some relief and restabilization. Understanding this principle within the therapy relationship releases the developmental potential of symptoms from their previously rigidified manifestations, while ignoring or suppressing symptoms misrecognizes the natural, reconstructive pressures on the individual toward a more fully synthesized resolution of traumatic experiences. The essence, then, of the posttraumatic recovery work beyond stabilization lies in the therapist's generating an environment of safety and trust where traumatic material and related affects can surface and be reexperienced and deconstructed, and where new meanings and relationships can be negotiated (Schwartz, 1994).

Posttraumatic symptoms represent, in part, the patient's paradoxical struggle to know and to avoid knowing (and reexperiencing). The therapist must validate, empathize with, and interpret both opposing positions. Reconstructive treatment, then, begins with observations and spontaneous and empathic disruptions of dissociative defenses and other characterological patterns toward their reintegration in the context of a more flexible identity and coping style. The therapist helps the patient to

- learn to grieve, face loss, and bear depression, despair, longing, and rage;
- reactivate and accept, within the transference, disrupted developmental processes (Atwood and Stolorow, 1984), sequestered self-esteem and attachment needs (Sands, 1994), and particularly the capacity for tolerating ambiguity, ambivalence, and paradox (Schwartz, 1994);
- develop a capacity for mutual and authentic positive regard and non-dominating power arrangements (as distinguished from compulsive dominance and submission);
- develop a capacity for reflectivity, especially in regard to understanding of the patterns that maintain his/her organization of dissociative self-experience and investment in separateness;
- develop a capacity for healthy dependence and independence (agency, self-assertion, aggression), as distinguished from the clinging, coer-

cion, manipulation, avoidance, or pseudoautonomy so common in this population;

- understand the role of shame and self-hatred and its internalization in subsequent personality adaptations. (These are the most immutable of the characterological aspects of severe dissociative disorders to work through in treatment—the painful feelings and beliefs that hold the entire dissociative system together);
- work through feelings of omnipotence and facilitate deployment of restorative fantasy (as opposed to catastrophic and crisis thinking, inflexible, reified imaginal productions, or trance logic); and
- recover his/her sense of continuity, personal narrativity, and historicity.

In sum, dissociative defenses are not developed or deployed in isolation; they are intertwined and interdependent with character-forming or -deforming defenses. The complex personality-disordered picture presented by severe dissociative conditions involves the variety of characterological positions located in different states whose roles and functions may vary and collide with one another. The alter personalities in an individual, like individuals in a dysfunctional family system, are locked into rigid positions that mutually reinforce and sustain each others' motivations and behaviors (Kluft, 1996a). In fact, about 50 percent to 60 percent of patients with DID meet criteria for paranoid, borderline,[2] and avoidant personality disorders (Ross, 1992).

LINKING AND DELINKING

Overreliance on dissociative solutions to trauma sustains a magical world that wards off anxiety and threat but simultaneously perpetuates the internal persecutory structure of experience and the absence of critical thinking, or a unified observing ego. According to Pye (1995), much of the clinical work with dissociative abuse survivors entails analyzing fears of linking one moment to the next, fears about the power of omnipotent fantasies, and fears about the significance of alterations in identity and affect states that surface in response to the events taking place in the therapy relationship.

In DID, as with many posttraumatic conditions, the omnipotence defense and other aspects of dissociative solutions are inherently attacks on the linking functions of the psyche (Bion, 1959). Effective psychotherapy involves recognition, interpretation, and at times confrontation with these often personified omnipotent defenses, which manage to keep emotional events and their possible traumatic meanings unrelated and disconnected in the patient's mind (and sometimes, through projective identification or other forms of unconscious influence, unrelated and disconnected in the therapist's mind as well).

Commentary on and interpretation and confrontation of omnipotent defenses and other forms of intrapsychic and interpersonal domination and coercion are central tasks of treatment. The psychotherapist's use of his/her own countertransference experiences of traumatization, intrusion, and betrayal is essential to a successful treatment outcome. The therapist's use also of his/her countertransference feelings of attachment, anger, hate, and love toward the patient both in self-reflection and in collaborative dialogue is crucial and complementary to the creation of a transformative relationship. The therapeutic posture and relational stance must be powerful enough to disrupt and neutralize internalized traumatic attachments and perpetrator identifications and to motivate the construction of a benevolent internal world.

Within the transference/countertransference matrix, it is ostensibly through the process of enactment—dramatizing or externalizing the patient's internal experience against the therapist's reality (Bromberg, 1993)—that empathic communication, useful knowing, and significant healing take place. Enactments involve the need to be known in the only way possible (i.e., intersubjectively) for Bromberg, through playing out with the therapist versions of the situations that led to the original needs for dissociation. Sharing the experience of replaying same behaviors with different responses facilitates the construction of consensually validated meaning "that allows the dissociated threat of potential trauma to be cognitively processed" (p. 154). Memories (of events, emotions, fantasies, family dynamics) that have never fully registered, never been linguistically coded into a meaningful historical narrative, can enter the psychic space between patient and therapist, first making way for the possibility of healing.

The joint discovery of, and awakening to, possible meanings of disturbing interpersonal and intrapsychic experience almost always involves confusing collisions and unusual convergences between the two parties. The manifestation of symptoms—the sudden intrusion of feelings of nausea, hostility, disgust, hatred; even a desire to withdraw from the interaction altogether—in either patient or therapist may be an important precursor to the emergence of memories, whose management will determine whether the intrusive feelings will illuminate or obfuscate the related psychic material.

Other kinds of abrupt state-changes in one or the other member of the therapeutic dyad or in the ambience between them may reveal or conceal underlying traumatic relational patterns slowly surfacing with the patient's growing tolerance for conflict and painful affect. Because severely dissociative patients are always alert to repetitions of the original traumas (which may be vigorously denied or dissociated when remembered) and because they are profoundly confused about the dynamics of trust and betrayal, unexpected and counterintuitive shifts take place between (and within) therapist and patient when they reach new levels of intimacy or when the clinician makes minor errors in empathy or consistency. In enactment their two psyches become tied in a knot; the process of untangling them is the essence of therapy. Sometimes, when new relationship experiences and insights develop swiftly, it happens rapidly, but when strong feelings of betrayal, retaliation, abandonment, and intimidation have entered the relational field, the disentangling process—understanding enactments, constructing meaning and identity, attributing responsibility—can go on for months, challenging the steadiness and resilience of the treatment alliance.

TERI

"I could die for telling you what I just told you," a dissociative patient claims anxiously. I do not negate (or become frozen and terrified of) her worldview, but explore its underpinnings, allowing her to experience the threat as real in the safe presence of inquiry that meets her subjectively compelling realities.

THERAPIST: You think I should send you away or beat you because you feel you've done something so awful here by telling me this secret; you actually believe you deserve to be treated badly even if you really don't want to be treated badly by me.

PATIENT: *[Nodding yes as if from several places at once]* I AM bad; that's why my parents left me with those people.

After a short discussion of her history and memory of being taken to various people's houses for prostitution, pornography, and sadistic abuse, the dialogue in the transference/countertransference resumes—now with more parts of the patient present.

T: Parts of you are afraid of my leaving you like the others did, parts of you want me to send you away so I will prove no threat to you in being like all the rest, parts of you want to get rid of me, and parts of you want to hang on for dear life. Some places in you think you deserve mistreatment, others don't know why you deserve such treatment, and some parts of you want to mistreat others. And all are welcome here.

P: *[Switching to another, more hostile and provocative alter]* You wouldn't say that if you knew some parts of me and what they've done.

T: You're just not sure I can handle all of you—who you are, what you've done, what you think you've done, who you think you are yet. Is that right?

P: Yes. *[Defiantly]* Can you?

T: Given your experience of betrayal, you can't just take my word that I welcome contact with all of your parts, and since maybe you know some things I don't know yet, neither one of us can be totally sure of what will happen next, so there's some risk. The real question is how will you go about finding out if I mean what I say; how will you test me?

P: What do you mean test you? I can test you? You would like that?

T: I imagine some of the ways you could test me would be quite stressful, but the point seems to be that it's hard for you to believe that I'd want you to have any power or say over what goes on in here.

P: Yes, that's right, and besides that I'm not sure if I'd want you to pass or fail.

T: Probably both at once, right?

P: *[Laughing]* Right, if you fail I'm back where I started from but at least I could gloat over that, and I would really like to gloat over that—and if you pass, I have to go forward, and I have to remember things and feel things and if I say some things bad things might happen.

T: What bad things might happen, for example?

P: I could be hurt. You could be killed. Or we could both be killed.

T: Can you say more about that feeling or idea?

P: *[After hesitating for a long time]:* Why aren't you scared to talk about this? Why aren't you scared of them?

T: When you say "them" I am not sure who you mean, but I do get the idea that you're threatened and you're wondering why I don't seem to be.

Staying close to her experience, and mindful of the dynamics of organized perpetrator groups, I do not automatically assume this concern about endangerment means the patient is projecting, deflecting her aggression toward me to some vague outside authority, or that she is simply fearful of her own aggressive impulses, although eventually, and in a different context, some of these dynamics involving fear of her own power and aggression will have to be addressed.

> P: There are things she [*referring to the host personality*] doesn't know and maybe can't know yet or ever, I'm not sure, and I don't like talking about it anyway.
>
> T: As I've told you before, you don't ever have to ever talk about anything until you're ready—if you're ever ready.
>
> P: Okay, that's good. I still don't know why you're not scared.
>
> T: When you feel or believe that I am not scared, what comes up for you around that?
>
> P: Three different things. First relief, like maybe there's protection and then I want to talk to you. Tell you everything, unload. Then there's the fear—a voice in my head says he doesn't know what it's all about, how dangerous it is, he's just a stupid therapist like all the rest and he'll never believe you anyway. Then I feel numb and confused and I think maybe you don't know what you're getting yourself into. I don't want to cause you to be hurt.

Following this discussion, Teri could begin to discriminate (and negotiate with) a variety of persecutor and perpetrator alter personalities as well as more clearly define a variety of external perpetrators—some of whom, using mind-control technology, had created hypno-programmed dissociative states to serve a variety of functions including prostitute, courier, and assassin. Distinguishing internal and external threats was a major precursor to Teri's beginning integration and to the systematic deprogramming of embedded triggers, commands, beliefs, and messages from her perpetrators.

Relational Perspectives and New Knowledge Acquisition

Certainly, given the blurring nature of dissociative processes, absolute knowledge and truth about the past may be unattainable. However, the methods of relational psychoanalysis and, to some extent, the cognitive/dynamic techniques of the dissociative disorders field foster the mutual construction of ever-changing narratives that at once make sense of the chaos of the patient's history and fragmented identity and leave room for the ambiguity of not knowing.

Along with interpretation from within the transference-countertransference matrix, and a focus on shared observation of reenactment patterns, psychotherapy for severe dissociative disorders always involves a degree of *witnessing* of survivors' testimony. Survivors have always needed not only to survive to tell their stories but also to tell their stories in order to survive (Laub, 1995). "There is in each survivor an imperative . . . to tell and thus to come to know one's story, unimpeded by ghosts from the past. . . . One has to know one's buried truth in order to be able to live one's life" (p. 63).

The intersubjective therapeutic environment promotes the patient's remembering, listening to, and tolerating the conflict among his/her multiple identities and diverse self-states without resorting to dissociation and subterfuge. Capacities for feeling, grieving, and critical thinking, shattered in the traumatic childhood, can be restored. One of the great paradoxes of treatment for the adult survivor is that trusting in the psychotherapy relationship means both that s/he might be hurt again and that s/he might finally feel safe enough to know how hurt s/he actually has been. That safety leads to awareness of the vulnerability and defenselessness long warded off and simultaneously to a realistic appraisal of one's true (as opposed to fantasied, omnipotent, identification-with-aggressor-rooted) power to survive and recover.

In the end, there can be a future for a patient who is no longer held captive to an unassimilated, unmetabolized past—a conscious, liberated, and participatory future instead of a lifetime of concrete traumatic reenactments and revictimization spirals.

Prior to involvement in such psychotherapeutic discourse, most severely traumatized patients either dissociate all human destructiveness out of mind or own and identify with it completely ("all me," "my choice," "my fault") in a childlike, omnipotent strategy to control and contain their malevolent childhood surrounds. Severely traumatized individuals have a particular incapacity to attribute responsibility properly: they impute everything that happens to their own actions or their own magical thinking (Van der Kolk, 1996), manifesting a profound omnipotent sense of responsibility not only for their abuse but also for subsequent problems over which they had no control.

The capacity to externalize cause accurately is an important element of healing, however (Alpert, 1995). Only when the dissociative conflation of past and present, the self and other, has been disentangled can a patient correctly identify and integrate his/her actual aggressive feeling, sexuality, and fantasies. Some of this work involves locating and developing entitlement feelings in the patient where none were allowed to exist before. Some of this work involves relinquishing or negotiating forms of entitlement and omnipotence developed in the abusive context and sustained throughout the survivor's life. (Cultural and professional confusion over issues of entitlement, reparations, and the protest appropriate to victims has led to incomplete treatments and in some cases retraumatization of patients within the systems designated to help them.) Some of this work involves linking personal psychological experience and character change with awareness of political and social realities that support and perpetuate child abuse and other forms of domination. And a good deal of this work involves developing models of personal transformation that promote resistance to merging with the dominant culture's unhealthy norms, a commitment to attend to one's own voice and integrity (Gilligan, Rogers, and Tolman, 1992). The purpose of psychotherapy is not only to soothe but to disrupt, not to adjust but to empower; this induces distress where formerly there was comfort, acceptance (Brown, 1994), complacency, and dissociation.

Recontextualization of DID symptoms as emblematic of the patient's adaptational and developmental needs in a sociocultural milieu of violence and betrayal is essential for avoidance of retraumatization (by means of subtly blaming the victim or potentiating disempowerment through ahistorical defense analysis). The wounded psyche of the adult survivor of severe childhood trauma must be attended to within a clinical framework that links psychological recovery of specific developmental processes with a progressive political awareness of the ways in which institutionalized systems of domination, including the family, can assault, damage, and pervert the individual. Without such an integrated approach to treatment (viz., Altman's [1995] three-person amplification of the two-person model of human development [Mitchell, 1988], where the larger social context is the theoretical third), the field of psychotherapy may participate in perpetuating a psychology of victimhood where learned helplessness, powerlessness, unmodulated rage and despair predominate in the minds of trauma survivors. The patient must be able to question ethics, morality, and responsibility in ways that help him/her find a voice of protest and outrage and a refined, conscious relationship with external authority.

Since severely dissociative trauma survivors have grown up under tyrannical and dominating family systems, the psychotherapy process must acknowledge the power of language and relationship and the psychopathologizing of subjective experience. In a context of abuse, the power to name, silence, and reverse meanings is a key tool of subjugation used by perpetrators in tandem with violence and intimidation to define the terms of reality and to exercise complete control over the victim and his/her mind. A central task in treating the severely traumatized patient—mind fragmented, reality testing permanently disrupted and confused by perpetrators—is interrupting and halting conscious and unconscious compliance with his/her own objectification and subordination, both inside and outside of psychotherapy.

RECOGNITION VERSUS DOMINATION

Dissociative identity disorder is almost always a disorder of internalized domination and failed recognition. There is too much identity and not enough identity; too much subjugated subjectivity and not enough agency; too much collusion with perpetrators and too much self-betrayal, insufficient autonomy and self-love. The too-much-identity part comes from elaborations of survival strategies, attachment needs, and the double binds of attachment inherent in child-abuse situations; the too-little identity results from developmental arrest, limited exposure to (or internalization of) benevolent interaction, and lack of integration of the disparate aspects of the self.

The inner world of the DID individual is riddled with both active and passive forms of aggression, coercion, and domination (Schwartz, 1994). The intergenerational transmission of violence and internalized oppression of perpetrating systems often results not only in internalizing the enemy/abuser and collaborator positions, but also in becoming seduced and mystified by their worldviews and messages, and ultimately in producing a set of alienated, disempowered (or falsely inflated) set of dissociated part-selves. Unconscious conditioning to fit into a pathological family and/or social system requires the development of distorted ideas about privilege and entitlement that alternate with self-deprecation, worthlessness, and alienation. (The ever-present values of the dominant culture are internalized below the level of awareness, where there is no possibility of their articulation

[Hertzberg, 1996].) In the unusual intrapsychic arrangements that evolve from chronic victimization experiences in pathological, violent families and in this culture in general, these belief systems usually emerge in treatment as cover stories along with dissociation (Waites, 1997): the patient's well-rehearsed narrative of the past (developed with the help of his/her perpetrators and collaborators and his/her own limited cognitions from childhood, plus his/her adult needs to pass as normal) obscures other versions of the past that are characterized by brutality and exploitativeness, subjectively experienced as the present, and usually sequestered in alter personalities whose voices are suppressed and "forgotten."

Neglect, violation, and duplicity have so marked the developmental experiences of the severely dissociative patient that s/he has come to embody extreme forms of human adaptation to a corrupt interpersonal world. In such deplorable and abusive interpersonal conditions, there is an almost complete incapacity for *recognition*, which—combining resonance and difference—is the response from the other that makes meaningful the feelings, intentions, and actions of the self (Benjamin, 1990). Recognition from caretakers allows the self to realize its agency and authorship in a tangible way (Benjamin, 1988). Children (indeed, people in general) come to know their emotional lives only to the extent that their emotions are recognized by others who can tolerate feelings and their corresponding representations in themselves, and who, moreover, can actually think about what they feel and can communicate to the child (or patient) something psychologically usable (Spezzano, 1996). From a contemporary psychoanalytic perspective, recognition is the central relational medium of healthy development.

From its roots in developmental psychology (Stern, 1985; Beebe and Lachmann, 1988), and developmental psychoanalysis (Winnicott, 1971), and from the self-psychological emphasis on empathic attunement (e.g., Kohut, 1971; 1984) to the emergence of theories of intersubjectivity (Stolorow et al., 1987; Orange et al., 1997; Benjamin, 1990 etc.) *recognition* has come to be seen in relational psychoanalysis as the essence of intersubjective exchange and as the primary vehicle for the transformative effects of psychotherapy (Ghent, 1995). In an effort to articulate what is at the heart of the relational perspective—even more definitive than mutuality—and to capture the nature of the mutative interaction that "reaches deep into the very essence of the patient's most private, and sometimes most unavailable, sense of self" (p. 110), Eisold (1999) has coined the term "profound recognition: . . . an experience in which the patient feels that some significant part of himself or herself, previously set aside, if not entirely dissociated, has been 'seen,' 'met' by the analyst in such a way that he or she can again come to know and acknowledge it as important"(p. 110). Rustin (1997) suggests that—leaving the patient with the feeling that s/he has been acknowledged and understood more deeply than ever before, and contributing to a feeling of unity with the therapist—such recognition leads to the development and consolidation of an enduring sense of personal agency in the patient that was not previously possible.

In sharp contrast to this model, sexual-abuse perpetrators are typically incapable of tolerating any affect or need on the part of the victim that does not conform to their own grandiose schemes for narcissistic gratification and the attendant imperative for secrecy; their interactions with the victim teach him/her to suppress all affects, behaviors, and thoughts that do not fit with the prescribed role. The mind of the perpetrator colonizes the mind of the victim and attempts to gain full recognition from the child without giving anything in return (although some children have perceived their perpetrators to have given them specialness, safety, succor, money, food, etc.).

The isolation of the victim's attention in child-abuse situations is the opposite of healthy recognition: the child must allocate most of his/her developmental resources to anticipating the needs and threats of the caretaker/perpetrators. Such marginalizing is accompanied by efforts to convince the victim to feel singled out—either as the recipient of the perpetrator's "love" or as someone worthless who "deserves" abuse. Because perpetrators withhold (or pervert) recognition experiences from their child victims (except the kinds that encourage compliance), and because the children develop state-dependent trust in untrustworthy authorities (which inevitably creates chronic doubt and confusion in their minds), the actions of the victims over time conform more and more with the ambitions of the victimizer (Nachmani, 1997).

Just as the double binds of the abuser foster division, camouflage, and self-evasion in the psyche of the victim, so the empathic and linking responses of the psychotherapist can promote internal or self-recognition processes—capacities born and shaped out of healthy mutuality in the parenting sphere of influence—to support the development and actualization of the healthy, feisty, and liberated self. The collapse of intersubjective experience and the eclipse of mutuality betoken a condition of domination, where there is refusal to accept the fundamental tension between the self's needs for assertion and the other's needs for recognition (Benjamin, 1990). A true sharing of realities presupposes appreciation for both one's own and another's (Benjamin, 1988; 1990), but in child-abuse trauma, there exists no such developmental dynamic—only the reality of a perpetrator with the power to induce fear, and the willingness to use the ideology of authority to justify abuse.

Sometimes the perpetrator uses the child's needs for recognition solely to silence him or her; at other times the perpetrator manipulates them for power—psychological inflation, sadistic gratification, or erotic stimulation. For example, some perpetrators tell the child-victim that when other people find out what s/he has done they will brutally reject and abandon him/her, while other perpetrators praise the sexual precocity of the child-victim, urging him/her to engage in even more bizarre sexual practices as proof of his/her special skills, or reinforcing his/her unique capacities to please the perpetrator and thereby gain monetary or other rewards. Through a combination of intimidation, coercion, and praise, some perpetrators are able to seduce some children to sexually abuse or violently turn against other child-victims as proof of their superiority to the other children, loyalty to the perpetrator, or entitlement to special privileges; in some instances, these events are part of the demented plots of child pornography and snuff films.

In the worst scenario, the child-victim's isolation and needs for approval and protection lead him/her to develop compliant selves that serve the economic needs of the perpetrator group, which—having deformed that child's psyche and sexuality—now profits from their accessibility. The perpetrator, the person who threatens the child's life, may also play on the child's natural empathy by claiming that s/he is hurting his feelings when s/he doesn't do as s/he is told. The highly dissociative child will then develop an ego state empathic to the perpetrator's hurt, and this state will be completely separate from the aspects of the personality that have knowledge of the abuse. Over the years, several severely dissociative patients (or specific alters within their systems) have described their awareness of (and psychological investments in) soothing their perpetrators during episodes of molestations, others have reported elaborate fantasies of *healing* the perpetrator while the perpetrator was raping him/her.

The domination experience—a variable-interval reinforcement schedule, as behavioral psychology would term it, of punishment, pain, and relief—that characterizes the life histories of almost all severely dissociative patients becomes internalized and then elaborated within the fabric of their dissociative worlds. Abusive parents/caretakers essentially use the child for primitive psychic-regulatory functions, demanding obedience and compliance, which are perversions of empathy and recognition. At the same time, they make recognition of the child's pain and needs for soothing and reality-testing, as well as moments of attention or comfort (release from pain or captivity or torture) conditional upon submission and compliance. In the most perverse child-abuse situations, such as those that obtain in most organized perpetrator groups, there is not only complete and intentional absence of recognition for the victim's experience but also the creation (and systematic inculcation) of new (false) identities and bizarre beliefs in the child-victim's confused posttraumatized mind.

Without a recognizing other to work out developmental issues of aggression and reparation from trauma-induced psychobiological dysregulation, the traumatized child, chronically jettisoned from the intersubjective, is left only with intrapsychic and dissociative phenomena to manipulate with any efficacy. Imitation (perhaps in caricature) of the most salient and powerful elements in his/her surround is sometimes the victim's only source of comforting fantasies and strategic dissociative identity formation. The psychology/ideology of the perpetrator(s)and often the collaborators as well is internalized in the child's psyche, regrettably, where the vulnerable self is treated by an increasingly dissociated self-abuser with the perpetrator's contempt and objectification.

In keeping with the operative levels of perpetrator influence and co-opting and the specific methods of torture and thought-reform deployed, self-abusers can become more and more detached from any reality other than the perpetrator's perverse desires and beliefs. In cases of internalized complicity and collusion, for example, the vulnerable, posttraumatized self is ignored, dismissed, or told by collaborator-parts either that nothing happened—that s/he is making things up just for attention—or that s/he deserved what happened. Patients who do not always (initially) remember their perpetrators' faces or names remember too well the names they themselves were called, repeatedly—names like Fat Ugly Pig, Stupid Cunt, or Worthless Whore. Words and the intent they convey are, for children, as impressive as actions, and hateful words hurt as much as physical violence, sometimes more. The internal persecutors who evolve out of chronic exposure to such contempt replay those words until internal identities actually bearing them as names emerge; thus devalued, they regularly submit to abuse and derision by the other internalized self-states. A behavioral psychologist would describe the dynamic as a conditioning paradigm in which increasingly distorted aspects of the patient's self and sexuality are systematically reinforced, while responses affirming autonomy, protest, and vulnerability are systematically ignored, punished, or extinguished.

Dissociation structuralizes the traumatized child by providing a soothing discontinuity between abuse events. (Also, it mirrors the massive denial and inconsistency inherent in abusive families or groups and echoes the state-changes perpetrators manage facilely as they switch from private to public spaces.) The result is a host of internal part-selves whose rigid roles and functions are never negotiated. As omnipotent fantasies replace restorative ones, feelings of omnipotence replace true mastery; the individual denies both inner and outer psychic realities, recognizes neither self nor other, remains desperate to sustain some sort of attachment bonds with the perpetrators, and sequesters, then vigilantly guards experiences in order to bind terror and annihilation anxiety. In short, the world has been divided into the dominators and the dominated, the potential for mutuality is lost, and dissociative limbo has become the only retreat.

Especially early in treatment, the dissociative patient will therefore attempt to convert all interactions with the therapist into repetitions of perverse power struggles with the perpetrator (including seductions, evasions, submission, coercion, and efforts to control the mind of the other), and inevitably the therapist will play out some of the expected patterns; if the patient is unable to exercise awareness of his/her dissociated past and his/her role in re-creating its dynamics, s/he will perceive the therapist as a victimizer. (Too many abuse survivors have, in fact, been exploited sexually by clergy or mental health professionals.) Some severely traumatized, dissociative patients polarize therapy interactions out of genuine confusion; others do so for secondary gain or to distract themselves from the need to face their own internal conflicts and pain.

Sometimes, early in treatment, a severely dissociative trauma survivor, often split off into a child alter personality, will refuse to leave the session or act in such a way that ending a session becomes extremely difficult for the therapist. The patient's behavior may represent true confusion in the alter personality about the nature and limits of the therapy relationship, an attempt to play upon the guilt of the therapist to gain special attention, a need to reenact boundary violations, or a need to create a power struggle with the therapist in order to deflect attention from emerging traumatic affects and memories or other disturbing needs and vulnerabilities. In a given dissociative patient demonstrating this particular behavior, all of these intentions and motivations may exist concurrently.

Extreme dissociative disorders, organized with varying degrees of narcissistic investment in separateness (Kluft, 1985) among alter personalities or self-states, replicate the dynamics at work between child and abusive caretaker(s). That is, all alter personalities dominate one another, though in different ways, being frightened of each other's power to destroy their selves or derail their pursuit of their goals according to reciprocal trance logic of the dissociative self-system. Some alters threaten, deride, and enact fantasied or actual violence on the other more compliant, complicitous, or childlike and victim-identified alters. The compliant ones exert control passive-aggressively, by disowning, disavowing, refusing to remember, and refusing to tolerate painful emotions, thus forcing those functions back onto other alters (Schwartz, 1994); enacting domination at another level, they claim innocence of aggressive impulses or behavior, preferring to feel either victimized or amnestic. Compliant alters also sabotage engagement with therapists by straining to maintain surface level dialogues, and they sabotage intimacy with other people in their lives by avoiding important self-revelation.[3]

Many severely dissociative patients insist on dictating their own treatment, being almost totally unable to tolerate the experience of another's power. In testing the therapeutic relationship, they attempt compliance, sabotage, and defiant seizures of power to determine the balance of that power. (At the same time, and paradoxically, most clinicians and theorists treating sexual trauma agree there is no group of patients more vulnerable to therapist boundary violations and other abuse than the dissociatively disabled). Toward gently disrupting the structures of internal domination that maintain the dysfunctional internal world, therapists must remember to relate all part-selves by recognizing their dependence on and domination of the others. Internalization of the benevolent, respectful, honest and mutuality-based interaction with the therapist is most subversive to the internalized system of domination.

Ultimately, a commitment to mutual recognition means reexperiencing traumatic affects and disturbing memories whose hallmarks are helplessness and betrayal, and, in turn, inevitably grieving and suffering profound loss. Therapists need to remember that it is easier for a severely dissociative patient to sustain the accustomed abusive relational dynamic in treatment (in reality or fantasy) than to risk allowing another form of relational awareness to threaten the security provided by the dissociative system. In the end (in order for a new, healthier systemic security to supplant the old one) the same gentle and gradual erosion of defenses that has distanced the patient from his or her suffering will have to be experienced by all the alters.

CLINICAL POSTURES THAT FOSTER RECOGNITION

Bringing about the *recognition* requisite to the treatment of severely dissociative patients embodies subversion of all forms of domination. Recognition is the product not of a set of interventions but of a cluster of attitudes that create an ambience—attitudes that mandate the clinician to

- Accept the intersubjective principle that the therapist's perceptions are not intrinsically more true or valid than the patient's, and that s/he cannot know the patient's internal reality directly but only through the perspective from his/her own window (Orange, 1995; Stolorow and Atwood, 1992).
- Notice and explore (and eventually diagnose and discuss as appropriate) the patient's patterns of dissociation and pathological multiplicity, maintaining openness and willingness to assess for factitious, malingering, and iatrogenic factors in a given presentation.
- Monitor his/her internal and interpersonal shifts between doubt and credulity, and balance skepticism with a willingness to believe (and to suspend disbelief) in the face of even apparently implausible or grotesque accounts of child abuse that emerge during the course of treatment.
- Access and work with alter personalities or other, less organized dissociative self-states in terms of their relationships with one another and relationships with the therapist toward apprehending empathically and articulating their roles in the individual's overall psychological and physical survival.
- Understand the paradoxical needs of most alters/self-states in a dissociative self-system to be perceived as voices at once desperately begging to be heard and having to hide and avoid recognition of any kind (Price, 1997).
- Balance the potential dangers of reifying the patient's dissociative self-system (through fascination, concretization, collusion, and reinforcement of narcissistic investment in separateness) with the dan-

gers of abandonment, neglect, and treatment stalemate due to failure or unwillingness by either party to engage in meaningful dialogue with the patient about his/her inner life.

- Be in touch with his/her own feelings as well as understand what the patient feels, what the patient has not yet felt, or what the patient may be unwilling to feel, and be open to feedback from the patient about what s/he feels the therapist is unwilling to feel, think, or believe.

- Tolerate ambiguity and uncertainty, appreciate the unexpected, and slowly cultivate these capacities in the dissociative patient's relationship to self and others.

- Face (and discuss) extreme human malevolence and be (unrighteously, but descriptively) willing to name it in the life of the dissociative individual.

- Create a climate hospitable to revisiting informed consent about different aspects of the treatment process and to reviewing responsibility and accountability in both participants.

- Respect how the patient's dissociative adaptations have served as a bulwark against overwhelming pain and distress, and explain how relinquishing dissociative solutions in treatment may lead to transitory exacerbation of symptoms in the process of coming to terms with painful recollections.

- Recognize what stage of treatment (e.g., stabilization, processing trauma, deprogramming, addressing intimacy issues, mourning/grieving, termination/resolution) the patient is ready to undertake, and help the patient learn to do so him/herself on an ongoing basis.

- Realize that patients may either be overideational, somewhat fantasy-prone, and highly invested in elaboration of an internal dissociative self-system—or fantasy-deficient, fantasy-phobic, and avoidant of any revelation or elaboration of the internal world. (Both extremes present diagnostic and treatment dilemmas, and in some cases both can exist in the same individual.)

- Explore, understand, and confront all addictions and self-defeating, self-destructive behaviors, especially those that jeopardize the patient's immediate well-being and obstruct the therapeutic alliance by cloaking and/or reinforcing dissociative strategies and impeding treatment progress.

- Foster the patient's observing ego functions regarding all internal and interpersonal patterns of dissociation, domination, collusion/complicity, and identifications with perpetrators.
- Discourage uncontrollable and exhibitionistic reexperiencing of trauma, and put safety and stabilization (and development of a strong treatment alliance) ahead of all other goals in treatment even in spite of the patient's protests to the contrary.
- Question, gently disrupt, and challenge all persona-restoring, avoidant, distracting, and obfuscating behaviors that culminate in the patient's lack of curiosity about him/herself and his/her relatedness and constrain the development of observing ego functions (respecting, of course, issues of timing, and pacing, safety, evaluation of patient's functional capacities, ego strengths, and abilities to engage in trauma work, and so on, in keeping with the dictates of treatment guidelines for DID consistently advocated by all the national experts including Ross, 1997; Kluft, 1995a; Putnam, 1989 and the recommendations of the International Society for the Study of Dissociation, 1994).
- Assist polarized self-states or alter personalities to encounter, understand, and ultimately embrace their affective, ideological, identificatory, or historic opposites.
- Discuss issues of memory and influence and address the current controversies about both in order to help patients take responsibility for deciding what in their memories and life histories is real and what is not, and also to help them tolerate the ambiguities involved in recovery of traumatic material. (This is part of facilitating an environment where the patients can eventually come to have confidence in their own gut feelings, reactions, and perceptions.)
- Investigate systematically whether the patient believes that s/he must adopt the therapist's viewpoint in order to maintain the therapeutic bond; accordingly, recognize the fact that all interpretations are suggestions that go beyond the patient's awareness of the moment and that they invite and encourage the patient to look at things from the theory-rooted perspective of the therapist (Orange, Stolorow, and Atwood, 1997).
- Name and describe double binds (and the feelings they engender) in the treatment relationship, in the patient's dissociative self-system,

and in the family system or perpetrator group. (The therapist's sharing of his/her affective responses to the double binds in a nonjudgmental way can liberate patients to express often forbidden feelings about binds they have been in throughout their lives.)

- Tolerate and allow the patient to hold two inconsistent perceptions of the therapist (or other significant others) in his/her mind at the same time, sometimes for a long time, without forcing him/her to decide prematurely which one is accurate.
- Represent, at times aggressively, the spirit of compassion, mutuality, democracy, dialogue, and negotiation to the patient (especially when s/he is intimidating, withdrawing, or polarizing).
- Maintain an atmosphere that encourages patients to (constructively) question all authority—including that of the therapist—and to express how they are experiencing the therapist and to ask how the therapist is experiencing them.
- Be emotionally available, emotionally vulnerable, and emotionally honest, and at times be very direct in standing up for him/herself against a patient's attacks, provocations, or unreasonable demands and protests.
- Be willing to be wrong, to apologize authentically to a patient, and to acknowledge personal (and professional) limitations.

RESTORATION OF PARADOX

One cannot choose between faith and irony, since both are real capacities. The rule in psychoanalysis is openness to the play of voices. (Eigen, 1998, p. 34)

The capacity to tolerate ambiguity and paradox are vital aspects of integration and maturation of the personality. DID exemplifies a developmental inability to tolerate contradictions, ambivalence, ambiguity, or the tension between opposites without splitting and collapsing into dissociative polarized identifications. As Pizer (1998, p. 52) states, "multiple personality can be seen as the failure to communicate between self-states, the burning of bridges between islands of psychic reality (thus, one person with multiple personality told me that paradox was a nonexistent concept for her)." The repudiation of contradictory self-experiences leads to an eclipse of inner conflict and an overreliance on defenses like projective identification that preserve the illusion of a nonparadoxical self. Although the dissociative patient is continually shifting between multiple realities s/he cannot effectively perceive the presence of multiple realities—his/her own, those of others, or the shifts taking place in the treatment setting (or in other intimate relationships). The goal of all therapy from this perspective is to shift dissociated multiplicity to what Pizer (1998) calls "bridgeable multiplicity" (p. 75).

For most severely dissociative individuals, the therapist remains one-dimensional, or many unlinked one-dimensional concrete things simultaneously—"an idea, a concept, an abstraction, safe as long as I keep you that way," in the words of one DID patient, Michael, after years of therapy. "I have never let you be flesh and blood to me," he said. . . . But there came a moment in Michael's treatment when he did, as we were negotiating a core layer of his autism and isolation, leaving him feeling dangerously exposed and then confronting him with overwhelming stimuli. It was as though a blindfold had been taken off after thirty years, or the bandages removed from a burn victim's charred skin of a long period of unconsciousness. Allowing me to be a flesh-and-blood human, which meant considering for the first time that I could be hurt, or that I might have been hurt or traumatized in my life, disrupted his entire mode of self-protection and shook the foundation of his remaining dissociative self-organization. By now, however, Michael was able to oscillate between keeping me as an abstraction and encountering me as a flesh-and-blood human being, because he had developed a capacity for paradoxical experiencing.

The essential process of negotiation that involves bridging disparate and seemingly unintegratable opposites—which Pizer (1998, p. 26) says "constitutes the intersubjective process that delivers the therapeutic action"— achieves its transformative power when a therapist finds his/her "own particular way to confirm and participate in the patient's subjective experience, yet slowly, over time, establishes his own presence and perspective in a way that the patient can find enriching" (Mitchell, 1993, p. 196)

Especially early in treatment, severely dissociative patients cannot make use of the therapeutic setting as a container of illusions because they lack the capacity for truly transforming intrapsychic conflict (as opposed to extending dissociative solutions) and for attending to multiple realities simultaneously, and also because danger is perceived as waiting around every turn. All illusions can trigger posttraumatic memories and affects for such patients, and any reality can be ignored. All transferences, since all—even positive ones—involve some illusion, are potentially traumatic: awareness of any strong feelings that might make the therapist three-dimensional is disturbing because they may lead to the patient's having to entertain multiple perspectives (about him/herself and others) at the same time in the central consciousness. In dissociative experiencing, there is no contrast among different levels of reality, but instead a collapse, or a figure/ground shift in perspective, where the relative importance or significance of one element is out of balance with the rest of the picture.

At one level this means the patient has difficulty discriminating between the transference and the objective dimension of the therapy relationship. That difficulty, in turn, produces confusion about the origin, meaning, and credibility of different voices in the severely dissociative patient's head competing for attention and authority. At the deepest level, the patient has difficulty with the very notions and the interplay of separateness and connection, symbol and reality, safety and danger. Innocuous events or dynamics can trigger defensive overcorrections in the same patient who responds to actually threatening or dangerous circumstances with indifference, a cavalier attitude, or even compliance.

In the severe dissociative disorders, instead of a healthy, vibrant tension between mutually informing psychological opposites, there is a collapse into a polarized experience of self and other. This breakdown of intersubjectivity originates in exposure to chronic trauma (i.e., in chronic traumatic impingements), and in the child-victim's helplessness in the face of abusive caretakers' extreme and nonnegotiated state-changes—the wellspring of what Pizer (1998, p. 92) defines as "intolerable paradox." Specifically, polarization results from the way trauma deforms the aggressive drive/response, inhibits use of fantasy, and disrupts cognitive development.

All intrapsychic defenses depend on the mind's capacity to minimize, magnify, or, as Eigen (1992) says, reverse valence. Chronic dissociation, more than most defensive maneuvers, interrupts the developing mind's capacity to be open to and imaginatively adopt the point of view of the *not-me* elements of the psyche (Schwartz, 1994). The radical breakdowns and/or failures in empathy among warring and mutually negating factions of the DID patient's internal world typify this problem with perspective-taking: the killers cannot see, often refuse to see, the worldview of the helpless child; the hypersexual prostitute addicted to high levels of stimulation cannot understand the need of the other functional and vulnerable part-selves for silence and retreat; the paralyzed child-states cannot appreciate the need for functioning in the world or physical contact. Chronic deployment of dissociative defenses also leaves the individual unaware of his/her impact on others and either overly empathic with them to the point of merger or absolutely insensitive to their feelings.

Both Kumin (1978) and Modell (1990) have described the pervasive fear of paradox where the child's only means of reconciling intolerable inconsistency is to split the ego defensively. In the spirit of Winnicott (1971), Modell (1990) emphasizes how the capacity to perceive and hold paradox is a function of a more advanced mode of object-relatedness that allows for effortless transitions between separateness and merger. In severely traumatized dissociative populations, however, the capacity for paradox is hostage to post-traumatic biphasic fluctuations and to a literalized imagination that experiences all change as dangerous, all symbols as real or potentially real, and all reality as alterable—except traumatic reality, which is viewed as continuous and unalterable.

Relational psychoanalytic treatment of severe dissociation must reflect efforts to restore the tension between opposites in a more unified consciousness. Dialectical therapeutic process is central to the successful reconstruction of the capacities for mutuality and healthy intersubjectivity. Bromberg, grasping the quintessentially paradoxical nature of dissociation, proposes a clinical ambience that balances empathic sensitivity with pragmatism toward creating transformative dialogue with traumatized patients. The therapist must understand their need to stay the same while changing (1995a), balance unity and multiplicity, and apprehend and act on the patient's need for him/her to keep one foot in the here-and-now, validating the patient's inner reality, while participating in "constructing a negotiated reality discrepant with it" (1993, p. 160).

Ross (1995b) expresses much the same thinking from a more classical MPD perspective and in more cognitive-restructuring terms: "It is essential to treat the alter personalities as if they are separate people, while stating explicitly that they are all parts of one person; doing so establishes the most solid treatment alliance with the parts who experience themselves as literally separate people, yet discourages secondary gain and evasion of responsibility" (p. 134). In Aron's (1999) summary words, "We need to be empathic to mirror and affirm our patients' subjective reality, and yet we need to confront their evasions and illusions" (p. 21).

In a dialectical relationship a generative tension exists between psychological opposites such that there is always movement in the direction of reconciliation. As Jung (1958) pointed out, the healing principle in psychotherapy, is to facilitate the transformation of conflict into a self-correcting play of those opposites. Siegelman (1991), writing from within the Jungian tradition, describes two methods for healing an individual's diminished freedom to "play" with opposites. First, by modeling, the therapist can help the patient juggle and creatively use multiple perspectives; in relational terms (Pizer, 1998), the therapist's recognition of multiple realities nurtures the patient's "synthetic facility for bridging the inescapable paradox of human separateness and connection" (p. 5). Second, the therapist can habituate him/herself to attending to psychic material in such elastic ways that the patient learns not from didactic commentary but "through active participating in the to-ing and fro-ing" (Siegelman, 1991, p. 165) and through experiencing the therapist's own ability to welcome more than one pole of meaning and more than one kind of outcome from the therapy and to tolerate the tension of opposites.

In thinking about trauma and its effects, neither the actual events nor their many meanings and associated fantasies can always be completely untangled. However, discourse about the myriad possibilities of meaning and identity can advance a patient's ability to come to conclusions about the past and develop capacities for self-validation—but developing appreciation for the complexity of the relationships between causes and effects and between conscious and unconscious beliefs and actions is a precondition. Rigid notions of both powerlessness and of omnipotence—often held simultaneously in separate trance states—must intersect and interact; rigid child- and adult-like responses that volley back and forth are difficult to learn to value concomitantly because they present so exclusively and dichotomously. Identity states must have a channel for dialoguing with one another, even if only through the therapist at first in the role of diplomat and interpreter. Confusion must come to be experienced as a natural part of being human rather than as merely terrifying and dangerous.

The relational psychoanalytic posture of analyzing enactments (e.g., Aron, 1996; Ehrenberg, 1992) contributes to the restoration of paradox, modifying Alexander and French's (1946) famous *emotionally corrective experience* to encompass the role of the therapist's struggle and his/her errors in the patient-instigated attempts to evoke a new model of relationship to emulate and internalize. The emphasis is on the therapist's *process* (not on the result of the struggle or even on the therapist's particular response), because it is the process of handling the challenge that the patient internalizes, symbolically, dynamically, interactionally, and transformatively.

For example, the therapist might empathically inquire into the delight with which intrapunitive alters reenact violence against helpless child personalities. By entering the omnipotent fantasy world of dissociative self-harm, s/he creates transitional space where fantasy and reality can intersect and interact. To approach the problem instead with a dialogue-quashing discussion of setting limits and making contracts around violence would be to miss an opportunity to model a nonpolarizing, nonconcretizing response to provocation or danger. (Sometimes patients unconsciously sponsor just such dilemmas for the therapist in order to create the conditions for generating a new learning experience [Modell, 1990].)

The underlying posture that guides the therapist in restoration of paradox resembles that of a negotiator among warring factions, except that the objective is not a concrete accord as much as it is the cultivation of mutual respect and of the patient's understanding of the importance of, and commitment to, taking multiple perspectives. As guardian of the tensions between opposites, the therapist manages paradox for the patient—representing minority positions and invisible points of view, exposing double binds for observation, disrupting trance logic and repetitive efforts at defensive concretization (Schwartz, 1994)—until s/he is ready to (re)activate his/her capacity for dialectical relationship, especially between the part-selves and the whole self.

In order to establish transformative dialogue, the therapist must hold and communicate to the severely dissociative trauma survivor all kinds of other paradoxes over time

- Severely dissociative individuals are both resilient and deficient: they demonstrate brilliance and density, capacity and incapacity, transparence and opacity simultaneously.
- Autonomy and differentiation, dependency and independence not only co-exist, but mutually enhance one another.
- One can be separate and connected, in communication and incommunicado, in the same relationship.
- One can be fantasy-prone, fantasy-phobic, and fantasy-deficient at the same time.

- One can be a victim, a collaborator, a perpetrator, and a rescuer at the same time.
- Overreliance on dissociative defenses simultaneously grants time to, and steals time from, the traumatized individual.
- New bridges between previously isolated or separated self-states or alter personalities lead simultaneously to relief and pain.
- Safety and danger can coexist in the same individual and within a relationship; one does not have to cancel out the other.
- Since shame is a key motivator of dissociation and shame is the emotion experienced when one feels exposed, then, as Wurmser (1987) points out, the very act of psychotherapeutic exploration aimed at reducing the patient's shame produces shame against which the patient must defend.
- Repetitions and reenactments represent developmental arrest, but they also create the conditions necessary for undoing the developmental arrest and restoring developmental progress.
- Repetitions in attaching to malevolent others (or objects) at once constitute omnipotent efforts to avoid letting go and avoid grieving and attempts to make relationships turn out differently (Russell, 1998).
- Psychotherapy is both a deconstructive and a reconstructive process: some old bridges have to be dismantled or blown up and new ones have to be built over dangerous terrain. "Tearing and building, falling apart and coming together are aspects of broader psychic rhythms, if one can tolerate the shifts" (Eigen, 1998, p. 33).
- The traumatized patient's need to be known continually meets the impossibility of being known; and the need to be known meets, as well, an inner refusal to be known (Grand, 2000). Grand calls this "annihilation's paradox" (p. 4): Although empathic understanding is critical for reparation of the trauma survivor's internal and interpersonal worlds, that very human experience threatens to renew his/her annihilation.
- Good things happen to bad people and bad things happen to good people.

PARADOX, DISSOCIATION, AND NEGOTIATION

Pizer (1998) sees the power of negotiation in psychoanalytic psychotherapy as "a jolting interruption of [the patient's] assumptions about a nonnegotiable universe" (p. 16), and he cites as end-products agreement about frame, boundaries, or fee issues; resolution of an intrapsychic and/or interpersonal conflict; a shift in the patient's representational world; a mutually sensible narrative construction of the patient's past; or a jointly accepted understanding of either a repetition by the patient or an empathic failure by the therapist.

What is extraordinary about a focus on negotiation and paradox in psychotherapy with severely traumatized, dissociative individuals—who truly do live, before treatment, in nonnegotiable universes—is that their traumatic fixity and dissociative rigidity may be consistently (and benevolently) disrupted. The whole process of working with these patients is encapsulated in a look at end-products of negotiations particular to their treatment:

- the revelation of a new alter personality;
- an encounter, an agreement to work together, or the integration of two or more alters or self-states;
- a shift from concrete enactment to symbolic representation;
- the release of traumatic memories from one encapsulated self-state into another or into a more unified consciousness. A disidentification with the aggressor and tolerance for the inevitable anxiety and disorganization that follow;
- an ability to discriminate between a perpetrator's injunctions or indoctrination and one's own thoughts and feelings;
- the shift from antagonism and self-sabotage to a firmer therapy alliance, and with it a willingness to confront attachment needs and longings;
- the capacity to contemplate the unassimilable polarities of human experience (i.e., benevolence and malevolence) without dissociating into mindless distraction, rabid denial, or extreme identifications.

JANINE

The male alter of a female patient with a history of self-mutilation is enraged by the fact that "the girls"—female alters who remember and narratively recapitulate abuse by the father—have criticized the parents, to whom "he" is loyal: "I want to blow those cunts away. I think I'll cut them up after the session today." The alter is also angry at me for allowing "the girls" to speak and for being willing to believe their version of history. ("They'd better stop criticizing our parents and you'd better not allow that or I'm going to cut them up.")

Bypassing the threat for the moment, I respond by moving to explore with the alter what happens inside him when the girls say hostile things about the parents. He, pressed to reach beyond his anger, briefly touches on feelings of sadness and loss. Here, the core of the patient's traumatic attachment to the perpetrator is beginning to be exposed and subverted.

In keeping with the expectable, paradoxical "staying the same and changing" (Bromberg, 1994; Russell, 1998), however, the male alter bounces right back into a power maneuver with threats of bodily injury in this first and very new contact with the therapist. If stripped of his repertoire of intimidation, he (and perhaps other part-selves) would be flooded with unbearable posttraumatic affect.

I make room for the alter to move back and forth between the two positions—defiant display, complete with threats, and feelings of overwhelming loss and disorientation. His very emergence heralds a new level of contact with the patient; I encourage his vitriolic verbalizing ("We hate you. You're taking us away from our parents") in preference to destructive action against the patient's body.

I make the observation that for anyone to entertain any view of the family or of reality in general counter to the one this alter holds seems to be tantamount to betrayal. The idea that the alter could remain loyal to the father but that the other parts (or the therapist) could have different thoughts and feelings comes as a total surprise to this polarizing part of the patient's self.

Introducing the question of how that dynamic has played out in the alter's relationship with the various parts—as well as the question of the therapist's role in facilitating dialogue between and among them, I speculate about the conflict between "the girls," who are angry at the parents and do not want to associate with them, and the alter ("Father's favorite"), who does not believe they did what the girls say they did. A brief discussion of the process among myself, this alter, and the self-system in general leads to clarification of each alter's position and the role of the therapist as both empathizer and disrupter.

The alter is relieved to hear me acknowledge that I am doing both things and I explain how different they are from the mutually exclusive demands or mutually inconsistent relational styles that comprised the double binds of childhood in an abusive family. The alter reminds me that he doesn't like to hear anything bad said about his parents, but does admit for the first time that he often felt confused watching them.

When I interpret the alter's threats of violence as mechanisms to ward off feelings or other conflicts with the other alters that are hard to tolerate, he resumes his defiant posture ("So what?"), on guard for any imbalance on my part that could come across as betrayal or abandonment and trigger more polarizing behavior. Rather than react by interposing the prospect of hospitalization or medication or by negotiating a no-harm contract, given the patient's history, I introduce the idea that different feelings don't cancel each other out but can coexist without competing and even intersect—a new concept in the trance logic of the patient's dissociative world. The patient, seeing me work honestly but not submissively with personal fear, can achieve a feeling of safety that can preempt the ongoing self-destructive behaviors long since transmuted into self-protective and even empowering ones.

Curiosity begins to replace threats and intimidation, to pave the way for the patient's experimenting with her experience. I do not push the patient to relinquish attachment to the perpetrator—nor do I try to become the replacement authority and object of a new traumatic attachment. Willing instead to take seriously the polarized subjective experience of the hostile alter, I make sense out of it for the patient as a whole.

Sometimes, describing—not reacting or polarizing—in a double-bind situation or enactment, and asking the patient to free-associate to the shared dilemma can effectively disrupt dissociation and concretization: ("How do you think we ended up in a lose-lose situation again?" "I wonder why we keep rerunning a play where one of us has to be hurt or humiliated or else we both have to be silenced?") The patient's alter is repeatedly invited to reflect and give me feedback on the aspects of the process that lead to impasse, stalemate, disagreement, or empathic disruption.

Sometimes, however, the therapist must disrupt polarization by confronting an alter's subjective experience of freedom (to cut the body, to block out memories, to sabotage work or school, especially to not feel) as costly to other parts of the self, and as based on commoditizing, objectifying, and dominating the self. Alters have to be nudged toward negotiating with, and ultimately embracing, their affective, behavioral, and psychological opposites.

The severely dissociative patient consistently urged to tolerate tension states begins to grow through paradoxical rather than dissociative awareness and begins the shift from holding contradictions in separate trance states to holding paradox. This process becomes most intense when the patient's love and hate for the abusers (as for the therapist), previously held in separate parts of the internal world—each almost with a life of its own—begin to collide. The patient learns that hating and loving can fight with one another and need not cancel each other out (or result in pain, humiliation, torture, or death), that they can find their way with their mixed feelings and that their mixed feelings can find their way with each other, when made conscious, verbalized, and placed in dialogue either in the inner world or (whenever appropriate, or possible) with the person who arouses mixed feelings.

The dissociative patient learns that paradox must be tolerated through bridging and bearing the irresolvable (Winnicott, 1971; Pizer, 1998). When the therapist models acceptance of and willingness to work creatively with psychological opposites, contradictions, and apparent inconsistencies (his/her own and the patient's), a developmental context is set that promotes the patient's achievement of the capacity to tolerate paradox. Then drastically incompatible emotions and perceptions that originally led to the unmodifiably dissociated organization of self (Bromberg, 1994) can be brought into conflict, negotiation, and dialogue—and ultimately some form of integration. Integration in this case does not necessarily mean resolution, for with paradox, the maturational developmental line has more to do with tolerance, acceptance, and creative reflection on that which may be irresolvable rather than with any kind of problem solving or synthesis per se.

In such a facilitating ambience there is, as Pizer (p. 65) says, "the feeling that the existence of the impossible is OK, even as it strains the accommodating embrace of the mind." Ghent (1992b) described the capacity for living with paradox as close to the concept of "acceptance" (p. 155). Significantly beyond the need for splitting and other defensive operations, the maturity implied in living with paradox involves the toleration and even the enjoyment of uncertainty, an ability to live in the flux of one's own and another's subjectivity, and the ability to maintain the tension between the need for discovery and the need for closure and privacy. In Pizer's terms, the developmental capacity for tolerating paradox is essential to bridging the disparate islands of self-experience that are the hallmark of the severe dissociative disorders. As Pizer writes, when therapists "are receptive to the multiplicity within their patients, they serve as transformational objects, sponsoring . . .

tolerance for paradoxical self-states by holding them within the unity of a single negotiated relationship" (p. 95).

LORRAINE

Lorraine, a polyfragmented DID patient in her late thirties, would bring one fascinating life crisis after another to therapy, only to drop each for its successor the following week. My inquiry about her experience of such discontinuity led to discussion not only of how her sequential abusers treated her when she was prostituted as a child (and especially of the humiliation after they finished with her) but also of how she related to her internal and interpersonal world on a first-come/first-served basis. Everything—topics, projects, people—was addressed as though here-today/gone-tomorrow, that is, without coordination, linkages, or sustained momentum.

So extreme a dissociative adaptation had allowed Lorraine to survive enormous abuses. Its central organizing principle—it's safest to keep moving—meant that having anything, showing someone that you had anything, or attaching to anyone or anything was dangerous; as a style of relating it made for quick shifting in response to interpersonal pressures. No one at work had any idea that Lorraine had a dissociative disorder: her behavior was idiosyncratic and sometimes even amusing, she "passed" as eccentric. The adaptive discontinuity served her well in certain ways, but it foreclosed deep feeling, deep attachment, and real emotional bonding in therapy and elsewhere.

Lorraine was unsure about whether she wanted to change her survival strategy, which I articulated as a natural response to survival imperatives during her years of sadistic abuse, adding that both her needs for relatedness and her needs for distance from people and from the pain of her internal conflict were valid. She became increasingly curious about her dissociative strategies and her effects on others and increasingly interested in monitoring the discontinuities that were her psychological process, often joshing about her follow-up or lack of follow-up and the complexity of her DID system.

In a later session and in a very playful way, Lorraine asked if she was driving me crazy. Before answering, I asked if her abusers had ever used that as an excuse or justification, and she replied that they did often blame her for their cruelty, saying at times that she was a terrible child who, indeed, was driving them crazy. When she asked me again if I ever felt that way I said yes, sometimes I felt dizzy and a little crazy from the shifts and the absence of follow-through.

Then I asked Lorraine what it felt like to hear me say that. Scared and relieved, she said, because people have rarely been so direct and honest with her, the intimacy of it felt new and uncomfortable—but she recognized my forthrightness as trusting, and that was a source of gratification. Finally, I asked if I was driving her crazy with my challenges to her way of being in the world; laughing, she answered in the affirmative. I speculated that we were reaching each other in deep ways by driving each other a little crazy, and perhaps breaking through barriers that couldn't otherwise be breached. Sometimes teasing, sometimes harassing, sometimes introducing one another to different sets of psychological rules, we were releasing aggressive energy in a safe way instead of just becoming irritated and frustrated.

Welcoming the mind-boggling notion that safety and aggression could coexist, and welcoming also my admission that her driving me crazy let me know some of how she might have felt as the child of deeply disturbed parents who misused, abused, and exploited her in every way imaginable, Lorraine reflected on the paradoxes and on the pervasive dividedness of her own mind. When she came to the conclusion that she could never see putting all the separate needs in different parts of herself together, I told her that they didn't have to fit like the pieces of a perfect jigsaw puzzle—that things could work out just as long as all the pieces were willing to touch, see, feel, and talk to each other some of the time.

In Mitchell's (1998, p. 55) terms, engaging and sustaining paradox "blows the old system apart, just enough for some new organization to emerge. For severely traumatized, dissociative patients the stakes of bridging (or negotiating) disparate facets of experience and tolerating paradox are high. Bearing—let alone standing in—the spaces between realities (Bromberg, 1994; 1998) is equivalent to embracing the almost inconceivable notion that the trauma is over, the self is safe, and freedom of (intrapsychic) movement is possible.

Negotiating attachment and identity, past, present, and future, and safety and danger in such a way can only take place when the severely dissociative patient is immersed for a long period of time in a therapy relationship where s/he faces and revisits his/her worst fears with outcomes consistently different from those that occurred during childhood. The therapeutic leverage derives from the therapist's allowing the patient to negotiate his/her experience of the therapist as both the person with whom the initial negotiation failed and the person with whom it might possibly be different (Russell, 1998).

As Leowald (1971) astutely observes, the only thing that works in psychotherapy is negotiation, and what negotiation actually means is whether things have to happen the same way this time. The ambience of negotiation can lead to the most significant redistribution of internal self- and other-configurations when the severely traumatized, dissociative patient recognizes simultaneously that s/he is totally responsible for everything that happens (in the present) and that someone else (namely, the therapist) can make a difference (Russell, 1998). For some extremely dissociative individuals, this amounts to the stunning realization that they are not alone in a barren, alien, or hostile universe, and that true benevolence exists.

CHAPTER 7

The Destruction and Restoration of Fantasy and Aggression

Perhaps it is awful to think of therapists as "experts" in awfulness. But it is part of one's job to turn awful situations around and around until unexpected pathways begin to open.
—Michael Eigen (1996)

The kinds of traumatic experience severely dissociative patients have lived through have led to significant derailments in the development of aggression, fantasy, and the use of transitional phenomena. Their psyches have been colonized by dominating others. When healing begins to happen, therefore, they must struggle toward new internal and interpersonal power arrangements. Treatment moves them toward democratic models of mind and relationships. This chapter explores two of the essential elements in the restoration of the fragmented lives and minds of severely dissociative individuals: fantasy and aggression.

THE RESTORATION OF FANTASY AND TRANSITIONAL EXPERIENCING

We turn wounds into dreams, poems, religion, art, law, social institutions. By feeding injury into dream work, primary process begins the endless task of making something of suffering, of working with pain through images, of discovering the joy of symbolizing what cannot be endured. (Eigen, 1996, p. 21)

It may seem paradoxical to conceptualize DID and other severe dissociative disorders as disorders of the psychological capacity for fantasy. The often theatrical elaborations of dissociative structures, the sheer diversity and complexity of their form and content, and the intricacies of patients' internal systems seem to suggest overinvolvement in, even mastery of, the use of fantasy. A more precise view, however, reveals that the severely dissociative individual is highly constricted in his or her abilities to imagine, play, and enjoy transitional space and transitional object relations.[1]

Traumatologists have described how chronic reliance on dissociation interferes with symbolization, keeping memory locked in iconic and somatosensory levels of experiencing (Van der Kolk and Van der Hart, 1989). Hence, what may appear as transitional or fantasy phenomena in DID to some theorists (Brenner, 1996) may upon closer inspection turn out to be epiphenomena of the maladaptive developmental line that moves from normal transitional objects to fetishism (Bak, 1974; Roiphe and Galenson, 1975; Weissman, 1971). Under conditions of extreme stress and fear, including danger to the body and annihilation experiences, a childhood transitional object can be treated fetishistically—rigidly and obsessively rather than flexibly and fluidly. In such cases, human relatedness and imagination are foreclosed and not enhanced by their use.

Essentially, illusions set up to mediate and negotiate the distinction between internal and external reality—transitional phenomena—may begin developing with the body (Smith, 1989) and shift to its soothers and caretakers, real and imaginary. Bodily violence and neglect from caretakers can severely disrupt developmental achievements that foster mind-body integration from infancy on, causing a split that disables the individual from accepting the separation of inner and outer reality by impairing the capacities to tolerate psychic pain and to experience the other as an independent object (Winnicott, 1971). The transitional space is an "intermediate area" between the infant or child's illusion of omnipotence and objective perception based on reality testing (Winnicott, 1971)—a sort of third world that is neither wholly subjective nor wholly objective, neither purely inner nor purely outer. Winnicott describes transitional phenomena as permanent facets of our mental lives, made possible when bridges over the gaps between self and other and internal and external reality are generated or supported by caregivers.

Transitional experiencing is, among other things, then, a child's way of handling the shock that results from the loss of omnipotence, according to Winnicott. In normal development this intermediate zone of experiencing continues to grow in complexity and richness and underlies the capacity to play and the process of symbolization associated with human culture. The absence of constructive experiences during childhood will be reflected in the patient's overall lack of integration and in the nature of the psychopathology to come (Giovacchini, 1978). Resulting disturbances in either primary or secondary processing functions of the psyche, or disruptions in their reciprocity can lead to developmental failures in the use of the transitional zone of experiencing.

Although complete mastery of intense pain and prolonged trauma may be too much to expect from any individual or any psyche, Eigen (1996) reminds us of the hope that rests in the primary processing capacity of the human mind: reworking of psychic injury in primary process may always be only partial and fragmented; however, by biting off bits of painful experiences and reworking savage wounds a little bit at a time, within transitional experiencing the psyche can grow its digestive capacity—absorbing terrifying impacts, shrinking masses of unmetabolized pain, and reworking states of shock and paralysis. But primary process itself can be wounded: when traumatic experiences (and/or biological predisposition) completely overwhelm, or damage the primary processor, the psyche's inability to process catastrophe inevitably becomes part of the catastrophe. The frozen states and chronic repetitions of posttraumatic conditions reveal a psyche that cannot develop images, fantasies, primitive narratives, or dreams able to effectively break up and rework psychic damage. For Eigen, psychoanalytic treatment involves more than making the unconscious conscious; it involves helping unconscious processing (of affects, ideas, and experiences) reset itself so that it can work effectively.

Dissociation, by segregating feeling-states and self-other perceptions, freezes and compartmentalizes experience, making it inaccessible to the dynamic restorative workings of the creative unconscious (Peoples, 1992). The resulting internal fixity and defensive commitment to the nonrestitutive deployment of fantasy among severely dissociative individuals severely challenges treatment committed to reactivating developmental strivings and aimed at cultivating transitional or potential space. While according to Goldman (1996), it is the "repeated cycles of adaptation, de-adaptation, collision, and negotiation that help generate potential space" (p. 355), these el-

ements so essential to any effective depth psychotherapy are hard for the severely dissociative patient to tolerate because they are inevitably associated
with imminent danger and often lead to emergency responses; further, constant immersion in the patient's concretizations and loss of symbolic functioning is detrimental to the therapist's own symbolizing capacities
(Giovacchini, 1978).

DISTURBANCES IN USE OF FANTASY IN DISSOCIATIVE DISORDERS

In severe dissociative conditions, the collapse of subjectivity and intersubjectivity is intricately intertwined with the developmental arrest in transitional experiencing. This is not to say that severely dissociative patients do
not engage in these adult forms of transitional phenomena; rather, their engagement is often limited and/or underscored by a desperation and
fragility that does not allow for a true contact with otherness or a release
from the alienation that marks the patient's entire mental and interpersonal
life.

For Marmer (1980), MPD patients create and use alters as "transitional objects forced inward" (p. 458); in a recent reformulation (1996),

> Because they can't make a coherent self, they make a polyfragmented self or
> selves, and they use their alters for the same purposes that non-DID children
> would use transitional objects, except that in normal childhood, transitional ob-
> jects are a way station on the road to establishing a coherent self, and in DID,
> patients are stuck with their alters. (p. 200)

Smith (1989), however, views MPD/DID as a complex false-self formation
and an inability to develop and use transitional objects; instead of representing an alternative form of transitional object, dissociative alter-personality construction may actually foreclose transitional experiencing. Alter
construction may in fact signal the incapacity to tolerate working in potential space where otherness may not always be omnipotently controllable or
playfully negotiated.

Brenner (1996) believes that attributing DID patients' deficits to impaired
use of transitional phenomena minimizes the importance of amnesia and altered states, and that "casual inspection of patient rooms in a dissociative
disorder inpatient program" yields indirect evidence affirming the use of

transitional objects in this population because they contain "more stuffed animals per capita than anywhere else in the hospital" (p. 157). In fact, however, the plethora of stuffed animals is probably evidence of DID patients' fetishistic and obsessive attachments to nonhuman objects.[2] Despite circumscribed manifestations of creativity consigned to specific alter personalities charged with distraction from pain, memories, and awareness of abuse, DID patients often have inhibited capacity for play. Some of their relationships with stuffed animals represent more of a collapse of the memory-imagination dialectic (Pye, 1995) than fantasy-proneness or effective use of transitional objects.

The issue is not whether severe dissociative disorders arise from fantasy proneness (as so many critics dismissively claim they do) or not, or whether the patients have overactive or underactive imaginations, or whether memories are only real or only false, but what kinds of limitations to fantasy and memory result from the trauma and defensive efforts at restitution of the self.[3] Working through the investment in some such efforts can even impact on the lifting of those limitations—as in each of three cases where Caucasian DID patients developed African-American alter personalities and strong identifications with African-American cultural icons. Their perpetrators had subscribed to White Supremacist ideologies and the victims had had to witness and participate in the kidnapping, torture, mutilation, and murder of kidnapped African Americans, sometimes children. Although the alters evolved to help the patients individuate from their traumatic environments and to master aspects of the guilt and shame associated with the atrocities, they also embodied the patients' respective capacities for protest, joy, and disaffiliation with the offenders—and, as the adaptive and defensive values of the cross-race alters were worked through in therapy, none of the three lost her affinity for African-American culture. That is, the capacity to play with adult forms of transitional experiencing actually increased while the more constricted need for specific alters to contain and isolate those patterns to particular part-selves faded.

In fact, DID and other severely dissociative patients vary a great deal in their use of fantasy and in their access to memory. When evaluating patients early in treatment, iatrogenic, fictitious, and malingering dimensions must always be taken into account. Some patients' dissociative systems show secondary and tertiary elaborations, and extreme levels of narcissistic investment in separateness with correspondingly high degrees of personification; others present very camouflaged, unimaginative, and constricted versions of DID.

Moderate- to higher-functioning DID outpatients tend to be disturbed by evidence of their multiplicity. Their investment in normal-unitary behavior leads to subtler presentations and less (at least for some time) elaboration of their personality systems (names, maps, personalities, definitions).

From a clinical standpoint, each subgroup presents its own difficulties: the inpatient's (sometimes flamboyant) narcissistic investment in separateness makes the working through of dissociative defenses more challenging, while the resistance to acknowledging the pathological multiplicity and the concomitant reticence to playing with identity construction and deconstruction in therapy handicaps intersubjective discourse with higher-functioning outpatients committed to camouflage. For the most part, the use of imagination among DID patients seems constricted even when they are obviously elaborating and personifying their systems for secondary gain. The themes of their fantasies are quite limited and repetitive, and any creativity polarizes into stereotypes and caricature qualities in many of their alters.

In DID, what may at first appear to be elaborate fantasy constructions turn out to be brittle and impermeable personified dissociative states that manifest in an unusually limited repertoire of behavior, affect, and cognition. Some alter personalities demonstrate more diversity, capacities, and elasticity than others—which is fortunate, because the by-products range from the potential for greater coconsciousness with other part-selves to the potential for greater participation in life and also in the therapy process. But other patients' alters excel only at specific tasks, functions, or attitudes that sustain the dissociative organization of self, as a result of the defensive development of parallel realities with limited internal space for the reconciliation of reality with fantasy.

From this perspective, dissociation can be conceptualized as another means of walling off experiences that cannot be transformed through fantasy—truly unassimilated, unassimilable experience. Alter personalities, then, are holding containers for pseudofantasy (*This is not my body. This is not my father. She made him hurt me. I am powerful. I don't feel. I wasn't there. I don't need anyone*), which operates on unmetabolized traumatic experience that has not been integrated by means of normal restorative fantasy.

THE SYMBOLIC REALM UNDER SIEGE

Repeated confrontation with mortality (Janoff-Bulman, 1992) and betrayal results in a massive disintegration of the symbolic world of the survivor of chronic child abuse, who has come to minimize contact with the external world in an effort to nullify the ideational, affective, and interpersonal effect of the traumatic spiral. Chronic trauma can thus be said to constrain symbolic elaboration and to sponsor a suppression or repetition of what limited symbolic functioning exists (Bollas, 1992). The disturbance in symbolizing capacity among sexual-abuse victims can severely constrict the ego's ability to represent elements of the trauma and its aftermath or to develop affective associative connections between the traumatic experiences and other sectors of the mind. In traumatized individuals the distinctions between reality and fantasy, remembering and reliving, and past and present, are either blurred or lost altogether as the innate capacities for self-observation and tolerance for ambiguity are overwhelmed by intrusions of powerful aggressive or sexualized transferences (Levine, 1990). These powerful transferences are rooted in posttraumatic reliving and also in how the trauma has deformed and perverted sexual and aggressive feelings and functions. The therapist may experience prolonged immersion in either affective deadness alone or in combination with volatile affect-states and sadomasochistic enactments before any of the patient's psychic material can be interpreted or mutually reflected upon.

At the very least, chronic trauma severely compromises a child's recuperative psychological capacities for fantasy, reflection, dreams, creativity, and play. (Even when the dissociative survivor has managed to maintain an outlet—or alter—for creative expression, and even when his/her artistic productions are ingenious and compelling, a constricted, repetitive character is, prior to therapy, consistently discernible.) In addition, chronic trauma survivors lose the capacity for wish-organized symbolic functioning (Auerhahn and Laub, 1987), and fail, because of traumatic impairment of the capacity for fantasy (Fish-Murray, Koby, and Van der Kolk, 1987), to use mental activity to transform traumatic experience. Fantasy, then, becomes conservative and preservative rather than mastery oriented and progressively constructive.

Where trauma cannot be transformed through fantasy operations, the child will resort to repetitive behavior and intrusive imagery in an effort to repeat or undo it. The world feels so fundamentally insecure that omnipotent fantasy solutions are not gradually relinquished but tenaciously retained. In the words of the main alter-group within one severely dissociative survivor of organized child abuse: "There is only me in a glass bubble watching and everyone else in the world who does cruel things. You [the therapist] aren't quite real, because I could have just invented you so you are really part of me. Or you could be one of 'them' in which case I cannot trust you. So either way I don't want to let you exist as a separate being I can't control."

Overexploitation of the imaginary to compensate for disappointments in the real interpersonal world after massive upheaval and chronic trauma is not the same as fantasy-proneness. The conservative, inflexible fantasy life of the severely dissociative individual is geared to preempting and controlling psychic damage; psychological survival is sustained at the cost of sacrificing most forms of intimate human relatedness and the freedom of psychological (intrapsychic) mobility. As Bromberg (1994) points out, the deformed imagination of severely dissociative patients is compounded by their continual reenactment of the experiential traumatic memory. Their simultaneous and steadfast avoidance of reflection upon and reexperiencing of trauma further restricts opportunities for both interpersonal and imaginal experiences of restitution.

Although Modell (1990) is impressed with the transformative possibilities inherent in symbolic and enacted repetitions of trauma in spite of their apparent impenetrability, these hope-inspiring notions of 'playing' with symbols and imaginary productions have given way in the severely dissociative patient's mind to other, more reified constructions. And the ability to create playfully has given way to fear of novelty such that behavioral discharge, amnesia, and numbing become the only options to having an inner life. In other words, the effort to work through and master trauma is replaced by massive efforts to (consciously) stay away from anything remotely resembling the trauma including fantasies, symbols, and dreams that bring reminders of the trauma to consciousness.

The severely dissociative patient's compromised imagination is fundamentally and paradoxically related to difficulties with reality testing, which involves more than merely intellectual and cognitive functions, according to Leowald (1974). He defines the relationship between the experiential testing of fantasy and an individual's full appreciation of reality as essentially interdependent, and defines the task of testing the "potential and suitability for actualization" of fantasy and "the testing of actuality—its potential for encompassing . . . and penetration [by] . . . one's fantasy life" as "a reciprocal transposition" (p. 368). The encapsulation of dissociative experiences and their impenetrability to modification by new relational and imaginal input lead to the atrophy of both reality-testing and fantasy capacities. Accordingly, both Leowald (1988) and Mitchell (1999) stress that an important goal of treatment is not simply the transformation of primary process into secondary process or the removal of the patient's distortions but the actual opening up of the potentially enhancing channels between fantasy and reality.

Bollas (1989) writes about the stylized, ritualized use of the internal world in extreme psychopathological conditions as the "ghostline world" or "playless space" (p. 129), a universe denuded of meaningful interplay between areas of mind that process internal and external reality. Forms of defensive concretization predominate, preserving or maintaining the dissociative organizations of self instead of promoting interactive transformative relatedness, such that the abused child no longer fantasizes escape or rescue or imagines retaliation, for example. Instead, s/he counts flowers on the wall, retreats to nothingness, or splits into part-selves that separately handle the hating, raping, memorializing, obliterating, and beating. The fragmented, dissociative self of the chronic trauma survivor, rigorously defended against intrusion or disruption and perpetually obsessed with its own imminent disintegration, does not have the luxury of entertaining renewal through nonthreatening forms of disorganization, regression, and recategorization.

Consequently, the patient may accuse the therapist of disloyalty and betrayal if s/he challenges dissociative solutions, sustains uncertainty and symbolic inquiry, or resists colluding with the patient's concretized responses to psychic pain and narcissistic or attachment needs. The patient may become enraged when the therapist proposes exploring why s/he wants to leave a small object behind in the office, preferring that the therapist accede without asking questions ("just do it"). The patient who tries to camouflage a potential reenactment of childhood sexual abuse or other boundary invasions as a simple request for empathic sensitivity, holding/containing, and/or generosity, becomes tyrannical when the therapist inquires about what is being concealed instead of addressing what is apparent. The therapist's inquiry is simultaneously perceived as rejection by the child-alters, as defiance by the internal perpetrators, and as irritatingly "therapist-like" behavior by the host/functional and collaborator-type personalities—all of which impressions may lead to a rupture (whereby the patient withdraws, ends the session, crawls under the desk, etc.) in the therapy relationship before the therapist can even determine what is fueling the affect storm.

INTEGRATING RESTORATION OF FANTASY AND
PARADOXICAL EXPERIENCING

The therapist may become the first transitional object the dissociative patient has ever experienced—"the first constant object, . . . the first lighthouse,
first North Star" (Marmer, 1996, p. 201). The therapist may be the first individual with whom all parts of the patient have relationships, the first to sustain an ongoing reality for all the alter-states. As each alter internalizes the
therapist's attitudes of inclusion and acceptance along with his/her challenges to dissociative modes of relatedness, the therapist is eventually experienced as a unified transitional object instead of as a collection of
transitional objects mirroring the patient's inner fragmentation and dividedness. In Marmer's analysis, the fulfillment of relational needs that will activate transitional functions is what allows the patient to reorganize
him/herself in a more integrated fashion for the first time.

To accomplish the formidable task of assisting the severely dissociative
patient with reactivating dialectical internal relations and developing transitional space, the therapist must adopt a posture that continuously opens up
avenues for restorative fantasy and play, especially with themes of destruction and attachment; s/he must resist unceasing seductive pulls toward
concretization—that is, replication of the dynamics of the original trauma—
and the collapse of potential space. The severely dissociative patient unconsciously strives for just that collapse of the therapy frame into a fantasyless
theater of concrete reenactments by enlisting alters who will not negotiate or
who insist they are the only ones, or that the multiplicity does not exist, by
generating threats and fears of violence, by requesting drugs, hypnosis, restraints, hospitalization, disability, by making demands for direct reparenting or excessive cancellations, extratherapeutic phone calls, and so on.
Inexperienced therapists or those intimidated by the patient, by ethical
dilemmas, by double binds and emotional blackmail (if-then proposals),
may even with the best intentions unwittingly participate in perpetuating
the central patterns and paradigms of pathological multiplicity—polarization, unbridled reenactments, concretization, domination, and false self-
construction.

Of course, the need for concrete intervention can on occasion eclipse the
need to restore transitional space in order for the therapist to protect the patient or the treatment or to jump-start symbolic processes and support the
working through of traumatic memories, and the patient's experience of

concrete protection to "survive destruction" (Winnicott, 1971) has the potential to enhance movement from concretized fantasy to symbolization. (For instance, internalizing the therapist's distress-response can lead to imagining rescue fantasies or to developing alternative approaches to the precipitating issues.)

There remains, however, the risk that the therapist will unconsciously participate in the maintenance of defensive multiplicity, omnipotence, and polarization, and under the rubric of effective intervention fail to steward the patient's advancement toward "potential space." This is most likely to occur when a therapist immediately seeks outside help because s/he is unable to contain—and too afraid to manage within the therapy dialogue—a patient's threats, self-destructive acting out, and aggressive energies. The patient's insecurity escalates with the mixed message of protection and betrayal/abandonment, which is reminiscent of the original trauma in which those elements were reversed in insidiously deceptive ways. Moreover, both parties may become increasingly dependent on outside support to manage their relationship.

For example, if a patient tells a therapist that s/he can only work through a disturbing memory in the hospital in restraints and if the therapist cooperates, especially without exploring the patient's obvious distrust of the therapist's capacity to provide containment and a suitable holding environment, the possible reenactment meanings of the request and the event would be buried. Or, more simply, if the therapist cooperates without examining whether the patient is actually ready for any such memory-processing (requiring concrete reenacting of the original trauma conditions), s/he may reinforce the defensive precocity and pseudo-autonomy the patient developed as a child to cope with overwhelming stress. Even by delaying action on the patient's suggestion while questioning, empathizing, and confronting at different points along the way, the therapist may become embroiled in a prolonged power struggle with the patient and the various alters who are advocating for hospitalization.

But by refusing to support the plan and insisting instead that the patient negotiate the different real and transferential meanings involved in the request, the therapist offers a new form of safety whereby the patient can discuss fantasies of restraint without having to enact them. Further, the dialogues that will ensue when the therapist opens for discussion his/her apparent failure to create the requisite climate of safety and trust in the treatment space can increase the intimacy and security of the therapy relationship and demonstrate the importance of reflection and multiple solutions to complex problems. The therapist thus models collaborative dialogue and mutuality in preference to dominance/submission and soothing through concretization, and still makes way for the patient's associations to childhood experience.

Similarly, when a patient makes unreasonable demands (for medications, physical contact, "special" privileges, multiple therapists, excessive or extratherapeutic contact) and the therapist agrees without extensive negotiation—perhaps out of his/her countertransference fears and anxieties, or perhaps because s/he and the patient have cocreated a situation in which the therapist, feeling like a victimized child, needs to enlist powerful authorities to protect them both—a collapse of transitional space is likely to occur independent of whatever crisis the patient has concocted to test the treatment or reenact traumatic patterns. Once again, the patient may feel unconsciously betrayed and will continue to seek the kind of holding environments where only concrete controls are believed to provide safety, where human beings are seen as helpless bystanders too afraid or too weak to confront and experience the patient's agonies directly.

From this perspective, effective treatment of severe dissociative patients must do more than suppress alter personalities with posthypnotic suggestions and ritualized integrations, perhaps reinforcing false-self organization and the collapse of symbolic functions (Smith, 1989). Rushing in prematurely to lower anxiety with action or directed fantasy to attain forgiveness, revenge, restitution, compensation, or even "safe places" without sufficient analysis, grief, and mourning can be tantalizing bait for therapists and patients alike. Therapists, too, welcome immediate tension reduction and soothing when immersed in chronically stressful conditions, and they may find themselves jumping into solutions they never would have dreamed of enacting with nondissociative patients just to avoid escalating the levels of fear and dread in the room.

Gaining the capacity to grieve or to fantasize retaliation and forgiveness and enjoy doing so is a major developmental achievement for most severely dissociative patients—an achievement that comes on its own when an ambience of mutuality, negotiation, and transitional experiencing is promoted through the implicit and explicit interventions of the therapist. Likewise, gaining the capacity for free association, a crucial element (often taken for granted) in the reactivation of restorative fantasy operations, represents significant realignment of developmental processes.

No such capacities can be foisted on the patient prematurely, however, to satisfy his/her or the therapist's need for completion of an abreactive or developmental process. Nor should alternative fantasies (i.e., alternatives to the trauma that the patient can hold on to) be cultivated by the therapist for, and foisted on, the patient to avert their having to sit with helplessness and despair. After doing just that, sitting with their pain, and experiencing its containment, witnessing, and even to some degree sharing, most dissociative patients begin without prompting to provide their own antidotes to the reliving of traumatic experience, having internalized the therapist's trust of their innate capacities to tolerate affect and restore fantasy.

The suggestion popularized in some of the early MPD literature to develop hypnotically induced "safe places" may work temporarily to create an illusion of safety but may leave the patient unduly dependent upon the therapist to do so and may actually foreclose the patient's own activation of restorative fantasy capacities, and may, in the end, fail to create any enduring fantasies of safety. In many cases therapist and patient have developed elaborate rituals—that sometimes take one-third of a session—for placing each alter personality in his/her own preferred special safe place. Such immediately helpful concrete enactments serve to manage other anxieties (usually hostile, sometimes erotic feelings in both patient and therapist) by submerging them; only on the surface do they support the patient's use of fantasy, and since repetitive rituals are tedious and boring they probably play to child-alters invested in reparenting.

The patient is after all an adult. Play therapy with child alters is not the same as play therapy with real children. Highly nurturant therapists who find this kind of ritual rewarding and soothing would be well-advised to examine their interactions and countertransference anxieties to guard against avoidant, constrictive, or destructive enactments that suppress the patient's maturation and development. By the same token, therapists who are reluctant to engage in safety rituals should examine whether they are acting out the role of the depriving or withholding caretaker of childhood.

In any event, a traumatized patient can derive feelings of safety by such other means as discussing insecurity and danger with the therapist, surviving making criticisms of the therapist, or interacting in other ways that articulate and disentangle the confusion between the past and the present. So the demand by a patient trained in the "safe places" strategy by prior therapists for help in imagining safe houses for each of his/her alters at the end of a session as a way of self-soothing, containing, and closing down is an invitation to wonder about its potential for mutating transitional experiencing into fetishistic experiencing and unanalyzed dependency. It is also an opportunity to ask about feelings of unsafety, about what might be going on in or missing from the current relationship to trigger a need for directed imagination. Further, the pain of separation and the processing of meanings and feelings about the ending of sessions may get eclipsed by these ritualized endings. Jointly surviving some of the power struggles that initially emerge from discussions of those issues both reduces the patient's anxiety and increases the ability to sit with feelings of pain, rage, loss, fear, dread, abandonment, helplessness, and endangerment that is the hallmark of integration.

The therapist must become the guardian of the realm of the symbolic. When his/her wishful thinking mirrors the magical solutions used by the dissociation-prone child to cope with massive trauma, the patient will continue to act out and engage in self-destructive behavior. The patient will not be able to internalize anything from relationship with a therapist whose "best efforts" entail, for instance, the exchange with the patient of excessive personal material to promote feelings of attachment and safety and the crowding of his/her office with examples of same. Indeed, objects from the therapist's office given to promote attachment, transitional experiencing, or help soothe immense anxieties about separation should become part of the ongoing dialogues. They are not magical tokens that should never be discussed again. Since DID patients can become fetishistically attached to objects, variously refusing to return them, developing very ritualized uses for them, or sometimes breaking them, the mere act of assigning transitional objects to DID patients hardly guarantees in and of itself the cultivation of transitional experiencing.

Negotiating from within the transference/countertransference dialogue is the clinician's best tool for monitoring the arena where reality and fantasy can blend and be articulated. When verbal expressions of terror, rage, hatred, and love replace obsessive requests for hypnotically created or concrete evidence of safety, progress is usually being made on all developmental fronts, and, more often than not, the patient's spontaneous use of self-protective and restorative fantasy follows naturally on the heels of restored affectivity. Psychotherapy must help the patient develop the capacity to bear and integrate anxiety and psychic pain and make room for an intermediate space, a space of illusion, while relinquishing omnipotent defenses and beliefs, addictions to substances, psychic numbing, and pathological identifications with perpetrators and collaborators. In this transitional zone, creativity, faith, and multiple meanings can be explored as the severely dissociative patient's urgency to concretize and to "know" gives way to a toleration for ambiguity, "not knowing," and the synthesis of new meanings for his or her personal history (Schwartz, 1994).

Within transitional experiencing, multiple realities being held by different self-states can find opportunities for linkage (Bromberg, 1994). Through the quality of language that emerges from participation in, and mutual reflection on, the patient's enactments, cognitive symbolization actually supplants the dissociative language often used by the patient to manage his/herself (selves) and avert the danger at once denied and anticipated. According to Bromberg, that cognitive symbolization becomes a new medium for transitional relating, and for the new, more flexible and imaginative self-narratives created in an ambience of such relating. Positing an important developmental trajectory where self-reflection and intrapsychic conflict-resolution achieve ascendancy over dissociation, Bromberg believes that a new experience of reality is also developed—one that goes beyond only the perceptual and interpersonal. By maintaining a therapeutic posture that values transitional experiencing, that protects the boundaries and frame of therapy in order to sustain what Moore (1991) calls "a sacred transformational space," the therapist becomes a "steward" rather than a director of liminal or potential space.

RESTORATION OF HEALTHY AGGRESSION

What a beautiful garbage dump therapy can be. Generations of psychic pollutants pour into therapy. The beauty of therapy survives them. How beautiful the ocean in spite of all the waste it metabolizes. Can it keep up with the toxins? (Eigen, 1996, p. 177)

Destruction of the natural and healthy aggressive, assertive, and self-protective functions of the psyche is one of the most insidious results of chronic child-abuse trauma. Some severely dissociative patients have absolutely no access to any anger—aside from virulent and repetitive self-hatred—that can be directed anywhere, especially toward any authority figure from the past. Other patients (or specific alters within them) remain perpetually angry with their therapists for real, imagined, and especially deflective purposes. They use anger to discourage dialogues about traumatic memories and affects, and, perhaps most of all, to forestall any implicit threats to their attachment to perpetrators. These patients seem unable to become angry at any of their family members until later in treatment, in spite of remembering or recovering and believing in their own abuse accounts, no matter how awful. Still other traumatized, dissociative patients engage in ongoing conflict and angry outbursts at a host of authorities in daily life—from bosses to employees and managers of hotels, restaurants, and car-rental agencies who in any way slight them or stimulate feelings of unfair treatment or betrayal. Never able to be angry at those who violated them the most, these individuals go about life making scenes, demanding redress and amends from vague or impersonal "power" figures, and end up alienating many people in their lives.

Untreated or minimally treated severely dissociative patients tend to be kind to those among their intimates who treat them abusively, inconsistently, or exploitatively; in their behavior to those who treat them caringly, fear, cruelty, and hatred alternate with moments of appreciation and recognition (usually when they sense that the other is fed up with their antics). Real emotional intimacy is extremely difficult to develop and sustain because aggression is completely upside down in the psyches of most severely dissociative trauma survivors. In keeping with the empirical correlation between how bad the abuse history and how long it takes for the patient to mobilize anger at the perpetrators, victims of organized child-abuse groups that relied on torture and mind control to co-opt their dissociative self-organizations are those in whom anger retardation reaches its zenith.

FORMS AND TRANSFORMATIONS OF AGGRESSION IN SEVERELY DISSOCIATIVE PATIENTS

- Despite being placed on a locked unit and closely monitored during her early treatment, Sara (whose host and functional alters remained completely amnestic) split off into sadistic perpetrator alter personalities who carved pentagrams onto her arms in blocks of odd numbers until she reached the number thirteen; once she had carved thirteen pentagrams on her arms and hands, she began the entire self-mutilation mathematics all over again.
- Following upsetting phone calls from her "former" perpetrator father, Diane split off into hostile and perpetrator alter-states, burned herself

with cigarettes, broke light bulbs and cut herself, and in one instance carved the words "I hate you" and "fuck you" on her breasts.

- Following a series of conflicts with her therapist, and experiencing extreme feelings of betrayal and distrust, Thea, a polyfragmented DID patient broke into her therapist's office and read the files of several patients, including her own. She did not reveal these actions to her therapist for several weeks.

- Whenever memories of coerced perpetration against animals and other children begin to surface in Justin's consciousness, he would fly into fits of rage and smash his hands against hard surfaces and valuable objects in a desperate attempt to contain and deflect the rage that was once co-opted by his perpetrators to be directed against others; Justin relies upon his hands to earn his living.

- Anna is a DID patient with severe diabetes and other health-related problems; she had hostile alters in her system who created amnesia barriers for the others so that they forget to take their insulin, precipitating recurrent medical crises.

- Stacey, a severely dissociative, ritual-abuse survivor reveals (or alleges) to her therapist that she is still actively involved in her family's intergenerational perpetrator group and has been reporting on the goings-on in her therapy through one of her mind-control-trained "informer" alter personalities; Stacey eventually declares that the group has been monitoring the movements of the therapist and his family and has people stalking his children at their school. Finally, her hostile alters announce that the perpetrator group is considering kidnapping and using one of his children in a ritual sacrifice.

- Deciding to use stuffed animals to communicate with her child-alters, Mira, a ritual-abuse survivor with severe dissociative patterns reveals that when she wakes up in the morning she finds the "children's" favorite one completely dismembered and disfigured; every time she sews it back together, hostile alters on the other side of an amnesia barrier emerge and cut up the stuffed animal again. These alters leave Mira and the therapist a note in red ink stating that the children must not be allowed to get attached to anything or anyone and that further efforts to repair the damage will only lead to more damage.

- Julia hears hateful voices in her head calling her "filthy slut," "worthless whore," and "stupid cunt"; she believes these names represent the hidden but ultimate truth about who she is. "Somehow" these

voices take over and leave burns on her body and make her beat herself with belts and whips—sometimes "against her will," sometimes
with her "compliance."

- Roberta, a DID patient with a confusing symptom profile alternately
  accelerates revelations of childhood violence and threatens, first subtly, then overtly, to report the therapist to state authorities and the
  False Memory Syndrome Foundation for willingness to believe her;
  some alters support, reassure, and plead on behalf of the therapist,
  while others continue to threaten and contemptuously deride the
  therapist for considering historical truth in the patient's material.

- Delia, a severely dissociative patient with a history of multiple hospitalizations, multiple suicide attempts, and multiple treatment failures
  reveals to her therapist that she has been in treatment with another
  therapist for the last 18 months of their relationship; Delia managed
  to obtain reduced fees from both therapists for multiple visits to each
  per week, has different parts of herself in relationship with each therapist, and has kept all of this a secret from both therapists for the entire 18 months.

- The hostile alters of Maureen, a polyfragmented DID patient, sought
  reprisals (for perceived neglect, abandonment, and other narcissistic
  injuries) against inpatient hospital staff and a particular patient on
  her unit. During the week when that patient was responsible for care
  of the unit's large aquarium, Maureen sneaked into the dayroom and
  took several of the fish out of the tank; she held them in her hands until they were almost dead, then returned them to the tank to struggle
  with shock and stress. At the next morning's community meeting,
  Maureen began a campaign against the patient charged with aquarium care and the director of the milieu program, accusing them of ne-
  glecting their duties and "murdering the fish."

Dissociative identity disorder represents, among other things, a thwarted
and fragmented aggressive response to chronic trauma.[4] Individuals subjected to prolonged, repeated trauma develop insidious forms of aggression
that invade and erode the personality (Eigen, 1992): hyperarousal to emotional and sensory stimuli (Kardiner, 1941; Krystal, 1978; Lindemann, 1944);
automatic and urgently repetitive destructive and self-destructive behavior
(Grossman, 1991); provocation of attacks on themselves by abused children
at play, and assaults on others (Galenson, 1986; Glenn, 1978), modulating ag-

gression by oscillating between uncontrollable expressions of rage and absolute intolerance of aggression in any form (Van der Kolk, 1987b). These extremes may be so polarizing that the same individual will have a history of multiple violent enactments against self and others and absolute intolerance for even the fantasied pain of, say, cut vegetables or flowers (Schwartz, 1994).

HOSTILE/AGGRESSIVE ALTERS

The DID individual, infused with chronic painful bodily and emotional experiences at an early age and isolated from soothing/restorative responses, is unable to direct the hyperstimulated arousal of aggression toward the sources of injury. The fear of abandonment by the abuser/caretaker forces the child into states of abject compliance and submission by developmental necessity—but as Freud (1930) so clearly stated, obedience does not exorcise aggression; rather it directs aggression against the self. In Freud's terms, authoritarian arrangements produce aggression that devolves into forms of self-domination, and the individual's own conscience becomes suffused with the hostility that cannot be directed at the unassailable authority.

DID/MPD dissociative solutions to this dilemma include the creation of alters who are fearfully compliant, proudly collaborative, or tenderly loving in relation to the psychopathology and tyranny of the impinging parent/caretakers; other defiant, aggressive alters are "secretly" constructed around counteridentifications to evade impinging others and eventually impinging memories (and concomitant fantasies), and still other alters are constructed according to elaborate rules of counterdependence.

Hostile alter personalities serve as a kind of trauma membrane in the multiple personality internal world (Putnam, 1989), and function aggressively like personified narcissistic and sociopathic defenses. They regulate the flow of information and memory; discharge aggressive and sexual tension states; maintain and protect remnants of the grandiose self; defend against the experience of hope, guilt, shame, vulnerability, disappointment; and attempt to prevent the reshattering of previously shattered fantasies of self in relation to self-object (Kohut, 1977). Deformed and derailed as they might appear, the severely dissociative individual's aggressive alter personalities contain much of the life force of the pretraumatized individual (Putnam, 1989).

Most experienced clinicians treating dissociative patients agree that it is essential to engage aggressive alters in a therapeutic alliance that recognizes their value and potential for healthy self-protection and differentiation; at times, it can be important to meet their force with counterforce. Hostile alters, usually the most underappreciated and misrecognized aspects of the self are not merely drive-derivatives of aggression or responses to empathic failure; they represent efforts—faulty efforts—at self-restoration, self-preservation, and shame avoidance. (The more they are identified with perpetrators—and the more they have been forced to participate in perpetration against others—the more shame they are holding and defending against experiencing.) Concretized and elaborated over time and in response to different developmental challenges, hostile alters are originally created by the child (in some cases with the direct help and shaping of the perpetrators) so that s/he could survive physically and psychologically (Putnam, 1989; Ross, 1989; 1997). When there is no soothing or ventilation of the injury, coping is accomplished through dissociation and personification of defenses paralleling identification with (or imitation of) the aggressor. These are the only tools of power left to the powerless.

Because the abused child's ability to sustain attachment (see Chapter 8 for elaboration of attachment dilemmas) depends upon the dissociative compartmentalization of aggression rather than on the direct expression or conscious experience of that aggression, the child comes to identify his/her own angry behavior and aggressive feelings as threatening rather than those of the predator/perpetrator (Howell, 1997); she may, accordingly, also dissociate unexpressed and inexpressible terror, pain, and helpless rage. The resulting protector self-state now must vigilantly monitor the child's behavior for anything that would be threatening to the attachment figure. "The fact that protection may require the vigilant monitoring, even persecution, of the ordinary self in order to curtail its potentially attachment-threatening behavior is what makes for the dual role of protector and persecutor" (p. 242). As the protector—who has been holding the rage and averting the provocation of dangerous others through preemptive persecution or criticism of his/her compliant and masochistic part-selves—becomes increasingly persecutory, its aggressivity can inflate into "cruel sport."[5]

The developing child relieves him/herself of rage, and knowledge of betrayal (Freyd, 1996), by placing (and reversing) thoughts and feelings onto other personality segments and then walling them off (Putnam, 1989; Ross, 1989; 1997). Since such alters come into existence to protect survival, their greatest fear is their own annihilation—being destroyed or literally killed by the therapist or others—often concretizing their anticipation of psychic disintegration in the face of powerful affects, dependent feelings, or any other kind of vulnerability.

Many internal persecutors begin as internal friends or helpers; some even evolve from imaginary playmates (Kluft, 1985a). Certain helper personalities initially created to suffer abuse have come over time to identify with the aggressor/abuser and to resent suffering for the other personalities (Putnam, 1989). Other aggressive and criminal personalities are specifically shaped through ongoing participation in organized perpetrator groups, where split-off aspects of the self, elicited and molded through behavior modification, torture, drugs, and elaborate mind-control procedures operate independently of the rest of the personality system and sustain ardent allegiance to the group and its ideologies. These hostile cult-type alters believe themselves guilty of complicity in all sorts of real and imagined crimes; silenced and enslaved by guilt and shame and sealed over by prideful identifications with the power of the group leaders—along with contempt for those outside of the group—they feed off the fear of other parts of the patient's system and of people (including the therapist) outside it.[6]

Frankel and O'Hearn (1996) identify subsets of hostile/aggressive alters in their classification system of alter personalities based on the social organization of the Eastern European Jewish ghettos during World War II (see Chapter 1). While some dissociated aggression manifests through help-seeking alters—essentially maladaptive role players who carry the burden of posttraumatic stress disorder symptoms and may be substance abusers or promiscuous or suicidal—most split-off aggression in DID is located in the "anti-bonding force," which consists of the following subsets.

Enforcers, often arrogant and challenging, are persecutory alters who are anesthetic to pain and amnestic for the circumstances surrounding their original emergence in the system. They control the system by force, threat, intimidation, and inciting acts of self-harm.

Deniers, self-blamers, and approval seekers divert and mislead the clinician and seek to discourage or distort the disclosure of newly emerging traumatic material. It is they who facilitate ongoing contact with perpetrators and instill denial both inside and outside the system, and it is they who create the internal conditions whereby all other alters are constantly questioning their reality. They use self-blame to create chronic doubt and to steer bonding with the clinician off-course.

Internal leaders, generally the most dominant group in the system, are often hidden behind the other groups of alters. They discourage bonding with the therapist for fear it will put the entire internal system in danger; they also distort and reframe information and experience to match perpetrator ideologies and belief systems.

Independence forces trust absolutely no one inside or outside of the dissociative system, including any of the sources to whom they report even though they may pretend to have temporary allegiances; they are completely self-serving. By warning of impending disaster to protect survival or guarding distrust as a survival strategy when other alters appear to be growing too comfortable with the therapy relationship, they can function to stabilize or disrupt at the same time.

According to Frankel and O'Hearn, these alters have a wide-angle perspective and "special dispensation to move about the internal system with a kind of limited immunity" (p. 501). While their observational acuity is potentially useful, they generally provoke chaos and havoc in therapy, at times *impersonating* alters from other groups. Personal clinical experience reveals that the greater a patient's exposure to a totalist, sadistic family system and/or to organized child abuse, the greater the likelihood that his/her dissociated aggression will mutate into Frankel and O'Hearn's diverse forms. All hostile alters, whether directly or indirectly shaped in response to perpetrators' messages, attitudes, and behaviors exist in a world of omnipotent rage and grandiose thinking. They can represent the extremes of collusion with the authoritarian paradigms of domination—and the only solution the traumatized self could develop to maintain the capacity to subvert authority through simultaneous maintenance and avoidance of attachments. Virtually all hostile alters are the terrorized, shame-ridden child- and adolescent-aspects of the personality who have seen and internalized the worst of human interactional patterns—those built on domination, betrayal, and duplicity. Their belief systems are based on particularly bitter and sardonic worldviews where sadism and control are the only pleasures left in a world devoid of protection or benevolent relationship.

Some hostile alters mutilate the body and set up dangerous situations including rape or other violence. Some sabotage treatment by convincing the patient to miss sessions, distrust the therapist, or drop out of therapy altogether, or by taking over the personality at certain specific times so the other personalities "forget" their therapy appointments. Some distract the patient's patterns of thinking and listening with chants, number-counting, headaches, or psychic fog to the point that they can interfere with the person's job and social functioning. However, by transforming themselves from the one threatened to the one making the threat, by shifting from passive into active modes of assimilating trauma and mastering anxiety-provoking experiences, hostile alters harbor the patient's capacity for healthy protest response and, ultimately, for separation from attachments to perpetrators.

A therapist's initial engagements with hostile alters may not be easy. And an alter's first contact with the therapist, beyond acting out or passively influencing other alters in ways that disrupt the treatment and the patient's life, usually entails some maneuver conceived to interfere with a genuine human connection. Created to deflect attention from traumatic memory and from revelation of the pathological multiplicity that concretizes their ongoing psychological mobilization for disaster, hostile alters seek to intimidate at the outset through displays of adolescent rage, obstinacy, and contempt.

SARA

Sara, who had managed to carve satanic pentagrams all over her arms repeatedly while "contained" on a locked unit in a psychiatric hospital in an astonishing display of dissociative aggression (and enterprise) following attempts to engage her hostile alters in dialogue, wrote me letters in the early stages of treatment.

"We think you are a sneaky slimy son-of-a-bitch who is out to get what you can. Maybe you think you're better than we are and you know more but you know NOTHING about us and how we are and how we work and you never will so you can just go fuck yourself and the whole fucking world. DO you understand? WE HATE YOU . . . We don't trust you, we don't like you. We don't trust or like anyone. We don't come to see you because there is nothing to talk about. We are just fine with hating everyone and everything and there's nothing wrong with that. We don't even trust each other and we don't have to. We're writing this jointly because we all think the same way on this. There is no reason why we have to like each other and we don't. So you can just stop being confrontative with that slut [the host personality] because we're never coming to you and we think that's just fine that she hates us too—this is mutual all the way around. Now she has to pay for trying to get through to us. And everything she tries, she will have to pay for it. We want her to hate us; we have no need for friends or understanding. All we want is for her and you to leave us alone. Goodbye from us."

In this case I chose to value what certainly appears to be a refusal to engage in treatment as an introduction to important parts of this patient that were based on radical self-sufficiency, intense shame, humiliated rage, strange bonds (but bonds nonetheless) to perpetrators, and a prideful refusal to trust anyone. By not backing down from contact with these parts and by insisting on the merits of communication while continuing to value the resistances to communication, I was eventually able to break the stalemate. In the end—and this is often the case—it was the patient's host personality and functional alters who were the most resistant to dialogue with the angry part-selves. Disrupting the dichotomies and internal polarizations they represent is a central task of treatment.

Restabilizing Aggression

Healthy aggression leads to essential developmental achievements in the areas of differentiation and capacity for love, play, mutuality, and fantasy (Winnicott, 1971). There is no way to avoid fury in childhood, according to Winnicott; the crucial factor is how this fury is met with by others. When all self-assertion, agency, and efforts at individuation (including thinking one's own thoughts) threaten the omnipotence and narcissistic equilibrium of the child's abusers, their reactions (rage, retaliation, abandonment) foster a developmental "freeze" in crucial areas. Everything related to aggression is experienced in omnipotent form, forced back into the intrapsychic realm, and fantasized as dangerous, and the victim keeps aggression dammed up in the internal dissociative matrix with no safe flow to the intersubjective world. With no expectation of welcome for, recognition of, or dialogue about anger, rage, or individuation strivings, the severely dissociative trauma survivor withdraws into excessive internalization and reenactment of abandonment/retaliation scenarios.

Since mental organization acquires some of its most significant characteristics as the child learns to express and regulate aggression (Grossman, 1991), working through the aggressive aspects of DID is a central reorganizing aspect of the psychotherapy process. It involves accepting and empathizing with the personified villains and demons and helping patients to apprehend compassionately these self-preservative shadow aspects of themselves—which, in fact, become destructive only when ignored or devalued (or programmed by perpetrators and split off from the agency and control of the rest of the personality system). Effective treatment also encompasses collisions with the therapist's power and value system, interpretations of the strengths and limitations of the alters' worldviews and methods of self-protection, and challenges to dangerous manipulations, cover-ups, and policies of deceit and omission.

Misconstruing motivations of hostile aspects of the self can be a major precipitant of violence and acting-out episodes. An overtolerant stance toward the dissociative patient's power plays can lead to regressive spirals of disorganization and disintegration of functioning—but the therapist committed to support restoration of a healthy protest response to welcoming all forms of anger into the therapy relationship is up against some difficult decisions. S/he has to determine when to empathize with what seems to be important communication about the therapist-patient interaction and when to confront blatant manipulations that enable sadistic acting out, replays of traumatic relational patterns, and most commonly avoidance of difficult feelings and conflicts, particularly about threats and challenges to attachments with perpetrators.

Successful treatment involves substantial engagement with hostile (and perpetrator-identified) aspects of the patient where an invitation into the intersubjective dialogue can be experienced as safely containing and negotiating aggression between the parameters of validation and limit setting. The accumulation of such engagements (e.g., where anger is dialogue rather than action, where fighting is safe, etc.), gently disrupts the sense of omnipotence that organizes and orchestrates dissociative life: aggressive alter personalities who boast about their sense of power will begin to admit feelings of vulnerability; compliant part-selves, cowering before conflict or any revelation of their own sadism, will become acquainted with the creative processes of diplomacy, assertion, resistance, and confrontation. Empathic acknowledgments of breakdowns in therapeutic rapport represent significant interventions because they demonstrate the therapist's benevolent use of power and solidify the patient's tentative expectation that restitution can follow disruption, an experience central to fostering healthy restructuralization of self (Kohut, 1971; 1977).

Negotiating with intrapsychic (and at times, interpersonal) terrorism is not a simple task, however. The dissociative patient's projections of, and seductive counterinvitations to, abandonment and retaliation can be relentless during some phases of treatment. Following Winnicott's (1971) assertion that the developing child must be permitted to continually create and destroy the other in fantasy to discover the durability of the other in reality, several psychoanalytic theorists (Benjamin, 1990; Eigen, 1981; 1996; Ghent, 1990) emphasize the developmental necessity of healthy collisions between self and other for establishing a sense of externality and engendering the capacity to maintain the tension between omnipotence and recognition of reality without constricting into the polarized identifications that are the hallmark of aggression in severe dissociative conditions. For Eigen and Winnicott, survival of the patient's destructive assaults (on self and others) leads to surrendering of false-self solutions and to the patient finally believing that s/he can really use another person for his/her growth. When the patient (or alter) systematically attacks the therapist's benevolence, the therapist must hold in mind that the patient deeply (often secretly) wishes for survival of the very goodness under attack.

Dialogues with hateful, vengeful, and demonized aspects of the self must take place so that the patient can deflate some of his or her omnipotent fantasies of aggression. For many hostile alters, the experience of having their hateful feelings symbolized, verbalized, and witnessed by a therapist who does not back away in disgust or fear from emotional contact is powerful enough to catalyze the building of bridges to other parts of the self. Curiosity, inquiry, and mirroring emergent aggression (in such forms as detailed, bloody vengeance-scenarios; joyous reveling in sadistic fantasies; colorful invectives directed toward the therapist) must guide the therapeutic process, supplanting the patient's passive-aggressive, acting-out, and self-injurious forms of expressing aggression.

Beneath the reenactments, the severely dissociative patient is seeking a new reparative object relationship to mobilize his/her derailed development. Effective treatment calls for a therapist who can empathize with and survive (without being overwhelmed by) deep and dissociated terror, rage, and hate, so as to render him/her at once less intimidating and less intimidated by his/her own aggression. Specifically, most people with DID have never learned how to say "yes" or "no" from a position of self-ownership and self-authorship. Traumatically induced compliant "yesses" and sequestered defiant "nos" (and extreme passive-aggressive behavior) have filled the void where no solid core self or will once existed (Schwartz, 1994). Organic protest responses have been disrupted and extinguished (Van der Kolk, 1987a).

Slavin (1997) writes about the importance of the patient's recovering a sense of agency from the process of recovering memories. Therefore, the pacing and timing of the regressive aspects of the therapy work and ownership of the memory retrieval process (including assessment of the relative veracity of the memories) must remain firmly in the hands of the patient. This approach will prevent even the therapist with the best of intentions from making the fundamental error of inadvertently subverting the patient's will and agency as a result of either overzealousness or intrusive skepticism or credulity. The therapist must encourage and respond authentically to all forms of the patient's protest responses, regardless of how provocative or camouflaged, in order to maintain an invitation for the patient to say no in every conceivable way while a therapeutic alliance based on mutuality rather than on compliance or defiance is being forged and strengthened.

The fractured developmental line of aggression can be recovered through empathic confrontation (Chu, 1992a), exploratory inquiry into instances of dissociative flight, and repeated successful collisions with the therapist and the frame of psychotherapy. The patient experiences the vulnerabilities and strengths of the therapist who remains unafraid of the patient and the patient's material and/or speaks honestly of his/her fears and concerns; concomitantly, the patient's omnipotent fantasies of destructiveness are worked through. The patient thus tolerates and sustains contact through conflict. S/he reflects on affirmative and negative responses and develops and delivers them with coherence, consistency, and space for negotiation. Formerly violent somatic communication on the body-self in the face of misrecognition, fear, or pain is transformed into verbal expressivity and the confident expectation of empathy in the face of hurts and disruptions in rapport.

One of the many ways concretized aggression manifests in treatment of severely traumatized, dissociative individuals—both inside and outside of the consulting room—involves weapons. Clinicians frequently have to work through issues involving dangerous drugs, knives, and guns with patients in order to establish firmer treatment alliances and to understand the inner dynamics of the their systems. The encounter with and mastery of fear, danger, and threat in the countertransference opens a channel for symbolic communication; variously, the patient may turn in guns to the police or unload and turn them in to the therapist (who then either turns them in to the police or safely contains them in accord with a joint agreement).

RENA

Early in treatment many hostile alters competed with the therapist for control of Rena, a particularly fragmented patient. When the therapist announced plans to take a vacation, a new alter—and the new issue of guns—emerged.

During the vacation this alter, who typically spent hours loading and unloading and stroking her guns as a form of self-soothing, convinced the others in the internal system that the therapist was dead. When treatment resumed, it took several weeks of reworking the fears and pain about the vacation for a number of the alters to realize how they had been "managed" by the powerful hostile alter, who had essentially created a set of false memories about the therapist's death (not an uncommon scenario).

The realization exposed further splits in the patient's system: parts wanted to keep the guns, parts found them an ever-present danger. Manipulating the guns (and manipulating other alters and the therapist about the guns) was the only way the hostile alters could protect flooding of affect and the release of too much dangerous information at once. It turned out that several were hidden in different locations; each was a secret revealed by some alters who angered the others by telling the therapist about it. Guns were clearly a preferred attachment alternative: they didn't talk back or ask questions—and they didn't take vacations. Frightened alters made desperate phone calls to the therapist, in whom great anxiety about suicidal possibilities was created ("The gun is in my hand, what do I do now?" or "He [another alter] is threatening to kill me, can you help?"). At the same time as patient and therapist were negotiating about power and the limits of the therapist's control and addressing issues of attachment and abandonment, suspense and morbid anticipation-reenactments were taking place.

After the therapist tried talking the patient down on the phone (unload the gun, put it in a new place, check in the next day), it was apparent that her agreeing to a no-harm contract would not work and that she had to turn in all her guns in order for treatment to proceed. This became a nonnegotiable condition, having to do with "safety first" issues and also with the impossibility of finding new solutions to self-soothing and self-protection needs in the presence of such concrete options. The therapist had personally to confront the subtle intimidation message, and to make room for some of the alters' feelings of betrayal about the vacation.

Standing firm about the absolute necessity that the guns be turned in before further treatment could take place, the therapist provided enough containment for the patient to persuade the hostile alters to try to go along with therapist's views of safety. After the guns were turned in, however, two more appeared: seeing a hole in the therapist's holding functions and feeling unsafe at some level, the hostile alters went out and bought others, generating another round of confrontation and negotiation.

When the therapist set a final limit, a deeper sense of balance was restored in the patient's system, where the hostile alters—sensing the therapist's strength and commitment and ongoing lack of fear and openness to dialogue, discovered a new and pivotal level of communication and bonding with the therapist. Giving up the guns did bring about more disorganization and disintegration besides—but increased contact with the therapist and the addition of very low-dose major tranquilizers to the medication regimen gave the therapist more access to more alters and led in turn to a higher level of integration and overall stabilization.

Before there was relief, however, the hostile alters, sensing the intensity of affect and pain, escalated arguments for the use of knives as a less dangerous but still soothing alternative to both guns and the current decline in functioning. The therapy dialogues then proceeded to take on the most difficult issues of all—trust, protection, attachment, and betrayal, and the question of whether or not any human being in the entire universe was big and strong enough to handle all of this patient's pain and aggression.

The fact that the therapist chose not to immediately hospitalize the patient or call the police but instead spent some time negotiating, inquiring, and assisting and then stepped in with a firm and rigid limit created the space between the therapist and patient where human relationship could be brought to conflicts the patient had only previously dealt with on her own. When patient and therapist continually relate in such a way that the concrete, literal quality of the patient's aggression is contained in a holding environment of shared responsibility and mutual reflection, the disparate self-states and full range of the patient's self-narratives (and the full range of his/her perceptual apparatus) are embraced within a single relational field (Bromberg, 1994). In this view, the dissociative patient's limitations in both the domains of aggression and fantasy and the constricted and repetitive narrative structures that maintain dissociation "as though the past

were still a present danger" (p. 539) are resolved by the creation of new realities between the therapist and patient. This therapeutic ambience honors
the patient's dissociative self-remedies of the past while forging more integrated protest—and imaginative responses to intrapsychic and interpersonal conflicts and challenges.

There is a small subset of hostile/perpetrator alters (and dissociative patients in general) who may impede treatment severely, sometimes permanently. Such alters represent one or all of the following: programmed, highly
trained perpetrator-identified part-selves created through torture, operant
and classical conditioning techniques, hypnosis, and the extreme manipulation of shame and guilt by organized perpetrator-groups; nonnegotiable
commitment to either a criminal way of life or an extreme or corrupt political or spiritual ideology; the products of repeated, failed, or abusive therapies in addition to massive early traumatization; personifications of what
Rosenfeld (1971) called "destructive narcissism," whereby they cannot tolerate the therapist's efforts to unmask their underlying worth or goodness because they experience shame for not being cruel or malevolent enough.

In this bizarre reversal, a therapist may be construed as a perpetrator, not
for hurting or empathically failing the patient but for indicating that s/he is
not all bad. When such strong identifications with criminality or evil exist in
a severely dissociative patient, the alters or self-states embodying them will
be nearly impossible to treat because they will see any sign of therapeutic
progress as weakening their diabolism and as an affront to their sense of superiority. Shame is so intensely defended against that coming into contact
with any vulnerability feels like a cruel death or dismemberment to these
extremely corrupted part-selves. Interestingly, Rosenfeld's (p. 174) description of the internal world of the "destructive narcissist" sounds quite similar
to the organization and dynamics of many perpetrator groups:

> The destructive narcissism of these patients appears often highly organized, as
> if one were dealing with a powerful gang dominated by a leader, who controls
> all the members of the gang to see that they support one another in making the
> criminal destructive work more effective and powerful. However, the narcissis-
> tic organization not only increases the strength of the destructive narcissism,
> but it has a defensive purpose to keep itself in power and so maintain the status
> quo. The main aim seems to be to prevent the weakening of the organization
> and to control the members of the gang so that they will not desert the destruc-
> tive organization and join the positive parts of the self or betray the secrets of

the gang to the police, or the protecting super-ego, standing for the helpful analyst, who might be able to save the patient.

In some hostile/perpetrator-identified alters the level of identification with pure malevolence, spite, envy, haughtiness, and callousness is so severe that their pleasure in assaulting the treatment and the psyche and spirit of the therapist (and the self) are endless. Yet sometimes, after years of confrontations and strengthening alliances with other sectors of the self, these extreme psychological positions can be systematically undermined and gradually eroded: in such cases the treatment is like a slow titration of light into completely dark chambers of the heart and mind of the patient.

When, however, these patients move among therapists or treatment programs, a set of seductively waiflike, victim-identified self-states often provides initial engagement (and hope); then, the set of powerfully malignant narcissistic/sociopathic alters finds ways to drive clinicians to get rid of them, taking perverse pride in their dark triumph over healing and goodness. They become predators in the mental health system. A few of these predatory, narcissistic/sociopathic alters might pursue malicious lawsuits against their therapists (sometimes in conjunction with their families or perpetrator groups); the ambiguities involved in diagnosis and treatment are manipulated by the patient to humiliate and ultimately destroy the career of the therapist and to extort enormous sums of money from insurance companies. (The wave of backlash against trauma therapy, MPD/DID, and "recovered memory" has created a cultural climate hospitable to such actions against therapists.)

More often than not, these unrelenting part-selves abort treatment or lead to patients' reentry into the criminal underworld (including the cult, perpetrator group, or family of origin) or to incarceration and/or suicide. Most therapists would like to believe that we can engage all aspects of a patient's dissociative self-system or that through a creative combination of empathy and confrontation we can eventually reach remote corners of the patient's shame-ridden and hostile self—but as Pizer (1998) laments in his work on negotiation and bridge-building in psychoanalysis, some things, some people, and some aspects of people are unnegotiable. While encountering this phenomenon of psychic nonnegotiability is exceedingly painful, awareness of its existence in certain hostile alters can help clinicians in the assessment and prognostic aspects of treatment; moreover, knowledge of such self-states can keep our own potentially inflated fantasies of rescue or redemption from leading us into naïve collaboration in our own victimization.

JOANN

Her last therapist promised her the world, then abruptly terminated treatment when Joann became suicidal and required hospitalization. The one before that got involved with her sexually. Given those therapy failures and others before them, Joann's fears of dependency—of being seduced and abandoned yet again in another therapy relationship—are quite pronounced.

Just as she had begun to open up an extremely traumatic issue from the past for the first time, a hostile male alter emerged to protect her from herself, that is, from trusting me. One of an unusual number of aggressive personalities who had manifested in Joann's self-destructive behavior (cutting, substance abuse, conflicts with coworkers, suicidality), he consistently preserved his separateness from the rest of her self-system. As soon as Joann's compliant demeanor gave way to his glaring defiant interruption, he said threateningly, "How would you feel if I cut her up into pieces?"

Acknowledging his power, I wonder aloud about whom the alter really wants to cut up into pieces—other part-selves, people from the past or present, maybe even me? He warns me acerbically: "If you make her talk about those things I will have to slice her up," and if I try any "shrink tricks" on him, he will slice me up too. This patient has provoked previous therapists into power duels, and I don't want to catalyze an acting-out episode—but I feel blackmailed by the bind he's tightening around talking. Recognizing it as a means of self-regulation and containment, however, I try linking it to his concern about the prospect of retraumatization in therapy with me, based on the earlier therapy failures. . . .

THERAPIST: I can see that your anger might be triggered by Joann's wanting to talk about what happened with your mother, and my encouraging her to express her feelings . . .
PATIENT: She's not my mother, she's her mother.

T: This distinction seems important to you. I think you're trying to tell me about what you're angry at yourself besides the fact that Joann and I are talking about painful things you feel might get out of hand.

P: Yeah, I am angry, so what. I'd just as soon cut you into pieces as talk to you.

Ironically, while trying to protect the patient from experiencing painful affects as well as from abandonment, and retraumatization, this alter is mimicking some of the threats of her perpetrators; he has probably caused more revictimization in the patient's life than he has prevented.

T: There seems to be a lot of emphasis on this cutting and threatening business; can we talk about it and get past all the intimidation in order to understand the meaning of the threats and the feelings that go with them?

P: Listen, mister, I just like to cut-cut-cut and tear and rip things. Cutting is better than talking. Get it!

Joann's history of severe self-mutilation had abated earlier in the treatment process when the DID diagnosis first opened up inter-alter communication.

T: How so? I want to understand how you see this.

P: It just is. I feel stronger and better and it keeps the others under control: when they begin to feel or get close to people, they get into trouble, and I can stop any feelings I want by telling them I will cut them or by cutting them or getting other parts to burn them and do stuff to them.

T: So you're in charge and you're protecting them by hurting and threatening them.

P: It sounds strange when you say it like that. . . . . I have to think about it. . . . . Listen, don't indulge yourself thinking I am here out of loving concern. I really don't give a damn about any of those others, so don't act like I care or anything. I don't feel like answering your shrink questions right now, I would rather go back to cutting; we haven't done that in a long time and I want to again. It's my body isn't it?

T: You're making a very important point, it's definitely your body—a shared body of course, but yours too.

P: Don't remind me about the other ones, I like to forget about them.

T: It seems like you can only cut and burn them when you forget about them, and forget that you're one of them.

P: You really like to rub it in. I've had therapy before and I know all about that stuff. I don't block them from knowing about the MPD anymore, but I still have to keep them in line. Reminding me that this is my body too and all of that therapy jazz—like I haven't heard some of this shit from your predecessors. . . .

T: You feel I am being sadistic now to remind you about your dissociation and the continuity of your body with your parts, like my reminding you that you're part of the others was some kind of attack. From your point of view, I'm pushing you around, hurting you, using power over you, just like everyone else always has.

P: The others are dumb enough to think you are different and trust you but I know you're just like all the other shrinks she's had. She always wants to trust them and she is always fooled in the end.

T: You're keeping them from falling into the trap of trusting me too much, is that right? You don't want them to need me and have me mistreat them, abandon them, force them into things. . . .

P: Without me, they'd have been in even more bad relationships than they have been.

T: I am going to say something that might also challenge the way you view things. It's possible that you even have a role in some of those relationships, including therapy relationships, not working out.

P: Yeah, right. People betray you and I have to take the heat for everything. I hate people, I hate you, leave me alone. I want to go away.

T: Let's talk about your hate and the betrayals. This is a safe place to do that. Don't just take your hurt and outrage and switch off or go away.

My invitation to dialogue openly about his hateful feelings—and only "for as long as he liked"—subdued the alter, who certainly wasn't expecting it and ended up focusing on superficial things he hates about the office and some clothes I have worn. When I pressed him to tell me what he really hated about me, the alter seemed to become hesitant, and in the middle of shifting states (as if really dialoguing about hate was beyond his capacity) said he hated that I seemed confident in what I was doing as a therapist. Not long afterward (and with no time to discuss the final comment), a slow switch took place and Joann returned, somewhat dazed and disoriented and with only vague recollections for the session. I proceeded to fill her in and explore why she had to dissociate it. My recounting of the session obviously disturbed her.

P: I don't know whether I am more scared of you or me right now.

T: What else can you say about your fears?

P: I don't like saying mean things to you. I'm afraid they'll make you go away like everyone else, and I'm afraid of what is inside of me. I don't want to know about it, but I do. I'm just mixed up.

T: You're afraid of ruining our relationship and losing me if these feelings get out of control, and you're afraid of not making any progress if you don't face this angry part of yourself and what he represents.

P: Yes, that's the bind. Things always get screwed up with me and other people, and I can't deal with it. Nothing ever changes.

T: Joann, have you ever considered that your not wanting to deal with your hate and aggressive feelings, your going away from them, is as much a part of the problem as the angry alter himself?

P: No, I never thought about it that way before.

T: Aren't you curious about what that part of you thinks and feels?

P: Honestly, no. I'm too scared to be curious. I don't want to start cutting again or being cut on or however it works in me. You can be curious for both of us [*somewhat sarcastically, which is unusual for the host personality*]; how about that?

T: There's a little edge to your voice now that you usually don't risk when you talk to me. What are you feeling right now?

P: Curiosity is a luxury. Don't you get that?

T: You mean this therapeutic ideal of knowing yourself that I represent and push on you from time to time is more difficult, more frightening than I understand.

P: Right. This angry part of me reminds me of people who really abused me and it doesn't feel like part of me, and when you try and convince me to deal with it I feel cornered and that brings up very scary feelings. But more than that, I don't want to lose my good feelings with you.

Since we are reaching the end of the session, I try to recap. I articulate the bind we seem to be in where neither talking nor not talking works:

talking with Joann's hostile alter about aggressive feelings threatens her attachment to me and triggers traumatic anxieties, memories, and fears of loss of control; not talking about these feelings keeps everything frozen, keeps our relationship limited, and keeps Joann at risk of spontaneously splitting off into self-destructive behaviors for reasons she doesn't fully understand. I also underscore an element of real progress: the aggressive aspects of her self are now in some kind of dialogue with me, and, whether for that reason or another, she was able to respond more assertively to my inquiries. Both the fact that progress could be identified and the fact that I found her directness and anger encouraging seemed to take Joann by surprise.

The hostile alter returned in the next session per my request, and after briefly reviewing our prior conversation, I patiently discussed the dynamics of protection, rigidity, and overgeneralization in an effort to define the costs/benefits of different forms of self-protection in relationship to the therapy, the various parts of the self, and to other people. Following several rounds of hit-and-run, his role in the system was also defined. Then he actually took me up on my offer of dialogue and shared inquiry, beginning by iterating his confusion about my approach to him, Joann, and some of the other parts.

P: You seem so comfortable pushing us around.
T: How do you feel pushed around?
P: You make me have to feel things.
T: When you say it that way, it sounds like force is involved.
P: No, you don't exactly force me, but you make me and them face things. I don't want to face what they did, how it felt, how it still feels, and then I start feeling weakened inside and it seems like it's your fault. You say you want me to talk and not cut and threaten and then I do and then I feel worse. And then it's all your fault.
T: By following my suggestion to talk instead of act out you're feeling something uncomfortable and painful. It's almost like you feel that I'm purposely doing something to make you feel bad.
P: First of all, talking usually does no good. Plus, here with you I'm starting to feel weak and you seem like you are enjoying yourself.

In my work with severely dissociative patients I do often enjoy "mixing it up" with hostile alters because I find that it leads to breakthroughs in resolving omnipotent thinking, models how aggressive feelings can safely be part of intimacy, and at times also releases pent-up aggression for patient and therapist alike. The accusation lands on more than a grain of truth, prompting me to reflect on what my motivations are, what I might not be aware of, what sadistic part from the patient's psyche or past or from my own I might be playing out.

T: I can see that I've been pushing you to deal with aspects of your dissociation, and actually I was feeling okay about doing that; it's not from wanting to hurt you or see you suffer that I was enjoying our work, but since you bring that up, I promise that I'll look at it and think about it. What I do know is that I was feeling frustrated with our conversation going in circles about the cutting, so maybe I've pressed you to deal with the dissociation too soon. But you know that sooner or later I would have asked you to look at the ways you stay separate from the other parts and how that affects the cutting and your history of self-destructive behavior.

P: [*cynically*] You're going to think about what I said. . . .

T: I will. And I can hear your doubt and skepticism, so let's keep talking. It seems as if you believe that if you're with someone else and feeling any kind of emotional pain, that someone is enjoying inflicting it on you.

P: That's how it's always been. And it doesn't seem any different with you: you're making us feel and look at what's causing the pain—so you must like doing it.

T: I can see how this is confusing. You don't really know what my intention is, and you have no reason to trust me. From your point of view I could be completely bullshitting you.

P: You probably are, because everyone does.

T: And you don't really know how to tell the difference.

P: Maybe I do and maybe I don't.

T: So if we get into any area where you or any other part starts to feel pain, or fear, or weakness, or vulnerability—which are places therapy eventually has to go—then you feel like I might be hurting you and enjoying having power over you or enjoying watching you squirm.

P: I don't trust anyone, so don't try and get me to trust you. People tell you what they have to just to get you to do what they want. That's what I think. No, that's what I know.

T: So what do you figure my motives are in working with you and the others, in questioning your dissociation or your relationships with one another or even in encouraging feelings whatever they might be?

P: I don't know what you're after, but I know it must be something. Maybe you're just taken with how smart you are or maybe you just like pushing your patients around, how am I supposed to know?

The alter started to dissociate and look uneasy. I asked what just happened.

P: I don't know. I can feel "they" don't like me talking to you that way.

T: You're putting your distrust and suspicion of me into words, and the others are more uneasy than you are with conflict and confrontation.

P: I don't care how they feel. I said what I said and I meant it. They like to be good and nice, as if that gets them anywhere. Nice sucks.

T: My feeling about what's been going on between us since the other day is that you were pushing me and threatening the others with violence and I was pushing you back, challenging you. I hoped we could both take that kind of struggle and get somewhere by putting the aggression in you between us instead of your isolating all of your anger inside and turning it on yourself as you usually do or maybe taking potshots at me. So, I was glad something different was happening: you're talking to me directly from your anger instead of doing hit-and-run. But, I also see how that was a risk, which could get us stuck in the replay of the past. You could think I am only trying to hurt you as other people have; then you get stuck and can't think about it any other way.

P: Well, I don't know if I can believe you, but you did say you'd be thinking about whether you wanted to hurt us or not. . . .

T: Yes, I did, and I will. I know I can be impatient at times and then push at your dissociative barriers too hard out of frustration to get through a stuck place, but I'm not feeling like I would enjoy watching you suffer. Since you keep asking, I'll keep thinking about it.

P: [Somewhat mockingly but also, now, almost playfully] Good. You think about it and get back to me.

T: It seems you're more comfortable with the idea that I'd want to hurt you than with what I have offered—a different type of relationship in which you would learn to integrate aggressive feelings and energies, and which would be inclusive of you and all the other parts of Joann.

P: Well, if I believe that you actually are enjoying being with me and pushing back and forth, and that it's safe to do that, then I'd have to trust you, and I don't want to do that because if I did then they'd all crumble into needing you too much and into feeling all sorts of things that I don't want them or me to feel, to remember, to think or talk about. It's easier to keep it locked up. That's what I know how to do.

T: So, it's all linked inside of you? One thing leads to another, and if one thing changes then everything has to change—and there's the dreaded dependency and betrayal waiting like a guarantee at the end of the road.

P: Right, and I don't like change. Or trust. Or dependency. It's weak. And I hate weak.

T: Playing with your anger with me and disagreeing is a kind of strength. How does it feel?

P: If I think you're trying to "get" me I don't like it, but if I believe that you actually like my pushing you and you can take it and you don't want to make me go away because of it, then I might really start to feel good about it and even enjoy getting angry with you myself, instead of just pretending.

T: Then we both would be safe and able to enjoy being with angry feelings and no harm would be being done to anyone.

P: It sounds too good to be true.

T: I understand that it's hard for you to believe things could be different. Why not keep talking and see what happens over time? If I do anything that doesn't feel right or fair, I want you to let me know.

P: But how do I know you are not tricking me?

T: That's a problem, isn't it? You aren't sure how to know the differences between words you can trust and words that are tricks.

P: I've been tricked a lot in my life and I swore that would never happen again.

T: Can we talk about that sometime—the deception you're referring to?

P: Maybe.

T: [*Playfully*] Since it's getting toward the last part of the session, let me ask you to think about it and get back to me on it, okay?

We both laugh at the same time and the atmosphere in the room shifts dramatically from an adversarial dynamic to alliance.

T: Before we begin to wind down this session, can I push you on this question of trust?

P: Okay. You're doing okay today, so go on.

T: What was going on between the Joann part of you and me the other day that made you come out in the first place?

P: Well, she was feeling just a little too comfortable with you and you with her. I thought you were just luring her in for the big kill and she didn't know it; she's so stupid about those things.

T: What was I doing or saying that made you feel that way from behind the scenes?

P: You were acting like you cared when she began talking about the grandfather-in-the-attic stuff. I thought you were trying to get her to open up to you by pretending you were interested and concerned like all the shrinks she had in the hospital who dumped her as soon as she got to be too much for them.

T: So you weren't sure if this was any different and you can't tell if I really care or just pretend to care as part of my job, so you came in to stop a catastrophe before it happened?

P: I guess you could say it that way. Anyway, I'd rather hurt them than have anyone else hurt them again.

T: You didn't want her to be seduced and encouraged by me into opening up and letting down her guard, only to be abandoned by yet another person promising to help?

P: Just don't give me that bullshit about how I do what I do because I really care about her, because like I told you, I don't care about anyone. I don't do what I do out of caring. I'm a survivor.

The alter was now attempting to reconstitute his initial position after softening some.

T: There's is a lot of cynicism and hurt embedded in what you're saying. Obviously a lot of the hurt, betrayal, fear, and rage about the past is coming into our relationship and we have to find a way to talk this through.

P: You can talk it through with other ones who like to talk. Me, I just keep them in line.

T: That's some pretty intense guard duty; you're always on alert aren't you?

P: That's my strength. Don't make me give it up.

I stress that except for our basic working contract prohibiting violence, sexuality, and confidentiality, no one in this relationship was going to make anyone or any part of anyone do anything against his or her will.

P: I'll consider that you mean what you say.

T: That also means I won't react well to you or any part of you threatening me or other parts of the self either.

[*Then, taking a leap*] Did you ever threaten your other therapists?

P: There've been lots of other therapists. And yes, I've probably done things to make a few of them feel uncomfortable and see how they reacted, but a lot of them pretended everything was okay even though I could see they were scared and then they found a way to get rid of me. At least you're telling me some of what you think and not pretending everything is okay.

T: On the one hand you're saying you value honesty, but on the other you like to test people without their knowing about it. I have some idea why you do that, but it can be confusing to be on the other end of it at times. It's even possible that you've had a role in the breakdown of some of those therapy relationships.

P: Okay, you're probably right about some of that, but don't tell me you don't know that a lot of those people in mental health just bullshit the patients all the time. Especially the ones they're scared of.

T: I won't deny that there's truth to some of what you are saying, but I think we need to put all the pieces together in one place to understand everything that's happened with you and the previous treatments to clear a path for some kind of different experience with me if that's still possible.

P: [*Sounding actually caring for the first time*] I don't think they can handle another therapy not working out.

T: I understand that could be devastating at this point and make everyone feel like giving up. One thing is for sure; it is hard for you to tell whether someone is or is not really there with you or for you, and whether someone is trying to hurt you, help you, trick you, or deceive you. That's a kind of "not knowing" we'll be exploring together for a while.

P: You mean you aren't going to try and convince me that you really care and that you really mean what you say and are totally trustworthy? The others always did.

T: With all you've been through, how could I do that and be believed? Anyway, I don't think real trust gets built just by what people say. You need to have enough time and experience with someone in order to know where they're coming from, and that's why I was suggesting you come back and talk some more and keep testing me and questioning me. Besides, it seems as if the too-trusting and the not-at-all-trusting parts of you aren't even in communication with each other.

P: It hasn't worked for us to know each other too well.

T: It's not working any longer for you not to know each other.

Just before Joann returns toward the end of the session (amnestic for large parts of the conversation), the alter offers, "And I think it will be okay for you to push me again sometime."

T: Maybe. That's giving a lot on your part. I appreciate your openness. Maybe, if it feels right. It's hard to know what will come up in a given session or what you or Joann or others will need to talk about. But, maybe next time I'll ask your permission to push you first about some things so you could be part of that decision.

P: It'll be a while before she can handle me and what I have to tell her.

T: I can see you don't want her to be overwhelmed, so I want you to consider that these things can happen slowly but consistently, a little bit at a time.

P: But she thinks your talking to me will make you not like her anymore.

T: Maybe we can both help her start to feel safe with angry, hateful feelings. Maybe she can enjoy getting angry, pushing me or you back sometimes, without having to worry about losing me or getting cut or threatened.

P: Maybe. I'm not sure how I'd feel about that.

T: Of course you're not because that would mean you and she would be closer, and you and I, and she and I . . . Some of your walls would be less thick. And there are so many feelings in there.

P: I've never been close to anyone. Just cutting and screwing and drinking and drugging. This is all new to me. Don't think anything is going to change all that fast, okay?

T: Okay. Nothing too much at once or too fast.

P: And don't give up on us either, okay?

When the therapist is enlisted as an ally, not only in processing traumatic experience but in "affect retraining," then therapist and patient will find themselves in the middle of repetitions of what has been experienced in the past and potential repetitions of what did *not* happen (Modell, 1990). The affects that surface in the transference include the re-creation of archaic feelings of love and hatred regarding the self as an object. Because of the compulsion to repeat, to reaffirm a perceived identity, and to engage the therapist in testing assumptions/perceptions, the severely traumatized patient may

> use the therapist's affective responses as a means of defensively re-establishing the false self . . . the hated aspect of the self may be a shell that protects a hidden, beloved sense of self . . . with the unexpressed hope that the therapist in her affective responses will interrupt this repetitive confirmation of archaic affect categories. (p. 69)

Effective treatment of the derailed aggressive and protest responses of severely dissociative individuals is an extremely arduous task, especially in today's litigious climate. As Barach (1999d) points out, many a therapist is so afraid of saying or doing the wrong thing that s/he rapidly falls into the tense and compliant role of the abused child in a disturbed family: when the therapist stays nice to avoid being attacked, or threatened, or sued and the patient stays nice to avoid being abused or threatening his/her attachments to either perpetrator(s) or therapist, then, "nobody trusts anybody and nothing is done" (p. 1).

RESTORATION OF DERAILED AGGRESSION

To sustain a therapeutic ambience that encourages the transformation of dissociated aggression, the therapist must

- Emphasize safety, stabilization, life functioning, and symptom reduction over memory processing, analysis of reenactments, or interpretation of the patient's dynamics.
- Review issues of informed consent on a consistent, intermittent basis so that the patient (and all of the alters) are continuously involved in collaborative decision-making and reflection about the directions and goals of therapy—with full knowledge of the potential risks and benefits involved in various aspects of treatment.
- Face, not avoid, all aspects of the patient's aggression regardless of form, content, or origin—which mandates confronting and negotiating with all intrapsychic and interpersonal threats, intimidation, passive-aggressive behavior, and blackmail. As Bromberg (1996b) states, a psychotherapy may not be successful or complete if the therapist has not gone head-to-head with the patient for a long period of time about a variety of issues; Pizer (1998) likens this butting of heads to a meeting of minds.
- Communicate empathy and respect for all, even the most extreme forms, of dissociated aggression and rage—which means assisting all parts of the patient to apprehend the survival-value of the hostile part-selves as well as the risks of maintaining their dissociation for the patient's future.
- Model diplomacy, mutuality, equality, reciprocity, and respect (including internal and interpersonal variations on "tough love").
- Teach the patient to observe him/herself and not to loathe and disavow what is observed (Wurmser, 1987).
- Confront all destructive uses of the therapy relationship and nonjudgmentally hold the patient accountable and responsible for his/her participation and behaviors.
- Develop an alliance with protector/persecutors based on empathizing with how much the patient as a child needed protection and how much his/her sense of attachment to caretakers/abusers needs to be protected (Howell, 1997).
- Encourage the patient's verbal and fantasy representations of hatred, revenge, and rage instead of concretizations, acting out, or dangerous reenactments, conveying the necessity to explore hurt, angry feelings while affirming that tyrannizing the therapist (or others, or other alters) will not be tolerated.

- Understand (and be able to communicate to the patient about) the complex issues of shame, guilt, and (coerced) identifications with the aggressor that many hostile/perpetrator alters represent.
- Focus on positive, life-enhancing, and creative aspects of the patient's aggression (or its potential).
- Recognize that the extremes of dissociative aggression—suicidality and homicidality—can emanate from any or all of three sources simultaneously: the patient's responses to real or imagined threat; identification with significant others; programmed messages and conditioned behaviors implanted by perpetrators.
- Help the patient discriminate between aggressive and perpetrator alters and self-states cultivated from his/her own ideas, imagination, and coping strategies, and those that have been heavily influenced by thought reform, torture, and training.
- Work through the therapist's fears of his/her own aggression and use of therapeutic leverage or power.
- Be willing to terminate treatment (in a thoughtful, nonretaliatory spirit) when a patient has refused to engage in cooperative management of safety and stabilization issues or when a patient has dangerously violated the boundaries and frame of the therapy. (Patients should be informed of these potential consequences as early in treatment as possible.)
- Emphasize restoration of the patient's sense of free will, sense of agency, and appropriate responsibility (and deflation of omnipotent fantasies of responsibility)—and, specifically, help the patient distinguish between having to do something and choosing to do something. (This theme, simple as it sounds, must be continuously revisited.)
- Focus on the patient's need for elaborate self-empathy, self-love, and self-forgiveness.

CHAPTER 8

The Destruction and Restoration of Attachment and Critical Thinking

Who controls the past controls the future. Who controls the present controls the past. . . . All that was needed was an unending series of victories over your own memory. . . . Reality control, they called it . . . double-think.
— **George Orwell,** *1984*

Attachment and critical thinking are two complex developmental trajectories that get significantly derailed in the inhumane environments where dissociative disorders are cultivated and elaborated. Victims' lifelong struggles to relate to others as well as their ongoing struggles for dominion over their own minds are particularly insidious consequences of chronic trauma.

REWORKING ATTACHMENT

Facilitating shifts from masochistic, self-destructive attachments to mutually respectful, loving, and empowering relationships must be a key emphasis in the treatment of severely traumatized, dissociative patients. All parts of the patient's dissociative self-system, from the most needy to the most disengaged, must enter into dialogues with the therapist about their intense fears, pains, and longings. Yet, due to the disorganized, anxiety-producing, and sadomasochistic attachment experiences that characterize the relational history of most dissociative individuals—and the corresponding expectations and self-fulfilling prophecies that have defined their lives until they started treatment—all aspects of human bonding have become threatening.

Chronic attachment to abusers throughout childhood leads to the phenomenon of *trauma-bonding*, whereby untrustworthy and destructive relationships are normative and innate protective mechanisms for discriminating safety from danger are turned upside down (Herman, 1992; Van der Kolk, 1989). Patients with highly dissociative psychic organizations demonstrate extreme vulnerability to revictimization—Kluft's "sitting duck syndrome"—because they block out danger cues, not by way of ignoring evidence of threat but as a product of activating dissociation to escape it (Waller, Quinton, and Watson, 1995). In turn, chronic reliance on dissociation actually deprives victims of vital access to signals of danger as resources for self-defense.

Survivors of chronic trauma may experience danger as fundamentally unavoidable, and in the absence of healthy aggression for self-protection, they are in fact quite vulnerable in all relationships. Most are "quite susceptible to declarations . . . of love . . . by unsavory types of people. . . . They often cannot tell the difference between the fools' gold of false promises and the real gold of sincere caring" (Howell, 1997, p. 243). Accordingly, all forms of intimacy are suspect for the dissociatively adapted. (And emotional involvement with them can be dangerous for others, including therapists, because of their emotional unavailability, seductiveness, inconsistency, intense neediness, and split-off sadism.)

Since prolonged captivity in abusive situations disrupts all future relationships, the dissociative survivor of chronic trauma will oscillate between intense attachment and terrified withdrawal (Herman, 1992), and approach all relationships as if questions of life and death are at stake. Lacking as s/he does secure, stable internal representations of other people, s/he will assign them roles (rescuer, bystander, perpetrator, etc.) that are subject to sudden and (to the outside observer) inexplicable change. ("There is no room for mistakes. Over time, as most people fail the survivor's exacting tests of trustworthiness, she tends to withdraw. . . . The isolation of the survivor persists even after she is free" [p. 93].)

Psychotherapy represents the proverbial dangerous crossroads where the legacies of old attachments are revealed and reenacted and where new forms of attachment can be negotiated. When significant attachment figures in a patient's early life are also predators, such that his/her very survival has been contingent on dangerous objects, the intrapsychic and interpersonal impact on bonding, trust, and intimacy are devastating. Clinicians can expect not only chronic distrust, intense avoidance, and endless rounds of testing, but also—as aspects of treatment challenge the patient's fundamental attachment to dangerous perpetrators—the upping of an ante that places them at personal and legal risk of reprisals. The reworking of the abnormalities of dissociative attachment mandates that the therapist believe and communicate

> how the individual is made and held within relationship, how there can be no such thing as an individual outside of relationship—that it is relationship (the fact that we are in relation with one another) that makes human endeavor, human individuality as we know it, possible. . . . Attachment, relationship, and the transmission of culture are unique human enterprises; without attachment to other humans, we cannot hope to be human let alone individual. (Orbach, 1999, p. 81)

Essential Attachment

Bowlby (1969) presents evidence that human infants are hardwired for attachment in the service of survival. Since attachment is not optional if survival is to be achieved, children become powerfully attached to whatever is available, for better and for worse (Main, 1995). The primary attachment process also plays a major role in forming character and in determining (and limiting) interpersonal repertoire; further, underlying attachment styles appear to organize emotional and behavioral responses (Bowlby, 1982; Main, Kaplan, and Cassidy, 1985; Stern, 1985).

Bowlby's attachment theory emphasizes the creation of an internal working model of relationships that guides people to re-create their original attachments throughout their lifetime; the more an individual replicates the old patterns of attachment, the more convinced s/he becomes of the viability of his/her relationship models. In order for severely dissociative individuals to maintain their old models, however, they must systematically misperceive discrepant aspects of their current reality; they must also continue to ignore evidence of, and continue to forget, their abuse and exploitation, and they must drive away (or keep testing) those who might support their individuation and emancipation from destructive patterns of relationship.

Since the abused child has no choice but to turn to the tormenting caretaker for soothing, protection, and assistance, Freyd (1996) suggests that s/he may need to stifle the ability to detect betrayal for the greater goal of survival. Not only is the (evolutionarily) adaptive mechanism of dissociation a defense against overwhelming trauma, overstimulation, and horrifying affects and events, but also it is a prime technique for maintaining attachments in the most brutal, inconsistent, and absurd situations. The dependent child protects (or minimizes harm to) him/herself both in fantasy and reality by separating out any thoughts, feelings, and memories that might disrupt idealization of the adults (Shengold, 1989) or provoke inner conflict or trigger more abusive attacks. In other words, s/he must sacrifice aspects of the self associated with perception of the malevolence of the caretakers. Freyd (1996) calls this *betrayal blindness*: the abused child maintains the relationship on which s/he is dependent by blocking awareness of feelings or information that reveal(s) betrayal.

As abusive caretakers persist in ignoring a victim's needs, the victim learns to be ashamed of those needs and the attendant perceptions and reactions. In some cases, they are literally beaten out of the child; many perpetrators physically force victims to stop crying (stop feeling), stop escaping, and stop resisting (stop thinking their own thoughts). In situations where a child is exploited and his/her anger and hurt are not recognized, the ability to sustain attachment will come to depend on the dissociative compartmentalization of aggression (Howell, 1997), and when it does, the child begins unconsciously to identify his/her own aggressive feelings and responses as the real (and perhaps only) threat. For the adult survivor of childhood abuse, the reemergence of normal needs and perceptions in other intimate relationships (including therapy) is blocked by intense shame (Benjamin, 1988), fear, or dread, curtailing any investigative curiosity s/he might have had.

An intense and perverse dependency evolves as victims become more isolated from people other than their perpetrators and as they come to depend, therefore, on the perpetrators for information, emotional sustenance, and in some cases physical and basic bodily needs (Herman, 1992). With increasing fear, victims bond even more powerfully to perpetrators, who understand the importance of destroying all old attachments. Isolation from them is not enough; even internal images must be demolished. (The most sadistic abusers tease their victims with temporary contact with a beloved person or object—only to dismember or destroy it before their eyes.)

Still more poignant and bizarre than a victim's eventual view of the world mirroring that of the perpetrator is a victim's quest for the humanity in the captor/tormentor (as per clinical communications in which survivors of sexual abuse report fantasies of healing their abusers/torturers). The counterintuitive form of captor/captive bonding first documented in 1973 as the Stockholm Syndrome (referring to the unexpected behavior of four bank employees held hostage in Sweden) embodies several such essential paradoxes (Graham, 1994). Hostages felt gratitude toward their captors for sparing their lives instead of anger at them for threatening their lives. Hostages remembered the small kindnesses shown them in preference to the larger picture of the captors' indifference to their terror and suffering. Hostages perceived the captors as the good guys and the police as the bad guys and would not have welcomed police-generated opportunities to escape lest the captors be killed in the cross fire. Some of the hostages became sympathetic to the political rhetoric of their captors, refused to testify against them, and variously sought leniency or developed legal defense funds on their behalf.

Investigators of the underlying psychodynamics of the Stockholm Syndrome (Soskis and Ochberg, 1982; Graham, 1994) conclude that *any* individual trapped in a situation involving confinement, isolation, and helplessness or inescapable violence will come to believe in the captor's capacity for kindness. When entrapment is prolonged, victims feel overwhelmed and appease, submit to, cooperate, and even empathize with their oppressors (Symonds, 1982). Soskis and Ochberg (1982) believe that since captors are the source of hope in an otherwise hopeless situation, the psychological adaptation to pleasing them preempts a collapse into futility and despair and activates escape fantasies when actual escape seems impossible.

When the victim believes his/her survival is at stake, s/he begins to determine what will keep the abuser happy and becomes hypervigilant to the abuser's needs, feelings, desires, and perspectives to the point of trying to think like the abuser, taking on his worldview (Graham, 1994). If the conditions of terror are prolonged, Graham says, the victim's entire sense of self comes to be experienced as through the eyes of the abuser:

> They will report how their abusers perceive them. If asked how they feel about something, they will report how their abusers feel about it. If what they are do-

ing is pointed out to them and they are once again asked these questions, they
will answer they do not know. (p. 273)

At one level, all children are hostages to their parents, totally dependent
on them for survival, which is threatened by parental abandonment or violence (Graham, 1994). In incestuous, sadistic-abuse, or criminal families or
cult systems, children are in fact literal and absolute hostages to their parents (Herman, 1992). DID—almost always cultivated under conditions of
prolonged exposure to sadistic abuse and cultlike conditions of isolation,
terror, and information control—is the Stockholm Syndrome run amok. The
paradoxes of helping-hurting, rooted in traumatic attachments, are repli-
cated in the internal world of pathological multiplicity, especially in the formation of aggressive/protector- or perpetrator-alters, who interfere
directly in the establishment of loving attachments while reenacting
parental abuses in the apparently contradictory services of self-protection
and self-punishment.

For the severely dissociative patient, hurting is helping and actual helping
hurts. Clinicians must fully grasp this elemental paradox in order to understand the subjective world of internalized violence, captivity, and torture.
The shaming, subordination, and submission to the will of the irrational authorities who once dominated the victim's interpersonal life now completely
color his/her intrapsychic life; they hold the fragile self together—by keeping the self divided. The healthy anger that might have supported differentiation from the traumatic attachment is now distorted to strengthen the
traumatic bonding, keeping the child—and, later, the mind, body, and soul
of the adult victim—psychologically annexed to the perpetrator's primitive
narcissistic self-regulatory functions. In the dissociative matrix of elaborate
intrapsychic compromise formations, self-sacrifice becomes the only instrument of attachment and the only way of life.

No Price Is Too High to Pay

The human need for an emotional bond with another person prevails at
whatever cost. If the only available relationship is an abusive (or seductive)
one, seeking pain (or seduction) becomes the vehicle for interaction. Children with histories characterized by violence and forced submission
"choose" the pain of contact over the pain of rejection and develop strange
forms of collaboration with their abusers in their own abuse. Eventually,

sadistically abused children become their own perpetrators and remain so even long after they have left home or their abusers have died.

One patient reported giving her mother the iron she was to be burned with. Another remembered signaling her father for sexual abuse by way of controlling at least the timing of the inevitable and quelling her intolerable anticipatory anxiety. Still another patient calls herself evil (as her father did during and after perpetration of emotionally humiliating, physically violent, and sexually abusive actions) whenever she recalls the incidents; some parts of her fractured mind say she must be awful to come up with these ("imaginary") ideas in the first place, while others say she deserved all of the abuses since she was so awful, and yet others—identifying with the father who repeatedly switched from TV evangelist persona to sadistic cult participant—believed that her abuse was justified by his benevolent efforts to cleanse her of evil.

When masochism is framed as an outcome of dissociation (and pain) rather than of volition (and pleasure), its victim-blaming connotations vanish, according to Howell (1997). Failure to understand the double binds of attachment reinforces the entrenched perpetrator-implanted conviction that masochistic behavior shifts responsibility for maltreatment to the victim. In fact, the masochist is not seeking pain or punishment at all; s/he tolerates both in the context of another priority. The desperate need for attachment supersedes even avoidance of pain as a guiding imperative.

Children raised in cults or criminal perpetrator groups and families are often forced to recruit other children by means similar to those used to force them into compliance. They learn to cultivate dissociative states and alternate identities when they are coerced into harming and killing animals and other human beings—often infants and young children.

> The final step in the psychological control of the victim is not completed until she has been forced to violate her own moral principles and to betray her basic human attachments. Psychologically, this is the most destructive of all coercive techniques, for the victim who has succumbed loathes herself. It is at this point, when the victim under duress participates in the sacrifice of others, that she is truly broken. (Herman, 1992, p. 83)

Identifying with abusers' ideologies and motivations not only sustains attachment possibilities, but allows victims to endure excruciating, otherwise intolerable guilt and shame. Dissociating the meaning, cause, and responsibility for the violence and rearranging all of those according to the perpetrator's psychological, political, spiritual, or even forensic needs, the victim becomes inextricably linked with protecting the perpetrator(s) or the family myths, ideologies, and delusions. The trauma bond is such that the perpetrator's agenda becomes the victim's, and the victim may cover more effectively for the abuser than the abuser can for him/herself. The trauma-bonding process is susceptible to manipulation by sophisticated perpetrators, who can, if all else fails, always count on their victims to be assaulted by incredulity, skepticism, and doubt—by them (the perpetrators) and by the culture.

With great shame and hesitation, several patients who were involved in sex-death cults throughout childhood and were forced to engage in ritual murder and dismemberment of infants and children have described their rage at the human sacrifices for not dying fast enough. Rage at perpetrators was unthinkable, having been extinguished as a possibility long before the child-victim was trained to kill. Slow deaths of those being sacrificed caused increased stress, shock, guilt, and horror for the child coerced into homicide—effects confirmed when the perpetrators criticized his/her killing technique, solidifying the child's belief in him/herself as evil, incompetent, or both. The perpetrators also defined the sacrificial victim as an enemy and a source of the suffering of the child-murderer, who thus deserved to die; not surprisingly, the child would come to develop alter personalities with no feelings (other than, perhaps, pride) about killing others.

No individuation is tolerated in the dominating and abusive families and/or perpetrator groups of severely dissociative patients. Any movement toward autonomy is accompanied by powerful anxieties about isolation, terror, and disintegration of self. Differentiation (much less escape) from one's caretaker/abusers would mean loss of ties to internal objects that have provided an enduring sense of belonging and identity—connectedness, albeit mediated by pain and desolation (Mitchell, 1988). Out of a desperate need for rescue and the maintenance of a good object representation, the child must repetitively split off what s/he experiences and must register the parent "delusionally as good" (Shengold, 1989, p. 26). Of course, such a mind-fragmenting operation requires strong and elaborated dissociative defenses, especially when the abuse is chronic.

The self held together by the dissociative tapestry is a very fragile one, so when old forms of attachment and bonding are threatened, extreme annihilation panic and narcissistic rage surface, accompanied paradoxically by numbness, psychic deadness, and compliance. The ensuing patterns of anxious and disorganized attachment, pseudocompliant attachment, sadomasochistic attachment (Barach, 1991), and fervent disattachment alternate in mutually exclusive, associatively unavailable presentations. When and if hope for another way of life emerges, it is met with a startling internal backlash and massive unconscious efforts to restore the primary attachment system. This aspect of treating severely dissociative patients produces enormous stress and particular pain for therapists.

In healthy development and attachment, where the child is constantly discovered and rediscovered in an ongoing process of satisfying recognition, contact with the environment is the source of his/her sense of existence (Winnicott, 1953; 1971). In situations of extreme impingement, however, it is only through withdrawal that an individual can feel allowed to exist: attachment is based not on recognition but on camouflage. To be found is to be humiliated, devoured, or destroyed by the caretakers' consumption-based narcissistic needs; the mere act of self-exposing is fraught with terror and annihilation anxieties.

Not surprisingly, the therapist's search for the patient's self is construed by the patient as a mission of destruction (or seduction), ultimately bringing the therapist into the triple transferential role of seeker-destroyer, seeker-seducer, seeker-betrayer. Simply sharing knowledge about the self/selves with the therapist (especially revelation of organized multiplicity), indeed any intersubjective discourse, can precipitate acute dread as the perceived demand for relinquishment of ties to one's internal objects arouses anxiety, and can even trigger emotional collapse akin to the psychic states that initiated defensive dissociation during and immediately after childhood traumas.

The patient's fear of, and resistance to, being known, so fundamental to the architecture of pathological multiplicity, must therefore be continually acknowledged by the therapist along with the patient's desires to be seen and contacted. Treatment must be informed by awareness of the matrix of interlocking double binds; it must recognize and affirm, and also dialogue with (but not pathologize) so-called resistance in all its myriad manifestations. At the same time, the expert dissociator's propensity for omissions and deletions must be systematically confronted: the subjective experiences of satisfying self-injury, positive identifications with violence, and attachment to totalitarian ideological systems must be understood and articulated from within the frames of reference of the alter(s). This posture stretches the limits of the therapist's empathy.

When a therapist decides to avoid contact with all or certain types of the patient's alter personalities for fear of being harmed or out of the mistaken assumption that s/he might be reinforcing a pathological multiplicity that would otherwise gracefully melt away, s/he conveys the message that s/he does not want to know the patient deeply. That message will be greeted with mixed feelings of relief and betrayal—and the core conflict of MPD/DID that needs to be worked and reworked in the transference/countertransference will be bypassed. The patient's ambivalent wishes to be attached and unattached, to be bonded both in old ways and new, must be attended to without one's being allowed to eclipse the other. If, because of his/her own ideological perspective or because of a personal desire to nurture the patient to health by ignoring the multiplicity, the therapist selectively supports only pieces of the paradoxical wish to be known and to remain hidden, dissociation will be strengthened. But if dissociative barriers are weakened and the patient struggles with his/her increased intimacy and trust with the therapist, a new sense of self can coalesce around this noble pivotal battle.

For traumatized dissociative patients, the psychotherapy process is in a sense an elaborate web of tests of the therapist. The object of the tests is to determine whether or not the therapist will relate in terms of the familiar pathological attachment dynamics mastered in the traumatic situations. For example, DID patients have a knack for regarding their therapists as simultaneously significant and irrelevant, replicating the original traumatic-bonding paradox whereby caretakers alternately disparaged and treated them as special; urgent demands for concrete rescue can coincide with strident disavowal of the therapist's usefulness—paralleling the patient's internal experience of a deeply conflicted and tormented relationship to him/herself and to the abusers of his/her childhood, when the inconsistencies of irrational authority became the focus around which predictive defensive strategies for survival were organized.

Behind the compliant, affable mask of the host personality's apparent accessibility lie layers upon layers of terror, anger, and humiliation-fueled rage resulting from compounded attachment failures. The therapist must recognize and continuously negotiate with the split-off extremes of traumatic compliance and virulent defiance—accepting both, questioning both, and introducing the patient to the notion of holding these voices in one central consciousness. When the patient can sustain the conflict among polarized parts of the self without resorting to remobilizing his/her dissociative defenses, s/he can begin to integrate attachment longings with attachment fears and develop the capacity to tolerate knowledge and feelings about past betrayals.

Relational psychoanalytic and trauma/dissociation theory share the conviction that the needs for safety, emotional contact, and (by fantasied extension) power to heal the disturbed caretaker synergize in the child-victim's mind to create strong unconscious bonds with malevolent perpetrators. From a traditional MPD perspective, the elaboration of separate identities as a means of maintaining attachment to dangerous caretakers is an epiphenomenon of the core dissociation that drives DID—a function, specifically, of the unconditional psychological survival need for someone to love: when there is no one on the outside, the DID child may create someone on the inside; essentially, the drive to attach drives the delusion (Ross, 1997).

Relationalists construe the fulcrum of DID to be an internally maintained and externally perpetuated repetition of power ties to bad objects or malevolent introjects (Fairbairn, 1952); the result is a personality structure whereby the processes of self-fragmentation aimed at retaining ties to bad internal objects operate discontinuously with other self-experience. Psychopathology is a cocoon actively woven of fantasied ties to significant others (Mitchell, 1988); relational patterns are the glue that holds the self together, the loyalties through which the child feels connected, devoted, and motivated to internalize the abuser and because of which s/he will inevitably confound loving bonds with sadistic behavior.

THEA

Thea, a polyfragmented DID patient became so adept at dividing her consciousness in relation to the only attachment figure with whom she could cultivate even an imaginary bond that she construed as entirely separate entities the father who carried her out to his truck late at night for delivery into group-abuse situations—and the father who picked her up after nights of prostitution, pornography, and brutal cult rituals and drove her home.

The latter, the one who "rescued" her from the multiple perpetrators, was her savior. Thea would not, or could not, connect him with the criminal lackey who sold, and sold out, his daughter—or with the father who raped her in the basement or the father who demanded sex in exchange for money for groceries for the other children or the father who just sat for hours staring into space stonefaced and drunk.

Traumatic relational paradigms are perpetuated in other relationships and become the *definition* of the self-in-relationship. As a consequence of the child-victim's chronic enmeshment in double binds—whereby counterintuitive givens abound, like the child's feeling safe only when the perpetrator is nearby (Ross, 1997)—the attachment circuitry is wired along lines that facilitate bonds with perpetrators (or, in psychoanalytic terms, malevolent introjects): nondominating, nonbetraying, and nonhumiliating relationships simply make no sense and bring on great anxiety. Healthier relationships, while longed for on the one hand, are so disruptive to the pseudoequilibrium of the trauma survivor on the other that the patient may repeatedly retreat from contact with the therapist to return symbolically or actually to the bond with the abuser. This can happen hundreds of times before any durable and transformative attachment is established.[1]

The dissociative patient, persuaded that no attachment contract can encompass differentiation, protest, or mutuality, becomes the best friend and collaborator of the perpetrator and his/her own worst enemy. Colluding with hard-won dissociated elaborations of the abuser's illusions has been a learned route to minimizing anxiety, and the contracts (tacit or explicit) between the psyches of victim and perpetrator become the basis—and disavowal of self the price—for other kinds of human contact. Thus, severely dissociative patients, whose capacities for trust are fragile at best, may continually ask the therapist to provide abuse—historically their only source of relational predictability. Perceived abuses, in any form, are experienced at once as intolerable violations and as treasured forms of relatedness (Lyon, 1992). This paradox can entrap patient and therapist alike in endless rounds of actual and fantasied trauma reenactments and double-binding tests of trustworthiness.

As Mitchell (1988) so aptly stated, psychopathology in its infinite variations reflects the unconscious commitment to stasis, to repetition of, and deep loyalty to, what is familiar. What is familiar in DID is layered in complexes of misidentification and dissociated belief systems. Loyalty to omnipotent, sadistic caretakers is a surrogate for self-cohesion; the necessary disruption of the ties to bad objects is exceedingly painful and disorienting for the patient. Therapists must appreciate how creatively grandiosity and idealized self- and object-representations are used to consolidate developmentally essential relationships, and must balance the challenging of patients' illusions with accepting and to some degree participating in them (Mitchell, 1993). Perhaps the most disorganizing experiences for the dissociative patient are facing the fact that s/he has created a whole texture of false-selves, self-deception, and illusion (including even invented memories of benign caretakers) to make life bearable and to avoid relinquishing the patterns that maintain familiar, destructive object relations.

When the narcissistic illusions ("I deserved it, I made it all happen" or "He loved me and that's why he did that to me" or "They're so awful they couldn't help themselves") are finally disrupted, the cement that has held together the whole labyrinthine construction crumbles. What results are apocalyptic anxieties—an immense and frightening sense of confusion, loss, and psychic nausea that often culminates in suicidal or homicidal urges. Only beyond them lies the transformative experience of freedom—freedom to protest and rage, freedom to imagine, freedom to question authority, freedom to trust, freedom to feel all the feelings on the spectrum (hatred to joy), freedom to love self and others.

THEA (CONTINUED)

When she first realized that her savior was her betrayer, Thea experienced a surge of virulent self-hatred: she was stupid for having needed and hoped for protection from her father and for not having put all the pieces into one single mind at the same time. She was stupid for needing and hoping. That was all there was to it. The father was not guilty of betrayal or criminal action. The patient was guilty and to be debased for hoping and trusting.

But the defense against grief and rage and against grasping the depth of her betrayal waned. A taboo image rose, an idea so long feared that it she could never before let it in. Thea was able to entertain for the first time the fantasy of punching her father in the face. (What made this particularly meaningful was that Thea's father used to punch her in the face whenever he thought her insufficiently compliant.)

Impairments in reality-testing and cognitive-processing abilities may protect traumatic attachments for victims and abusers alike: with the internal abusing parental introject (now the victim him/herself) as well as the actual parent of the adult abuse survivor usually denying, minimizing, or amnestic for the abuse, neither the victim nor the perpetrator wants to relinquish the trauma bond. The therapist, immersed in contradictory representations, can be in a precarious legal position in addition to a frustrating clinical dilemma. A severely dissociative trauma survivor may misrepresent the therapy relationship—out of genuine confusion or in the context of a seduction/betrayal enactment—when communicating with his/her family and thereby ignite retaliatory actions, for example. (In a worst-case scenario, a patient actively involved in a criminal family, cult, a perpetrator group, or a false memory advocacy group may explicitly set up a therapist.) Ultimately, the therapist's job is to assist the patient in holding in one consciousness contradictory ideas and feelings about attachment to primary caretakers/ abusers and in tolerating ambiguity and conflict, but not to decide for the patient what his/her reality is or what his/her future relationships with family members should look like.

RECOVERY OF CRITICAL THINKING

We only become what we are by the radical and deep-seated refusal of what others have made of us.

—Jean-Paul Sartre

All forms of sexual, physical, and emotional abuse of children involve the destruction of the child's capacity for critical thinking and psychological reflection. The more intense the abuse, the more extreme the conditions of the victim's captivity, and the more profound the isolation from other sources of attachment and information, the more serious the damage to the essential functions of agency, autonomy, introspection, reflectivity, self-differentiation, and so on, that give rise to, and sustain, what is commonly referred to as free will.

The assaults on the minds and free wills of children by perpetrators occur in a whole variety of forms from subtle and unconscious influence and suggestion to cunning mind manipulations orchestrated to control their lives— all the way to formal brainwashing by means of mind-control technology for the manufacture of a supply of psychic slaves to support criminal, political, and spiritual cults and perpetrator subcultures. It is hard for most of us to accept that while some parents and caretakers pour their hearts and souls into raising and loving their children, others deliberately feed off of children's innocence, use them as psychic dumping grounds, and/or systematically break children's hearts, minds, and spirits—sometimes for the fun of it, sometimes for profit, often to unconsciously perpetuate intergenerational forms of captivity, subjugation, and sacrifice.

Abused and neglected children are easy to manipulate. Their undeveloped sexuality can be easily shaped and perverted to match a perpetrator's appetites and their affectional needs can be completely sexualized; their sense of their own innocence and worth can be completely undermined and corrupted, and their needs for comfort, protection, and attention can be systematically exploited to get them to behave in perverse, destructive, and self-destructive ways. Psychological usurpation can be so thorough that the perpetrator's agenda can be substituted for the child-victim's spontaneous desire, initiative, and worldview with the complete eradication of the child's sense of self and invalidation of his/her sense of reality.

When chronically abused children are coerced into having sex with or harming other children (or animals or other adults) for the entertainment or economic profit of the perpetrators, or into kidnapping (or otherwise seducing) other children into doing so, overwhelming and intolerable shame can dominate every waking moment of their lives. They have to identify with evil in order to maintain their psychological equilibrium. Malevolent authority has succeeded in creating the developmental conditions where inflexible, automatic, and unreflective psychological organizing principles (Stolorow, Brandchaft, and Atwood, 1987) govern everything from the child's inferences and convictions to his/her behaviors and sense of future possibility. Perpetrators' exploitation of shame combined with self-disgust can "destroy self esteem with a ferocity unequaled in human experience" (Nathanson, 1992, p. 463). When a child's sense of self has been totally annihilated to this extent, all forms of mind control are possible.

Most children will work hard without much training and prompting to project that everything in their lives is normal: they devote enormous efforts to covering their confusion, despair, and psychic injuries of immense proportions, so even in our putatively enlightened era most children's torment goes unnoticed. Adult survivors of severe abuse describe how as children they moved among sadistic family systems, criminal cults, public schools, neighbors' houses, and religious institutions without generating the slightest awareness that anything was awry. Adult survivors also consistently report no reaction, much less any investigation whatsoever into possible abuse, from the medical professionals who treated their physical injuries over the years.[2]

A remarkable characteristic of trauma is the blindness and indifference of "authorities," the purposeful lack of curiosity, the denials of family and relatives. These are the denials of the editors of the communal text. Most atrocities have not begun with the slaughter of the innocents, but with the selective silencing of narrators . . . what makes trauma traumatic is not simply the violation of a person's rights and expectations, as in the violation of a taboo, but the deadly fact that nobody notices, labels, categorizes, talks about it. (Nachmani, 1997, p. 194)

Psychotherapy must become a vehicle for restoring critical thinking. The role of the therapist is to help the patient organize and reorganize experience in less painful and more creative ways—but, as intersubjective theory reminds us, all clinicians must be sensitive to the influence and impact of their own thinking and psychological organization. To the extent that a therapist does not understand the dynamics (or believe in the existence) of mind control/thought reform and of the survivors' accommodations to this particularly insidious element of their trauma, s/he will fail to cocreate the transformative vehicle of liberatory intersubjective discourse for repairing the patient's shattered critical thinking. Toward preventing even inadvertent reinforcement of a mind-control victim's isolation and despair, the goal here is to help clinicians to pursue the ultimate intersubjectivist agenda—creation of a spacious intersection between the unique subjectivities of patient and therapist where the unbelievable, the unfathomable, and the unspeakable can be explored together and known, and can begin to be integrated (Orange et al., 1997).

RON

Extremely charming and high-functioning in a way that obscured his severely dissociative (atypical DID) organization, Ron had been in the mental health system for a number of years prior to beginning therapy with me. He had attained sobriety through 12-step programs and had left a physically abusive relationship with a male lover of almost two decades after completing a Victims of Domestic Violence program. Sexually compulsive and acting out in dangerous ways, he had also been misdiagnosed with bipolar disorder and overmedicated accordingly. His unconscious attachments to perpetrators were thereby sustained and his silence thereby perpetuated.

Analyzing the unusual intensity of his sexualized attachment to me from the beginning of therapy is what led to broadening his awareness of his dissociative process and the emergence of memories of incest. Once Ron was able to recall and face his victimization by his father—who regularly slept with him—and his abuse by multiple perpetrators in an all-male pedophile group, he came off all of his medications and began to reveal the complex traumatic bond whereby fantasies of specialness and exhibitionism substituted for real love and attention.

Ron's father would take him to the perpetrator group and trade him for access to other young boys. Ron eventually disclosed that the men in the group anally penetrated him with a gun following his first serial rape and molestation. No words or threats were necessary to elicit his compliance or guarantee his silence: the gun was sufficient. All thoughts of escape or rescue were dissociated behind layers of fear and intimidation, feelings of deep shame about his complicity, and in the end behind perpetrator-identified self-states cultivated to defend against guilt at harming animals and having sex with other children on command.

During the middle phase of treatment when elements of his malignant attachment were being exposed and deconstructed, Ron spontaneously remembered what he called his father's tacit "ten commandments":

1. You will never be strong.
2. You will excel but you will never enjoy your success.
3. You will give without receiving.
4. You will not resist.
5. I own you.
6. You exist to please me.
7. There's not enough to go around and you lose.
8. You will never love or be loved.
9. You must give sex on demand.
10. Betrayal equals death.

Ron's articulation of these injunctions and other aspects of group and paternal programming allowed him to develop a firm protest response and to begin differentiating himself from the traumatic bonding matrix.

Ron was soon able to establish the first mutuality-based, loving, intimate romantic partnership of his life.

THE DISSOCIATION OF MEANING

All persistent child sexual abuse involves boundary violations, coerced compliance, and disruptions in the victim's relationship to his/herself—all damaging the child's delicate but emerging capacity for intentionality, self-reflection, and free will. Chronic sexual abuse also creates changes in consciousness and in the victim's identity and invents pseudo-identities (that may or may not evolve into alter personalities) based on self-betrayal, shame, and identification with the perpetrator as well as on the silence of the colluding family and social system.

When the family or subculture is extremely sadistic, cultlike, and/or part of a criminal organization, the power of meta-communications (Bateson, 1972) to silence and to shape personality and behavior will eventually have effects as powerful as torture. The natural automaticity of being—the knee-jerk, nonconscious links between our goals and our perceptions, evaluations, and self-regulating activities that function to make us behave in consistent ways and effectively pursue our objectives (Bargh and Chartrand, 1999)—can be corrupted in environments where volition is systematically undermined.

Patterns characteristic of incestuous family systems make them crucibles for the isolation, confusion, and dependence on mythology that set the stage for subversion of the minds of the child-victims. They feature closed-group, cultlike dynamics, being socially separate, unusually enmeshed, resistant to change, and dominated by authoritarian leadership; their communication style is distinguished by secretiveness, inconsistent or unclear messages, infrequent discussion of feelings, little attentive listening, and lack of conflict resolution skills (Trepper et al., 1996). Other indices of dysfunction include minimal nurturing activities, lack of healthy attachment, and a large role for substance abuse as a precipitant for episodes of abuse.

The relationship between autobiographical memory and sense of self is a dynamic, interactive process. Language serves to organize what to remember, and how it will be remembered and for how long. Dissociative experience, which reorganizes self-structure after massive upheaval and annihilation anxieties, adds, deletes, compartmentalizes, and distorts aspects of the original traumatic events. Since severe dissociative conditions are created through the double-bind process, the language of multiple personality is a language of contradictions that can never be spoken (Rivera, 1996): "Your father loves you; your father rapes you; your father never touched you, and if you say or even think he did, he will hurt you again harder until you learn that he never hurt you" (p. 60).

Children in particular are profoundly influenced in thought, action, and reflections about events by both direct and indirect pressure from authority figures. Waites (1997) describes the many ways in which, throughout a lifetime, external or internalized authority figures serve gatekeeping, reminding, or censoring functions. Extremely powerful others, when they are excessively rigid and absolute, may govern all narratives that shape memory in a child's life; they may also implicitly and explicitly forbid questioning and impair critical thinking. Definitions of reality by perpetrators and collaborators imposed on a child's natural strivings to make sense out of abusive incidents and their aftermath can disrupt healthy observing ego and critical-thinking capacities.

When people in power provide misleading or false explanations about traumatic events, they not only reinforce denial but also supply alternative narratives to define the victim and the victim's relationship to the world (Waites, 1997). Variously by silencing protests, labeling actual experiences as dreams or fantasies, orchestrating elaborate cover stories, dismissing accusations as products of wild imaginations, or insisting that the victims are guilty and will be punished for disclosing anything to anyone, perpetrators manipulate malleable posttraumatic psyches and the dependency of the children they abuse, encouraging the rapid internalization of false beliefs that will reliably regulate victims' identities and camouflage the perpetrators' crimes. The victims' compulsive self-doubting, confusion, and recantation patterns support the impression that they are not competent sources of information; both publicly and internally, they compare unfavorably to the confident attitudes of the perpetrators.

Increasing the complexity of the memory-suggestibility issue is the fact that reality and fantasy interact. An individual's encoding of external events as well as his/her reactions to them can be seriously distorted by the need to substitute acceptable self/other representations and less threatening narratives for unacceptable impulses and disturbing experiences; one result will be the quashing or editing of truthful reports (Waites, 1997). More benign or bizarre narratives may be created, their coherence dependent on the non-conscious incorporation of inferences to fill in blanks in an effort to make sense of or adapt or transcend painful aspects of reality. In some cases the details of a memory are inaccurate but the gist of the story or event is correct; in others the details may be quite right but the overall interpretation skewed (Siegel, 1997). And once the capacity for fantasy construction has been developed, false assumptions are integrated into the fantasies ("Things like that don't happen here," "Adults are always trustworthy," "I am worthless," "I deserve punishment," etc.), and the fantasies become integrated into memories (Waites, 1997).

The beneficial dimension of suggestibility is the opportunity to internalize the messages and belief systems of trusted authorities under optimal conditions. This salutary process can lead to learning when and how to ask for help and how to detect candor or deception in others. However, in situations where hierarchy is valued (and/or eroticized) over equality, the development of the critical thinking faculties necessary for evaluating the influence of other people will be inhibited by toxic interpersonal and cultural (power) arrangements. Further complications derive from the fact that victimized children may have only limited tools for analyzing and limited repertoires for categorizing their own experience.

Vulnerability to undesirable suggestion and an overreliance on external authority as arbiter of truth and reality are consequences of a reduced capacity for critical analysis, and they culminate in excessive self-censorship, overcompliance, and failures to discriminate between appropriate and inappropriate demands. As Waites (1997) points out, "Instituting the self as a distinct authority who can override other authorities is a complex aspect of individuation that is typically not fully achieved until adulthood and, in some individuals, never achieved at all" (p. 81). When psychotherapy fulfills its mandate to support the individuation process, the patient's emerging capacities for critical thinking may coincide with access to previously unavailable knowledge about traumatic personal history—both in its details and in its meanings. When psychotherapy betrays its essential functions, however, it can suppress the patient's autonomy and critical thinking and train the patient to lean on the therapist's power and perspective (and/or reinforce the patient's false self adaptations and submission to familial, societal, and/or perpetrator group belief systems, cover ups, and denial).

A double injury is inflicted on the child's fragmenting self at the moments of chaos and self-disintegration when the hunger to make sense out of experience, to stave off annihilation anxiety, is most desperate (Schwartz, 1994). The victim's matrix of meaning, order, and predictability is shattered—and, ironically, it is to the victimizer's worldviews and definitions of self that the victim will adhere. Internalizing the offender's cognitive distortions by buying into responsibility for what s/he did, what s/he did not do, and what s/he could not and did not know how to do is actually a way of preserving some hope of controlling the abuse—an investment in the prospect that if the victim caused it, s/he can prevent its recurrence (Salter, 1995).

"Trauma echoes" (Rasmussen, Burton, and Christopherson, 1992, p. 43) are the perpetrator messages that continue to resonate beyond the period of the abuse—messages that the victim adopts as his/her own beliefs. Binding victim and perpetrator in a sadomasochistic attachment and also to a distorted worldview,[3] these are the most likely of all the disturbing, insidious, and far-reaching effects of trauma to lead to despair and self-destructive behavior. The enduring residue of dissociation is such that the *meaning* of traumatic events for which patients finally retrieve memories, details, and fantasies continues to elude them. Thus, individuals surrounded by the intentional cruelty of malevolent caretakers throughout their lives may be unable to feel, name, and react to it, even as they project the malevolence onto innocent others in their worlds. Basch (1983) refers in this connection to "alterations . . . that prevent the union of affect with perception" (p. 137).

ALEC

Alec, who indeed separated perceptions from affects was entirely without access to the inconsistencies in his memory and their stunning implications. His parents had drugged, raped, and handed him over to strangers involved in organized criminal activities—but they also programmed him during hypnotic daytime "training conversations" to invalidate his experience of reality ("You're a good boy, you know what to remember and what not to remember," or "We're your parents and you know we would never do anything to hurt you").

Plied with cognitions that destroyed his critical thinking and his curiosity about himself and his own history, this Ivy League graduate fluent in Holocaust literature and leftist politics developed alter personalities that maintained that people who are parents could never do awful things to their children. So simplistic and magical an equation of family and benevolence from a sophisticated, highly educated, and politically astute man is emblematic of the construct Basch (1983) labels "disavowal of meaning" (p. 137).

In keeping with the foregoing, dissociative patients frequently remain more resistant to relinquishing their trauma-based belief systems than to reexperiencing traumatic affects and imagery. That is, long after recalling gruesome details and confronting some of the previously dissociated mind-body pain attendant on childhood abuse, a survivor may feel incapable of separating from tenacious attachment to systems of meaning that transpose a hurt self into a bad self, a helpless and victimized self into a willful and powerful agent of harm. The shocking absence of any anger at the perpetrators is entrenched and stays intact, as though prolonged immersion in sadistic abuse and extreme trauma bonding have almost completely reversed the self-protection system of the survivor.

"BRAINWASHING" AND MIND CONTROL

The shaping of captives' thought patterns and belief systems—called "brainwashing" in reference to the Chinese indoctrination techniques discovered in the 1950s—leads to some of the most pervasive and devastating sequelae of child abuse. As documented by a CIA and Air Force sociologist (Biderman, 1957), the coercive techniques for eliciting individual compliance resemble those used in Ewan Cameron's more recent CIA-sponsored research on mind control (Weinstein, 1990; Bowart, 1994). The basic methods for developing dependency on, and obedience to, the captors have been generally accessible for at least the past forty or forty-five years, and they are the same ones described by people who have been indoctrinated into mainstream cults or underground criminal cults, including satanic groups.

- isolation;
- monopolization of perception (sensory deprivation);
- induced debilitation and exhaustion;
- threats (to self and family, of endless isolation, etc.);
- occasional indulgences;
- demonstrations of omniscience or omnipotence (complete knowledge of victims' activities, control over their fates);
- degradation (reinforced helplessness, lack of privacy, insults, taunts, imposition of incontinence, disregard for human dignity);
- enforcement of trivial demands (obedience to detailed rules governing all aspects of daily living, even simple and menial).

Long before *The Manchurian Candidate*—Richard Condon's 1958 novel of an American army sergeant captured during the Korean War and hypno-programmed to murder on cue—brought mind control to the attention of the American public, the psychological techniques it describes had been used by various groups as the "blueprint for the creation of an army of hypno-programmed zombies" (Bowart, 1994), many of whom were assassins prepared to kill on cue; others were informers, hypnotized to remember minute details of events and conversations; some were couriers, carrying illegal messages outside the chain of command, their secrets securely hidden behind posthypnotic blocks. In all cases, posthypnotic amnesias were installed to ensure the disappearance of secrets from the minds of those who "no longer had the need to know" (Marks, 1979; Bowart, 1994). The essential goal of mind-control programming is the creation of a population of subconsciously programmed individuals, motivated without their knowledge and against their wills to perform in ways in which they would not otherwise perform. Bowart claims that, although forms of brainwashing and mind control have existed for centuries, complete control of the human mind was only managed in the late 1940s by the U.S. government through the use of pain- and trauma-based classical conditioning paradigms.[4]

Many political, religious, military/paramilitary, and cult groups deliberately program ideas and beliefs into their victims during overwhelmingly painful torture sessions, or during periods of shock, and/or following periods of sensory isolation and incited terror.

ALEC (CONTINUED)

After a period of sensory deprivation and confusion, Alec was forced to witness a gruesome infant sacrifice that he was told was conducted for his benefit—that the sacrificial victim was chosen to die while he was chosen to live; because he was to be forever indebted for his life, his loyalty to his perpetrators was impenetrable for many years. The dissociative split in his personality thus orchestrated became the basis for elaborate assassin training involving myriad obedient, perpetrator-identified, cult-alters, who were specifically instructed to distrust all therapists and law enforcement agents, and to deflect or argue against any mention of multiple personality disorder. Over many years in treatment, Alec observed the emergence of a consistent, ego-dystonic type of hatred toward me whenever the subject of child abuse or multiple personality disorder was discussed.

SONJA

While being repeatedly raped and sodomized by a group of men from a satanic/Aryan cult in the basement of a local church, Sonja was told that she was Satan's child whose special position in the cult hierarchy made her worthy of such treatment, and simultaneously that she was a worthless whore who was good for nothing but being excreted upon. (She went on to develop isolated islands of specialness and worthlessness, loyalty to the group, and vehement self-sabotage.) Following other torture sessions, Sonja was repeatedly indoctrinated with beliefs that God hated her and had rejected and abandoned her (how else could such satanic abuse be taking place?), and that whenever she entered a church she would be reminded of her torture and would not hear or remember anything being said during church services. Not surprisingly, Sonja developed a complex set of phobias and traumatic reactions to churches, clergy members, and crucifixes. Reinforced by and intertwined with preexisting and ongoing everyday life experiences like so much other programming, Sonja's embedded beliefs in her abandonment by a benevolent deity were highly resistant to change.

CLARITA

After being removed from a sensory deprivation situation in extrafamilial ritual abuse, Clarita was repeatedly raped and told that her old self died in the "death box" while her new self, an obedient and compliant alter, was being born to serve her masters. This new self was given specific hypnotic instructions to wake up in the middle of the night, go into the kitchen and get a butcher knife, and go up to her parents' bedroom and murder them in their sleep. The perpetrator group had Clarita's cult alter practice with various animals, dolls, and possibly in one case with an infant. The double murder was averted when Clarita's abuse came to her parents' attention just as she was being trained to respond to the hypnotic triggers. For many years in treatment, Clarita remained terrified of her own angry and aggressive feelings, secretly (and unconsciously) fearing that any expression of fury would lead to homicidal behavior.

Automatic responses to the trigger cues embedded in the victim's unconscious mind (activated by strategic words, sounds, phone messages, hand signals, etc., and/or sometimes by a message with encoded information passed along by an unwitting sibling, relative, or friend) can cause switches between personality states and amnesias, and can lead a victim to follow directions to attend a gathering or ritual against his/her will.

ROBYN

By means of commands implanted during and after torture sessions when she was in robotic self-states of whose existence she had little or no awareness for most of her life, Robyn had been hypnotically trained to open her front door when she heard a specific sequence of footsteps. She often let cult contacts right in through her front door only to be transported to rituals where she was retraumatized and reprogrammed. Some of this took place while Robyn was in her first stages of contact with the mental health system. At that time, and prior to her being correctly diagnosed with DID, she was almost completely dysfunctional and unable to communicate about most of her experiences. When she tried to tell her psychiatrist and the staff at the mental health center about people entering her home at night and her agitation about footsteps, they told her she was paranoid and administered antipsychotic medications. Because her perpetrator group knew that Robyn was in treatment during that period, they initiated intense supplementary silencing programming. Caught between two destructive subcultures, Robyn ingested massive quantities of Valium and gin and repeatedly attempted suicide.

Most survivors report that while the torture is going on they are given specific instructions on how to behave outside the group, whom to associate with and whom to avoid, and of course the consequences for talking about the abuse or group subculture. Inevitably, programming in these cult contexts indoctrinates into children beliefs in their superiority over others, isolating them from identification with healthy human beings (Smith, 1993), and bonding them by means of the perverse sense of specialness that is the only allowable form of recognition—and the pride of membership in the elite group that is the only allowable form of belonging.

Although many people find the ideas of brainwashing, mind control, or posthypnotic suggestion hard to believe, theories and research on the physiology of psychological trauma, extreme stress, and state-dependent learning (Elin, 1995; Van der Kolk, 1987b; 1995; Rossi, 1986; Rossi and Cheek, 1988; Krystal et al., 1996), the processing of dissociation in response to trauma (Foa and Hearst-Ikeda, 1996) as well as the literature on hypnosis (Nemiah, 1985; Whalen and Nash, 1996) suggest that information offered during and after torture may be encoded at deep psychobiological levels, sequestered from mainstream consciousness. Such information may then become state-dependent to specific psychophysiological stimuli and/or triggers; memory and learning may become apparently dissociated or lost (or retrieved) when there is a shift between states (i.e., alter personalities).

Foa and Kozak (1986) note that pathological fear structures, including the unrealistic elements that may become associated with states of absorption and heightened arousal often attendant on extreme stress, are *extremely resistant to modification*. Hence, the power of all statements made during and immediately after abusive episodes while the victim is in an altered state will be enhanced by the absence of an operative critical consciousness (Conway, 1994) and by the indelible connection with intense fear, intolerable anxiety, or mind-shattering dread. Psychologically sophisticated abusers who have mastered the methods of mind control know how to induce state changes, how to elaborate and encapsulate them, how to provide the cues to trigger them, how to tap into and alter the victim's motivational and belief systems, and how to layer amnesias within a personality so that a polyfragmented DID individual can appear to lead the life of a normal hardworking citizen, yet can function undetected (by himself or by others) as a mind-controlled operative or marionette-operative and remain available for service to malevolent individuals or groups.

The motivations behind the extremes and excesses of perpetrators who use mind control may be

- *psychological*, and include sadism, psychosis, paranoid fantasies, reenactment, tension reduction, primitive envy, omnipotence, externalization of primitive states of inner torment, and so on.
- *economic*, involving the supply of labor for prostitution, pornography, drug running, arms trafficking, and snuff-film industries, and so on.
- *political*, entailing espionage, sabotage, propaganda, assassinations, indoctrinating ideologies, and so on.
- *forensic*, aimed at silencing victims, protecting secrets, evading detection, confusing the public and the authorities, blaming victims and other innocent people, and so on.

- *spiritual*, in the forms of hatred of God, hatred of humanity, assault on Creation, destruction of society, mockery of culture à la Charles Manson, defiling innocence, archetypal envy, and so on.

But there is more to understand. The mother of all addictions is the addiction to power, particularly power over others. The axiom that "power corrupts and absolute power corrupts absolutely" is central to apprehending the extremes of human malevolence once power over others appears to the perpetrator(s) to be unlimited. Those who have not been personally exposed to those extremes may be unable fully to appreciate the compelling, corrupting, degenerative spiral of extreme power obsessions. History has shown that once an individual or group becomes inflated with power (Hitler, Idi Amin, Pol Pot, the Duvaliers, Stalin, to name a few), a pattern of extravagant sadism, wanton cruelty, and irrational and ultimately self-destructive binges of exhibitionistic violence leads to eventual explosion or collapse. History has yet to reveal that these same diabolical dynamics are at work outside the context of war and politics—in perpetrator groups inflicting their power on children worldwide in the form of unimaginable abuse.

JENNY

Like other survivors, Jenny reported deliberate assaults on hope and mastery at the hands of particularly sadistic parents and in perpetrator groups whose training program mandated complete breakdown of the personality to facilitate the substitution of their agenda for her own. Jenny's mother's sadism was so extreme that it is difficult to fully understand her motivations to inflict such ongoing torment on her daughter. Although Jenny's mother received money from the pimps and handlers who came to take Jenny to houses of prostitution in the evenings, on weekends, and during school holidays, her own sadism was so unbridled and so twisted that she tortured her daughter in the regular "preparation" process and inflicted ongoing torment the rest of the time. It is impossible to know whether she learned her methods from upper-level perpetrators or came up with them on her own—and impossible to imagine what kind of internal state she herself must have been living in.

Jenny's mother created a cruel game to "purify" her hours before she would be serially raped and sodomized. She purportedly filled three enema bags with water, two of them with household cleansers mixed in. Jenny, four to ten years old during this period, was told to choose the one that would be used to clean her out; if she picked one of the solutions that would burn her insides, it was her decision, her responsibility, and, of course, her fault. While struggling with the effects of the painful enemas, Jenny would be beaten "to help her make the right choice next time." The mother, when handing her over to the men looking like a wreck, would tell them that Jenny had resisted her enemas, for which they would administer extra punishment. It took years for Jenny to realize that the Russian roulette with her intestines was bogus and that her mother had always set it up so that all three bags contained the painful solutions. Jenny's mother was head of the school PTA during some of this time.

Jenny's personality was annihilated, her self-hatred consolidated and intensified. She was completely confused and devoid of any sense of hope, agency, or mastery. The tortures amplified her sense of numbness and isolation, and eventually fostered increased compliance with both mother and perpetrator group. The constant double binds escalated her vulnerability to extreme dissociative adaptations, which were exploited by the group to shape alter identities who could tolerate extreme pain and horror, and participate in destructive activities without any feeling or caring.

CLARITA (CONTINUED)

Like many groups trafficking in child prostitution and pornography, Clarita's perpetrators were also involved in satanic ritual abuse, part of whose programming necessitates a rupture in the child-victim's relationship with a benevolent Divinity. Accordingly, Clarita was told by her handler that she was going to a special place for a surprise (which only a highly dissociative child would believe after multiple rapes and betrayals), and then ordered Clarita into the confessional booth in a Catholic Church where a costumed "priest" (either a child prostitution customer or a member of the pedophile group) was waiting for her. He demanded that she perform oral sex, he raped her, and during the molestation he locked in her view of herself as damaged, evil, dirty, and abandoned by God, saying that she was very good at "this"; that "this" was all she was good for; that God knew she liked "this"; God knew this was what she was good at; that God was coming through him as he was inside of her and that God wanted her to always be like "this" and do things like "this"; and that he was planting God's seeds in her.

After ejaculation, the "priest" pushed Clarita out of the confessional into the waiting arms of her handler, who typically gave her some kind of drug-laced candy or ice cream to induce sleep between the traumatizing events and the posttraumatic programming. (Of course by early adolescence Clarita had a raging eating disorder). On the way home, the handler reinforced and expanded on what the "priest" had begun: God wanted her to do this for other men, God knew what she liked and who she really was, and this was all she was good for; God would reject her, God had raped her, and since God would have nothing to do with her, she belonged to the group who would protect her from God's cruelty.

Clarita remembered that when she awoke later that afternoon in the home of her neighbor/perpetrator he was telling her that she had had a bad dream, that things like that don't happen, could never happen in a church in broad daylight since so many people would be coming in and out.

During this session, the perpetrator had his arm around her as he assured her, "you are still special to me no matter what." He taught her some breathing techniques to suppress the emergence of bad feelings and implanted suggestions about how to manage them. Dissociation training and pain- and affect-management are essential parts of most perpetrator groups' programming methods to increase the victim's dependency on them and enable the victim to cope with the pain they inflict.

When her primary perpetrator grabbed her by the shoulder in the midst of an altered, drugged state, looked her forcefully in the eye and repeated, "I am the only one who can protect you," Clarita concluded that you have to protect your protector and that the man influencing her then was not the same person as the man orchestrating her abuse. She went home to her parents' house later that day feeling awful and condemned but not knowing why, since she had no memory of the events; later, whenever any memories began to surface, a voice in her head would remind her it was only a dream; things like that never really happen.

THE CONTINUUM OF
MIND CONTROL AND THOUGHT REFORM

In the lives of severely dissociative individuals, attachment to the sources of trauma has taken precedence over self-gratification and self-actualization. This is not surprising since the resources of the traumatized self have been devoted to survival and avoidance of painful feelings and memories, and since some stability has been achieved through identification (including rehearsal of false historical narratives, cover stories, and lies) with the perpetrator's worldview, belief systems, and representations of the victim. Even more disturbing than vulnerability to collaborating in one's own subjugation by establishing traumatic attachments with oppressors is the exploitation of that vulnerability by those oppressors, possessed of the know-how to capitalize on human desperation in the face of stress, chronic shame, and isolation. And more disturbing still is the evidence of persistent denial among mental health professionals that precisely these species of thought reform and mind control are realities to be reckoned with.

From military and paramilitary brainwashing to the criminal and ritual abuse of children in cults and incestuous families, from Stockholm Syndrome situations to television advertising that plays on people's fears and low self-esteem, the mechanisms of thought reform and mind control operate on a continuum whose points include subtle influence, coercive persuasion, traumatic bonding, orchestrated terror, torture, and indoctrination. While in cases of child abuse specifically, the more organized the context, the more central will be the role of explicit programming, the distance on the continuum between the myth making and denial characteristic of the enmeshed, secretive incest family and the systematic tactics of the most "professional" groups is more of degree than of kind. If the former embodies entrenched identification with the aggressor and the absolute collapse of critical thinking, the latter can involve greater dissociation as well as the encapsulation of layered trauma and belief systems in a complex psychic organization that can take years to dismantle.

Salter (1995) likens the thought-reforming process to footprints left by the perpetrator on the victim's heart and mind. She also distinguishes between two types of denial, both of which shape the victim's experience of reality. *Explicit denial* applies where the offender "attempt[s] to groom, persuade, instruct, bribe, and/or threaten" (p. 123) the victim before, during, and/or after the abuse to control the characterization of reality. *Implicit denial* refers to the tacit message conveyed when "rape in the night [is] followed by breakfast with family [members] who act . . . (for different reasons) as though nothing happened. Upon leaving the house, [the victim] face[s] an entire world of implicit denial. Everyone—teachers, friends, coaches—all act . . . as though nothing happened" (p. 123). Different types of abusers leave different footprints on the child-victim's identity, memory, feelings, and worldviews, consistent with their different imperatives—sadism, hunger for power and control, fantasies of the child's arousal, or impulses to participate in evil behavior. Motive notwithstanding, however, abuse always attacks and sometimes suppresses the child-victim's sense of reality, recall, and capacity for critical thinking.

THOUGHT REFORM AND SUBJECTIVE ORGANIZATION

Things will happen to you from which you could not recover if you lived a thousand years. Never again will you be capable of ordinary human feeling. Everything will be dead inside you. Never again will you be capable of love, or friendship, or joy of living, or laughter, or curiosity, or courage, or integrity. You will be hollow. We shall squeeze you empty and then we shall fill you with ourselves.

—George Orwell (1984)

Linked to the literature on incestuous families, thought reform, cults, and the Stockholm Syndrome, is Brandchaft and Stolorow's (1990) important theoretical statement about the defensive encapsulation of mental life in the service of sustaining primitive object ties to malevolent caregivers. "Developmental traumata derive their lasting significance from the establishment of invariant and relentless principles of organization that remain beyond the accommodative influence of reflective self-awareness or of subsequent experience" (p. 108). Similarly, Stolorow and Atwood (1994), though not addressing incestuous families and organized sex rings, describe the primary developmental motivation of the self to be maintaining the organization of experience by consolidating pathological structures that rigidly restrict the individual's subjective field. These inflexible structures allow traumatized individuals to predictably order their experiences to prevent the emergence of emotional conflict and subjective feelings of danger; in the case of more profound thought reform and pathological attachments to violent perpetrators, the constriction exists to prevent any free thought and feeling that can disrupt the rigid belief system internalized during the prolonged immersion in the abusive relationship and the totalist milieu.

When traumatized individuals develop cohesive psychological structures whose primary goal is to prevent the consolidation of new structures, the thus-enfeebled core self is as trapped intrapsychically as the captive child was in the malevolent caregiving system. So when highly dissociative patients begin in therapy to demonstrate increased self-reflection, observing ego, and critical thinking abilities, powerful internal voices emerge almost immediately to sow profound doubt and confusion, and fears of repeating traumatic childhood experiences plant unconscious defensive resistances to change. The fears arise unpredictably in the transference as the process of therapeutic inquiry illuminates and therefore threatens "the matrix of emotionally enslaving early ties" (Brandchaft, 1994, p. 67).

Recantation of child-abuse claims are easily explained by the tenacity of the entrenched principle of self-organization whose primary feelings and cognitions are in complete compliance with the delusions, cover-ups, omnipotent fantasies, and threats of the perpetrators. The constituent losses of inner cohesion, subjectivity, affectivity, authenticity, agency, temporality, continuity, and self-differentiation are articulated by Orange, Atwood, and Stolorow (1997). The following self-destructive beliefs and invariant organizing principles internalized by the victim accumulate in proportion to the frequency and intensity of abuse, the number of perpetrators, and the degree of organized cult or criminal involvement:

- You deserve punishment and condemnation.
- Resistance is futile.
- There is no escape and no hope, and hoping will cause you more pain.
- You can do nothing to effect any change in the situation.
- No one can hear you scream, no one cares; faith in any person or in God is useless, and continued screaming will elicit more torture.
- No one will believe anything you say, no matter what you tell them.
- Feelings are dangerous; stay away from them or you will be destroyed.

- Weakness and vulnerability are disgusting; they merit punishment, torment, and humiliation.
- You will do and think and say exactly what you are told, but you will think you are doing as you choose.
- Your choices have made all this happen.
- You have and will have no memories but the memories I/we authorize.
- We are always watching you; we know your every thought, feeling, and action.
- You can hate and be angry only at yourself or those we direct you to hate and harm.
- Something is deeply wrong with you and you must constantly hide it from others.
- You must always act normal and fit in as though nothing out of the ordinary has ever happened to you.
- You belong to us; we will protect you.
- Any power or success you have comes from us and belongs to us; should you seek anything on your own you will endlessly self-sabotage until you collapse into utter futility and self-hatred.
- You will die if you tell anyone or if you try to leave us.

The Systematic Destruction of Critical Thinking

First you take a child and confine it in a box. Then you add worms, bugs, and snakes and place a lid on the box. The child will kick and scream in terror. You ignore the child until no noise comes from the box, at which time you remove the top of the box. You then check the muscle tone of the child. If the tone is relaxed, you have caused a dissociated switch, and you can now train this new personality to be who you want and to do what you want. The child will obey without question. (Fraser, 1997, p. 195, paraphrasing the instructions of a patient raised in a Satanic cult)

Once the cult-indoctrinated alter—sometimes given a new name[5] that the perpetrators can use to elicit learned (state-dependent) behaviors—is further separated from the pretrauma self and directed to perform certain acts, its sense of isolation from the rest of the personality (and from humanity) is concretized, and its identification with the group continues in a mindless and robotic pattern.

Singer (1995), defining the tactics used in cult contexts, identifies three staged preconditions for thought control: *destabilization* of the victim's sense of self, *indoctrination* into the leader's re-vision of reality, and *dependency* on the group. (In psychoanalytic language, that paradigm translates as disruption without restitution, faulty or deceptive restitution, and identification with the aggressor.) Hassan (1990) labels the same phases *unfreezing*—by means of drugs, hypnosis, torture, shock, or trauma (which last can be accomplished in children through seduction, shaming, or sexual arousal alone); *change,* commonly registered with the deliberate inculcation in the victim of a special belief, for example (see *Clarita*, below); and *refreezing.*

CLARITA (CONTINUED)

Molested in a child-care/baby-sitting context for two years beginning at the age of seven along with her little brother, who was then two and a half, Clarita was conditioned to believe that she was sexually excited by death. The perpetrators purported to murder her brother and then (exploiting her rivalry toward him and his favored role in her family), claimed they had done so as a gift to her. After carrying him away (temporarily unconscious), they unleashed a particularly sadistic man on her who raped her brutally. Her "handlers" told her that she enjoyed the sex more this time because it followed her brother's killing—but that they would keep her secret, since she would be publicly humiliated if people found out that she was THAT kind of person.

Nachmani's (1997) basic scenario for eviscerating the capacities for self-witnessing, memory, and narrativity in interpersonal trauma cuts across incestuous families, ritual-abuse cults, and military mind-control programs.

First, victims are isolated, their credibility and judgment are destroyed, and their shame at their own helplessness is exploited along with their humiliating degradation on finding themselves powerless to make any choice other than to collude in their own captivity and subjugation, unwittingly, by identifying with the aggressors. Next, victims are deprived of what they care about, whereupon the abusers create double binds around pain avoidance and their attachment needs to cultivate dependency and engender betrayals of self and others. Then victims are deliberately confused, forced to reassign responsibility and to subscribe to a new worldview, according to which pain is pleasure and pleasure is pain; feelings are bad, numbness is good; vulnerability and resistance are bad, power and compliance are good; keeping secrets is praiseworthy, speaking openly is stupid and dangerous.

CLARITA (CONTINUED)

Consistent with extremes of abuse that included gang rape and burial in a mortuary chamber along with threats to harm her family or expose her to the authorities and also the intermittent administration of drugs, usually in ice cream or other sweets, Clarita was subjected to extremes of confusion in the form of the "dichotic listening paradigm" dating back to mind-control methods of the 1950s.

Two men on either side of her would simultaneously whisper different messages in her ears. When, for instance, the perpetrators coerced her little brother on top of her naked, one man said, "You must lie with your brother," and the other said, "It's a sin to lie with your brother." And in another set of double binds, when Clarita was forced to have oral sex with several men, she was told at once how specially good she was at and for doing it, and what an awful pig of a child she was for wanting to have sex with all those men—and her little brother. . . .

Years later in therapy, the patient reported that her anxiety became so intense that she felt as though she would agree to do anything they asked just to make the feeling stop. The continuous shifting between self-images of specialness and despicable worthlessness is common practice among perpetrators seeking to "break" a child by fomenting dissociative splits in his/her psyche.

For Feiner (1996), the knowledge taboo—being forbidden to know—underlies mind control, thought reform, and brainwashing of all kinds, independent of the sophistication of the particular technique. Negating that edict wreaks intrapsychic havoc on a dissociative system set up with not knowing as its central organizing principle. (Not knowing contributes also to the susceptibility of abused children to "the inauthentic, the con, or the adulterated" [p. 419].)

When a victim is able to transcend the pseudo-safety of Freyd's (1996) aforementioned *betrayal blindness* and surmount the anxiety involved in breaking the unconscious contract with the perpetrator, s/he can count on him/her to attempt to reinstate the original subjugation by means of a letter, a phone call, a look across a courtroom, a hypnotic preprogrammed trigger word or signal, or a direct threat. If that fails, the perpetrator will switch to debunking the victim's narrative. And if that fails, the perpetrator will reverse cause and effect to make the victim look like the victimizer.

Lifton (1961) notes that thought reform has a self-perpetuating momentum, and indeed patients' accounts confirm that organized mind control is consistently, if unintentionally, reinforced by the family and culture at large. The bizarre creeds of ritual abusers and cults that culminate in counterintuitive self-sacrificing totalism emanate from the same conditions and the same dynamics that apply in incestuous and sadistic family systems. In each context, the group is valorized over the individual, the expression of feelings and the use of language are severely constricted, the power of the leaders/parents is magnified by the failure of the authorities to intervene; outsiders are regarded as worthless, protest is suppressed, autonomy is associated with danger, and escape is portrayed as futile. Most DID patients have been exposed to the extreme end of the continuum—and it is once again, emphatically, a continuum—of totalist environmental conditions.

The combination of brutality and sadistic sexuality with harsh, punitive, and fear-based fundamentalist religious practices that can devastate any child's self-esteem and create constant guilt and shame makes for a not uncommon kind of additional doublespeak. Conformity to conventional dogma by day is perverted by explicitly forbidden abuse by night—sometimes ritualized in satanic ceremonies conducted by the same individuals who conduct socially sanctioned religious services; the perpetrator's use of (pseudo) religious terminology to justify the abuse compounds the child-victim's mystification.

Many patients who have been victims of mind-control cults have reported experiences of good cop/bad cop scenarios in which one perpetrator asks personal questions in an accusatory manner, inflicts pain, and/or makes derogatory statements while another acting friendly, speaks comfortingly. Like the dichotic listening paradigm, this model seems to have the effect of arousing high anxiety and psychological states of terror, eradicating memory for the specifics of the event, and fracturing the psyche in such a way that the perpetrator's messages, beliefs, or directives may be implanted beneath the layers of the victim's conscious awareness. Later in life, such patients experience great panic whenever anyone asks even innocuous personal questions, and they do not understand their intense reactions even to filling out forms.

Several patients who were trained for long-term participation in sex/death cults or criminal groups making snuff films had to undergo various forms of classical and operant conditioning in order for them first to be able to tolerate witnessing animals, children, and adults being tortured, raped, and killed, and then to become sexually aroused by these stimuli. By the time they were responding automatically (against their own inner moral imperatives) to the torture with sexual arousal, their memories of having been conditioned had disappeared from consciousness; they knew only that they were filled with unbearable shame and an inexplicable mix of specialness and awfulness.

The victims' belief in their new identities is reinforced when perpetrators recount their involvement or replay the events on film. One thing is certain in these conditions: the now dissociative child will virulently hate him/herself and not the perpetrator and will become highly invested in covering his/her own tracks, believing s/he is and has always been evil. When a therapist, often later in therapy, uncovers such an elaborate perpetrator-identified dissociative matrix in a patient, s/he is likely to be disparaged, ridiculed, and emotionally (sometimes physically) assaulted in a variety of ways, in an analog to the predictable responses of an exposed perpetrator.

Some patients have described the day-by-day breaking down of their personalities through exposure to impossible ethical or psychological conflicts and double binds. Organized perpetrator groups have learned how to induce antisocial behavior in otherwise moral and ethical individuals by using hypnosis, blackmail, forced choices, threats, coerced participation in perpetration, and other brainwashing techniques. The use of chronic pain, electroshocks (high voltage to hurt and fracture the personality, lower voltage to implant suggestions and shape the emerging self-state), drugs, sleep deprivation, physical exhaustion, incited terror, isolation, and starvation further help break down victims' personalities to make them reliably receptive to programming (Bowart, 1994).

JULIA

Julia was five years old when one of her primary pimps in an organized sex ring threatened that if she did not initiate oral sex her siblings would be spirited into the group's sexual adventures too. When, after much hesitation, she complied, her perpetrators built the case that she had chosen to participate in the sex that was to brutalize her body. They even forced Julia to watch films of her "volitional" sexual activity to lock in her identification with that choice. Of course these same films had another value—on the black market—after they were used to cement her indoctrination. When her perpetrator group later wanted to punish a transgression (an imaginary one, in this case, meant more to break her down than to actually punish her) and teach her that she was completely powerless, and to gain complete compliance and submission, they raped her sister in front of her and threatened to do it again if she ever strayed from the group again (which she had not done to begin with).

When Julia's perpetrator/trainer lost his erection he would rage at her for not "doing it right" and then penetrate her with objects that made her desperate for a method—any method—to sustain his and then the paying molesters' erections. The same perpetrator taught this five-year-old that his penis was a person who could read her mind and see what she was doing so that when she was misbehaving his penis would know it, become erect, and have to come find her and rape her. Even late in her therapy, Julia had difficulty comprehending the basic facts of male sexuality; she was nauseated by almost any sexual contact.

Victims report literally being driven out of their conscious minds—losing their free will and their ability to reason and question. One objective of mind control is the victim's conviction that s/he has made the decisions; when personalities are thus strategically subdivided, they can be harnessed by "invisible reins" (Bowart, 1978; 1994). Reworking the attendant assumptions in therapy can be among the most difficult tasks of integration and recovery from chronic trauma.

JENNY (CONTINUED)

Late in her therapy, Jenny and I stumbled into a major piece of torture and programming related to hope, futility, ambition, and despair. It came about when a series of extended medical complications thwarted her plan to complete her education (one of the by-products of her success in treatment), whereupon Jenny fell into a massive depression unlike anything we had previously encountered.

A defiant, detached, depleted, and deadened set of alter personalities emerged in response to both present concerns and unmetabolized trauma, though how much to which was for a time unclear. The density of Jenny's reactions was threatening a dangerous psychological paralysis such that for the first time in our years together I was feeling like giving up on her. Only when I shared that feeling with her was Jenny's psychic deadness and our paralysis punctured: the intensity of our discouragement, the depth of our mutual caring, and her gratitude for the honesty and the wake-up call were powerful enough to surface fragments of the story that follows and give us access to programmed beliefs and alter personalities.

Jenny had been incested, tortured, and used extensively in child prostitution, pornography, and ritual abuse before entering first grade—but once she started school, her handlers had to preempt the prospect of her exposing that world/life, wittingly or not. Jenny's extravagantly sadistic mother was a natural ally at coming up with ways to break Jenny's spirit and destroy her soul to condition her to remain a pawn of the group twenty-four hours a day. Aside from outlets for her own sadism, Jenny's mother received money from the group for her efforts and at times participated herself (for money and possibly for her own perverse amusement) in prostitution and pornography. Jenny was, in effect, a major financial support of this extremely poor family.

In Jenny's school, each child had to bring a cigar box filled with crayons, pencils, scissors, a ruler, and other school supplies. Jenny's eagerness to put her "gift box" together was matched by her mother's perverse pleasure in alerting the head of the child-abuse ring to report it, and his response was to rape Jenny anally and vaginally with the precious objects in her special cigar box, tainting them and conditioning an ugly association.

Only a couple of days after that incident, on the eve of the first day of school, Jenny's mother went into a rage, scribbling all over the precious box and systematically ruining the contents. Jenny was horrified the next morning when she opened the box and was so anxious about what the teacher might say that she closed it and, as she remembered in therapy, put her head on her desk and refused to talk as the teacher approached her desk. She gave up fighting the inevitable, took her hand off the box . . . and adamantly denied responsibility for the destruction—whereupon the shocked, angry teacher telephoned Jenny's mother, who beat her on her return home both for her alleged behavior and for "lying" about it.

The school authorities branded her a liar (and she carried that label in school from then on); her perpetrator group, meanwhile, brutalized Jenny for "bringing attention to herself." She was also taught to never draw pictures like the other kids in class, to never follow the teacher's directions to draw objects or people but to ONLY draw scribbles. Reinforcement of these conditioned inhibitions throughout her school life ensured that Jenny would produce no artwork that would cast suspicion on her extra-school life.

While Jenny looked forward to a good start to second grade, having completely "forgotten" the details of this initial incident because of her already fixed dissociation, her mother by then had to make the game more complex. She threatened Jenny with no food or sleep until she actually participated in the destruction, helping to break up each pencil and crayon and make at least a few scribbles of her own on the new, clean cigar box. Now her complicity was assured; this time, if she denied doing the damage when confronted, she would indeed be lying.

By the end of third grade, Jenny dreaded school and had a deep distrust of her own memory. She had come to believe that she had "somehow" destroyed her own school supplies—after all, everyone agreed, her parents, the teachers, the aunt who had paid for them and to whom Jenny was forced to apologize. Her reputation as a liar and as a "hard-to-reach child" preceded her year after year. Meanwhile, Jenny had become so highly dissociative that she often did things she could not remember doing, which added to her overall confusion.

This took place in the late 1950s and early 1960s in a midwestern small town where there were no school psychologists. Jenny remembered hating herself for believing life would or could be different. She hated herself for hoping. She developed alter personalities to defend against hope and to denigrate those who believed in a brighter future. Some forty years later, it was still hard for Jenny to conceive of how much energy her perpetrators had put into abusing her and shaping her mind and belief systems, and also to recognize her mother's role in orchestrating the concentric double binds with the perpetrator group—to make Jenny an expert dissociator and correspondingly excellent performer for the group. Any hopes of escape were systematically shattered.

So much rigorous training had gone into consolidating Jenny's memory-loss programming that whenever, early in her first inpatient hospitalizations, she would begin talking with mental health workers or her psychiatrist about her childhood traumas, she would immediately dissociate, become mute, and lose complete memory for what was going on in the conversation. At times, the entire musculature of her body would freeze and she would enter into dissociative states of paralysis, completely unresponsive to all stimuli. Incorrectly diagnosed, and greeted with rage, frustration, and retaliation by various caretakers, Jenny earned a reputation as a difficult, noncompliant patient. As she eventually explained to me once her dissociative patterns were recognized and correctly diagnosed, she needed someone to help her learn to talk, think, and remember all over again—from scratch.

Basic Forms of Organized Programming

Although not an exhaustive list, the following represent the essential forms of organized programming used in all mind-control situations, and are the foundation upon which all other more complex and sophisticated forms of indoctrination and structuralized dissociation are based.

Memory Loss.   This most basic of programming objectives maintains the secrecy of the group, cult, or individual perpetrator, ensuring the ongoing viability of the abusive situation. From the molester of a single child to government-sanctioned operations, all use amnesia techniques (hypnotic suggestions, threats, shaming, drugs, classical conditioning, dissociation training) to erase victims' memories of incidents, names, even faces. (If you ever begin remembering you will . . . fall asleep, immediately think of something else, cut yourself, walk into traffic, etc.) (Related programming may include silencing training, shutdown training, confusion, recantation and false memory training, etc.)

Cover Dialogue.   While the purpose here is also the containment of perpetrator identity, the method is not merely obliteration of actual memory, but in fact the implantation of phony memory. In the simple cover-story situation, the child is programmed to recall incidents that never happened and to recount them when asked by outsiders for explanations. (Fresh bruises, for instance might be described as by-products of a fall on the ball field.) In cults, the cover programming is far more complex: children are often trained to dissociate and feign ignorance on hearing such trigger words as "child abuse," "multiple personality," "Satan," "sacrifice," "rape," and "torture"; or the demeanor of abject confusion itself becomes the cover.

At a simple level, many survivors use the repetitive story that they are "crazy," "damaged," or "awful" when any traumatic memories are emerging; the shame of exposing their defective self becomes motivation to guard secrecy while sustaining a plausible (and ego-syntonic) narrative for deflecting further introspection. If anyone gets close enough to become acquainted with the survivor's internal process, these negative self-affirmations will seem part and parcel of a problem in self-esteem and will more than likely be accepted as neurotic symptoms rather than suspected to be the tip of a posttraumatic and brainwashing iceberg.

In other situations, a child is taken to a local pickup point, say in a shopping mall or at a theme park, and used for hours in prostitution, pornography, and rituals and then programmed to tell about his/her day at the cover location when anyone asks where s/he spent the last period of time. (When Jenny was sent away for entire summers the cover story that she spent her summer with her "uncle" in the country was implanted and trained into her mind, and told by all of her family members.)

In long-term abuse, cover-dialogue programming becomes an intricate and well-developed part of the child's identity and world. The programming can be so extensive that nothing of the original child's personality remains and, instead, an outer shell is built that functions in the outer world. This pseudo-identity can eventually become, and indeed is intended to become, more real than the child's personality. With time, the innocence of the original child is stored in a sub-child-alter personality. Like a prisoner who has been kept in isolation for most of his life, this personality often remains autistic and unable to function in any place or setting without the help of its guard: the hostile alter. It is important to note, however, that the innocent alter is a source of hope for successful treatment—evidence that personality integration may in fact be possible.

All of the cover stories can surface as such when retold during therapy: they begin to unravel under scrutiny as factual improbabilities, insufficient detail, and false meanings become clear. The very revelation of ill-fitting pieces may lead to a breakthrough. Often, the cover story emerges simultaneously with other traumatic memories and competes for attention and allegiance within the mind of the patient. Many therapists preferring to believe innocuous stories over trauma memories are seduced by cover dialogue.

Task Programming.   Programming children to perform tasks—from stealing money for a parent to delivering messages or drugs on to committing harmful acts including kidnapping, murder, or political assassination—involves some form of abuse to ensure compliance. That is, the victim is repeatedly victimized in whatever specific way that will break him/her to do whatever s/he is asked to do; s/he is eventually rendered not just malleable to the perpetrator but actually a "willing" collaborator. One way this occurs is when a child is forced to choose between being (once again) tortured or torturing someone else. Once the child "chooses" to harm another, s/he becomes ensnared in guilt and shame and "willing" to do what the perpetrator asks.

In other situations, following complete breakdown of the child's personality through electrocution torture, for example, opiates combined with hypnotic commands are given so that pain relief becomes conditional on compliant performance of specific tasks and functions. Medical professionals trained in torture and personality restructuring may monitor the breakdown and reconstruction process through noting optimal levels of arousal, dissociation, breathing, heart rates, various brain waves, and so on, in preparation for conducting inductions and personality shaping. In the most sophisticated child-prostitution rings, victims are trained and conditioned under threat of pain, terror, and death, to discriminate among and fulfill the fantasies of different types of child molesters.

One DID patient explained how she was trained to stalk and lure children to waiting cars with the promise of candy or a toy. By means of films and on-site observation such as at parks, playgrounds, and beaches, she was taught to detect parents who let their children wander or children who seemed lost. She learned how to approach the potential kidnap victim and begin to play with him/her to gain his/her trust. Once in the car, where a perpetrator would immediately drug the kidnapped child, she was to contain him/her on the floor of the backseat until the vehicle arrived at a transfer point. Such training took place with an already broken, highly dissociative, compliant child with a considerable history already in underground activities. She was told that if she did not comply she would end up as one of the "van children," who never went to school, had no records, and had no life outside of the perpetrator group; they were shuttled about in trucks to be repeatedly prostituted, raped, used in pornography, and eventually murdered in a ritual or snuff film.

Suicide Programming.   In most cases where an abuse victim has witnessed the victimization of others, or where s/he has been privy to illegal actions of other kinds, suicide is encoded into the child's programming as a mind-control safety net for the perpetrator(s). Lifelong, very specific, and often designed to pass as something else, the suicide program could entail becoming dissociative and walking in front of a moving bus or falling out of a window.

(In cult or governmental/military assassination programming, of course, the individual is programmed to kill himself after killing the assigned subject(s) and in some apocalyptic cult groups the individual is programmed to commit "random acts of violence" prior to self-destruction.)

Many survivors are programmed to cut themselves with razor blades, to drive off the road, or to overdose with drugs and alcohol when they are about to remember and/or reveal the traumas or group secrets. Very urgent, peculiar, and often ego-dystonic thoughts disconnected from major life concerns—an impulse to slash one's wrists, for example, in the middle of washing the dishes—may be exposed as the result of suicide/self-injury programming.

Some survivors have described being cut with knives or razor blades by their perpetrators following rape or torture as a "demonstration" accompanying hypnotic suicide programming. The combination of hypnosis and cutting creates repetitive, powerful state-dependent imitations very difficult to undo even when the survivor becomes aware that the operative thoughts, intentions, and actions are not his/her own. Ritual-abuse victims report implanted commands to enact suicide on birthdays, anniversaries, and special "holidays."

Hostage Programming.   Intended to keep the victim bonded to the perpetrator and thereby insulating the group's inner spheres, hostage programming inculcates a false form of loyalty—as when an incesting parent convinces the child (using threats, physical abuse, manipulations, seduction, authoritative/authoritarian influence), that disobedience or disloyalty—or displays of anger or disagreement, indeed any expressions of independent thought, which are part of all children's normal development—would victimize the perpetrator. So a father abusing his son might explain that he has every right to touch and even hurt him, that all adults have the same right, that telling anyone will bring more pain on him and will be tantamount to hurting the whole family.

In its most extreme form, hostage programming becomes a form of total personality removal. That is, the victim is programmed to feel no anger, no thoughts of revenge toward the perpetrator and/or is programmed either to not have the desire to escape or to not even know that escape is a possibility. Normal, healthy self-protective reactions are obliterated; what is left to the victim is only a shell. Systematically taught that all hope is lost, separation from the perpetrator impossible and maybe not even desirable, and that attempts to escape will either cause more torment to the victim or else be futile, the victim will run up against a corresponding block in therapy and will contend, after assembling most of his/her shattered memories, that s/he cannot do anything with them, that s/he will NEVER be able to get away from the perpetrator or the cult. At this intersection with hostage programming, the patient usually becomes highly resistant to the therapist s/he had learned to trust and may want to quit treatment; s/he may become agitated, resentful, depressed, and/or suicidal, entrapped in the conviction there is no exit from the allegiance to which s/he is internally programmed for life.

LINA

Painful genital torture was administered in conjunction with messages telling Lina that she was being filled with poison and toxins. They would infect anyone she would ever get close to or love (and indeed they affected all her intimate relationships), and her entire life would be a failure regardless of any efforts she made. When repeated therapies that focused on intimacy issues (but did not address trauma or programming) failed to produce the desired results, Lina became increasingly depressed and suicidal, feeling impotent and incompetent to change her life in any significant way. Various forms of learned helplessness had been essential parts of the breakdown and conditioning of her personality—and Lina was also repeatedly hypnotized to have an inexplicable urge to find a razor blade and cut herself whenever she was about to reveal anything about her trauma. The ongoing malignant synergy between the unconscious narratives inculcated during torture and the naturally occurring reenactments of trauma in everyday life created a virtual-reality psychic prison for Lina; many survivors can never escape.

DEPROGRAMMING AND THE RESTORATION OF CRITICAL THINKING

It is virtually impossible to disrupt such programming in therapy without restoring affectivity—having the patient recount and find feelings for the specific traumas that were used to create the dissociative identity splits in the first place. This is extremely difficult and laborious because the abusers usually layer mind-control programming with suicidal and homicidal thought-behavior patterns, encapsulate dissociative states in drugged conditions that block access in the therapy setting, and leave the patient terrified of recalling the points where splits under torture were created. The goal of thought reform, whether in the incest family or in the organized child-abuse group is the same: gaining control over the individual and his/her identity and dissociative states to establish the greatest degree of compliance and the greatest degree of silence. The more complex the actions required of the victim, the more elaborate is the shaping and structuring of the dissociative system.

The goal of therapy where mind control and malignant attachments are concerned is to enable the state-bound commands, beliefs, identifications, and physiological and affective reactions to be accessed, deconditioned (unlearned), and integrated (Conway, 1994). Deprogramming, correcting cognitive errors, breaking trauma bonds, illuminating unconscious organizing principles, reversing brainwashing . . . Brandchaft (1994, p. 57) felicitously calls the process "freeing the spirit from its cell." By whatever name, it presupposes belief in the fundamental priority of individual autonomy—including a subjective sense of agency, critical thinking, and the capacity for protest.

> Whatever new identity she develops in freedom must include the memory of her enslaved self. Her image of her body must include a body that can be controlled and violated. Her image of herself in relation to others must include a person who can lose and be lost to others. And her moral ideals must coexist with the knowledge of the capacity for evil, both within others and within herself. If, under duress, she has betrayed her own principles or has sacrificed other people, she now has to live with the image of herself as an accomplice of the perpetrator, a "broken" person. The result, for most victims, is a contaminated identity. Victims may be preoccupied with shame, self-loathing, and a sense of failure. In the most severe cases, the victim retains the dehumanized identity of a captive who has been reduced to the level of elemental survival: the robot, animal, or vegetable. (Herman, 1992, pp. 93–94)

In order for healing to take place, relationships with oneself and society must be regarded as more important than those with family or any other group, including any religious system and also including the theoretical system of the therapist. The therapist must create an atmosphere of safety so that the patient can choose to begin crossing the amnestic barriers constructed by the perpetrating agent(s) and the colluding social systems. Unless s/he understands and repeatedly contextualizes the patient's unavoidable existential shame over his/her victimization and loss of free will, the working-through process will be stymied and the reciprocally reinforcing protection racket between victim and perpetrator will not be exposed and undermined. The therapist must apprehend and help the patient to apprehend the reversals of trust/distrust and safety/danger produced when perpetrator-manipulated shame is at the root of dissociative identities. The therapist must take the position that feelings must be valued at least as much as thoughts; doctrine and logic must be circumvented by exposing double binds and the explicitly deceptive practices of the captor(s).

Of course, the therapy relationship must be simultaneously exposed to the same scrutiny. Any doubts or fears the patient has about the therapist or the practices must be immediately and sensitively addressed and when possible the patient's perceptions must be validated. Unprocessed injunctions from the perpetrator continue to control the victim-survivor's identity and self-esteem and to some extent his/her behavior until these messages are verbalized and the context of their inculcation recalled (when possible). Beyond the restoration of affectivity—the capacity to sob, to rage, to feel gratitude and to hope, and to tolerate helplessness and despair—the essence of "deprogramming" involves accessing perpetrator-shaped dissociative identities and belief systems and linking their existence to the observing ego capacities of the self as a whole.[6] The cognitive dissonances stimulated in therapy dialogues inevitably lead to great anxiety and turmoil in the survivor which, when navigated ineffectively, may propel him/her into a speedy retreat into the security of the old belief systems regardless of how absurd or destructive the beliefs might be (Brandchaft, 1994). Hence, this reparative discourse must take place in a relationship ambience where the therapist consistently communicates that the individual's free will and free choice are to be respected at all times. Even the freedom to return to his/her abusive original group/family or to sustain a particular belief system must remain an option so that new forms of indoctrination and coerced compliance are not being used to replace the old system.

The attempt at integration of mind-control programming will require that patient (and therapist) face disturbing realities about the existence and nature of evil, raising intense anxiety and unsettling fears about self, security, and the world. Most difficult to confront is the deep shame that surfaces when the patient becomes fully aware that someone has literally stolen his/herself or mind (sometimes subjectively experienced as something s/he has given away, sold out, or "sold to the devil"—or as abandonment by God). The realization that one has been thoroughly and completely deceived and subjugated leaves in its wake a haunting recognition of the self's vulnerability. Survivors of mind control tend to be angrier at the absence of something in themselves, something they imagine should have been there to protect them, than at their families or at society for perpetrating or colluding in child exploitation.

The therapist and patient must not only empathically understand and disrupt cognitive distortions, mutually reflect on the methods and intentions of the captors/perpetrators, and help the survivor understand his/her adaptations to totalism, but also learn to tolerate the ambiguity whereby the therapist is regarded as simultaneously or alternatingly a potential liberator and a new form of captor/perpetrator/torturer. Similarly the therapist will have to tolerate the patient's shifts among moments of self-liberation, threatening and intimidating enactments, and efforts to make the therapist the object of thought reform and mind control.

The treatment of thought reform and traumatic bonding cannot simply take place on the cognitive, didactic, or insight levels, important as they are. Essential for providing the framework of a powerful "new object" or "emotionally corrective experience" are the therapist's consistent disarming of the dissociative self-protective system through empathic resonance and empathic-introspection; authentic and spontaneous use of his/her emotional presence and authenticity; a sense of humor; persistent challenges to automaticity of both patient and therapist's response patterns; use of language that enlivens rather than deadens therapy dialogues; and maintaining a therapeutic posture that welcomes protest, disagreement, and discourse about the patient's experience of the therapist.

Therapists unfamiliar with the dynamics of perpetrators, abusive groups and subcultures, or authoritarian systems may be at a disadvantage in understanding the thinking and relationship patterns of survivors of chronic childhood trauma and DID patients; they may misrecognize the common patterns of impermeability; they may misunderstand the layering phenomenon where self-generated dissociative identities strategically mask the existence of perpetrator-structured dissociative states; they may directly or indirectly disparage (or submit to) the patient. They may become so frustrated at the other end of dialogue with dissociative mind-control victims who do not know they are mind-control victims that the inevitable (and potentially useful) transferential assaults on the therapist's hope, faith, and capacity for critical thinking become unbearable. They may find it difficult to avoid frustration, rage, and the impulse to encourage the patient to restore observing ego functions rapidly when states of mindlessness and robotism emerge in an otherwise responsive and/or intelligent individual. DID patients working through complex mind-control programming, however, need to pass in and out of the states of mindlessness and deadness that occurred as a result of the original trauma and mind control in order to link up all of the previously separated self-states.

To be effective in disrupting thought reform, the therapist must begin relationships and facilitate dialogues with these unfeeling, unreflective parts of the self (including the "cult alters") and help the patient as a whole to own—and to not avoid or disavow in fear of losing the therapist's respect by revealing part-selves who are automatons, prostitutes, couriers, or killers— these mentally impoverished and thoroughly indoctrinated self-states. Many dissociative patients are afraid to think out loud or mention the cues, triggers, trainings, directives, and specifics of their mind-control programs, lest doing so lead to their acting on suicidal or homicidal feelings or to their regressing to mindlessly enacting the structured identities or behavior patterns. They are also afraid the therapist will abandon them after the horrors (and identities) are revealed. It is only by directly facing these fears that a patient and therapist can cocreate an environment of sufficient trust, safety, and shared power to overcome in the patient's mind the real and imagined power of the perpetrators and their coercive influence on the patient's cognitions, affects, and consciousness.

Therapists who treat severely dissociative patients solely with fantasies of restoration and reparenting are forgetting that they have experienced repeated failures of attachment and meaningful, protective, well-boundaried relationships, and that in some cases they suffered explicit torture aimed at altering their core personalities. Avoiding the individual's distrust and rage with reparenting strategies is only a temporary and, in fact, doomed effort. Both overnurturing and overdirection reinforce compliance, eclipse paradoxical experiencing, collapse intersubjectivity, subvert mutuality, and perpetuate embedded sadomasochistic relationship patterns. These therapeutic extremes also foreclose sitting with (and sharing) the patient's dread, despair, and helplessness in the face of extreme human malevolence.

As bad object ties are slowly given up and risks are taken for new kinds of relationships, the cast of characters in the dissociative patient's subjective world changes and the possibility of a new kind of life emerges. The patient will experience both a new sense of connectedness with others and a new sense of aloneness. Critical thinking replaces betrayal blindness, dissociation, and knowledge isolation of all kinds. The fact of human malevolence and evil is faced consciously for the first time because the reality of human benevolence—including someone willing to witness atrocity without turning away—is experienced by the patient, creating the kind of inner strength necessary to hold knowledge of his/her history. Rigid beliefs and thought reform based on viewing the self through the eyes of the perpetrator, the collaborating family members and society, or the misrecognitions of the unenlightened mental health system are replaced by an ability to more accurately detect deception, betrayal, and self-deception in interpersonal affairs, and most of all by an ability to consider multiple perspectives. This includes tolerating the anxiety of not knowing without collapsing into rigid, arrogant, and other defensive postures learned in the perverse context of traumatic captivity.

"Deprogramming" should not be considered something outside of or adjunctive to psychotherapy or psychoanalysis, nor should it be mystified or associated solely with cult-related phenomena. Critical thinking, healthy assertion and agency, and the capacity to belong and relate to others out of choice and not out of desperation or direction are goals of therapy that cut across all modalities. So is establishment of a strong empathic bond and relatively stable trust (i.e., where distrust can be discussed) with a therapist who is seen as both powerful and compassionate. Indeed, the power of a healthy therapeutic relationship is usually underestimated not only by those who abuse and program children, but by the patient him/herself.

Deprogramming then involves deflating omnipotence, restoring affectivity, activating the patient's critical thinking abilities, remembering and systematically analyzing as many of the perpetrator's inculcated messages, identities, behavioral chains, secrets, and values as possible, and cultivating an informed protest response. Grieving, mourning, and some depression will inevitably follow as the dissociative survivor recovers memories of myriad deceptions, betrayals, and manipulations against his/her will. Survivors need an enormous amount of patience from therapists in working through the intense shame that accompanies recognition of mind-control subjugation while taking responsibility (without guilt, blame, or judgment) for the creation of traumatic bonding as a survival solution and for the resulting vulnerability to thought reform, alongside accepting the truth of their helplessness and powerlessness in the authoritarian or abusing system. Ultimately, all patients must be helped to realize that recovery from mind control and separation/individuation from the traumatic matrix is a potent form of self-love and is also the most constructive, permanent form of retaliation against one's abusers.

However, the ultimate transformation of severe dissociative disorders and all traumatically bonded individuals takes place when the mystification of the omnipotent is replaced by a healthy respect and valorization for the more mundane but enormously powerful forces and struggles involved in human love, respect, and mutual regard. More than any technical procedure or therapeutic stance, the enduring power of a passionate and compassionate human bond that survives the vicissitudes of traumatic transference/countertransference enactments and polarizations leads to the disempowerment of the internalized traumatic bonding and to the disarming of mind-control programming. It is a relationship, not a technique, that results in the trauma victim's empowerment as a thinking, feeling, protesting, witnessing, working, remembering agent.

Part Three

Survival, Transformation, and Transcendence

CHAPTER 9

Surviving Dissociation, Surviving Destruction: Transcending Secondary Traumatization and Reclaiming Faith

The first rule of therapy is that the therapist must survive the process.
—**Margo Rivera**

One may need to sink a long time into the limits of capacity, into what cannot be done, for bits of movement to begin, for unexpected openings to occur.
—**Michael Eigen**

Psychotherapists find themselves trapped in double binds of inconsistent and contradictory demands and expectations from the culture at large, and from patients, their families, the professions, the legal system, insurance and managed-care companies, and from conflicting personal, theoretical, and political loyalties and attachments. Emotionally embroiled in the suffering of those they treat, therapists sometimes feel like victims to the destructive forces operating within severely dissociative patients' psyches and family systems, and sometimes feel as though they are losing themselves to the clients they serve (Figley, 1995). They sometimes feel impossibly sand-wiched between the needs of their traumatized patients and the needs of people in their personal lives, particularly those who do not comprehend the enormous demands of clinical work with severely traumatized people. They sometimes end up feeling like bait for predatory, avaricious lawyers, or like pawns in the burgeoning, dehumanized, mega-business of adminis-terial health care. They may be compelled to take sides in polarized profes-sional controversies against their better judgment or torn apart and more confused than supported by factionalized commentary of the elders of the field. Heartbroken by their patients' accounts of pain and torment, they may also be worried, even shamed, because being heartbroken might be an un-professional response. In the face of intense object-hunger, greed, selfish-ness, insensitivity, distrust, and demandingness, subtle and overt, from severely dissociative trauma survivors, therapists can come to feel like units of flesh are being torn from their bodies. Sometimes they wonder about just giving it all up for almost anything else. "[M]any of us who started out hop-ing to make a difference in the world have ended up hoping simply to make it to the end of the day" (Grosch and Olsen, 1994, p. ix).

FROM THE TRENCHES. . .

A young therapist treating her first MPD case seeks consultation after experiencing generalized anxiety, nightmares, and flashbacks to the pa-tient's grim memories of sadistic sexual abuse and forced dismember-ment of animals in the family basement. Her marriage is at risk because of her overinvolvement—which now includes daily extra-session read-ing of the prolific patient's journal tracking her exponentiating alter personalities as well as nightly phone calls to manage panic attacks and suicidality. Initially fascinated by the disorder and committed to em-pathize and avoid retraumatization at all costs, the therapist has agreed to a reduced fee for longer and now more frequent sessions. She cannot bring herself to change the status quo lest the patient repeat the accusa-tion that anything less than adherence to the needs and goals the pa-tient asserts makes the therapist no better than another sadistically abusive perpetrator.

An experienced therapist, already struggling with increasingly fre-quent periods of depression after listening for years to survivors of in-cest and egregious sadistic violations in childhood, now faces a feeling of overwhelming futility on learning that the police declined to take action against a family he reported for abusing the young cousin of one of his patients. The therapist alternately fantasizes transferring all his trauma cases and quitting clinical practice altogether.

Late one night the husband of a difficult, long-term DID patient with a history of dangerous acting-out calls her therapist to report that she didn't return home after that evening's session. Mindful of the time the year before when the patient had sliced her wrist in the bathroom of his office suite, the therapist rushes back to see if she might have locked herself in there again. She hadn't, so he roams nearby streets looking for her, checking in periodically with the husband, who informs him sometime after midnight that the patient has just sauntered in and said there's nothing for anyone to be so upset about. When confronted by husband and therapist, she complains that she's a victim of unfair questions and undeserved hostility; furthermore, she insists that the therapist's concern about a suicide attempt is his agenda, not hers, and rooted in his unconscious wish to get rid of her. (The year before, after the therapist contacted the husband to go after the patient in response to an actual suicide note, she temporarily dropped out of treatment, enraged that the therapist hadn't cared enough to come and stop her himself.)

After twenty years of clinical experience, several of them treating trauma survivors, a therapist finds herself silenced, unable to respond inquiringly or empathically, let alone identify reenactment themes, when a patient describes in childlike voices alternating between terror and flamboyant eroticism the roles she played in pornographic films. The therapist switches rapidly in and out of skepticism, nausea, numbness, and sexual arousal while listening, feeling out of control and sometimes overcome by drowsiness and the sense that her brain has "turned to cotton candy." Mostly, she cannot collect her thoughts to make coherent interpretations during the clinical hour; when she can, she feels that the patient would be devastated by their content if she were to share them.

About a year after starting to treat a woman suffering from classic posttraumatic stress symptoms including bizarre nightmares of rituals, orgiastic sex, and human sacrifice, a veteran therapist reports finding bloodstains on her office porch, a dead bird in front of her house, and one of her tires flattened five times in a six-month period. She sometimes felt she was being followed by a car that resembled the patient's, and began to feel haunted by a barrage of strange messages on her answering machine accompanied by lengthy musical passages. Agitated and afraid, the therapist felt guilty for connecting the traumatized patient to this sequence of events. . . . By the time she asked for consultation, she was seriously considering buying a gun.

TRAUMATIC TRANSFERENCE AND COUNTERTRANSFERENCE

Trauma survivors' emotional responses to people in authority have been so deformed by their experiences that they are prone to transference reactions unparalleled in ordinary psychotherapy (Herman, 1992). Shengold (1989) refers to the "galloping transference," Loewenstein (1993) to the "flashback transference," Ogden (1992) to the "tyrannizing transference," and Rosenfeld (1987) to the "lavoratoric transference." The shattered trust and deep-seated expectation of imminent abandonment and betrayal that pervade all of their relationships causes trauma survivors to challenge every aspect of the therapist's identity and integrity as well as the value, dependability, and efficacy of psychotherapy.

Correspondingly, their therapists' experiences stretch the usual notion of countertransference to its philosophical limits, incorporating the phenomena of emotional contagion, covictimization, secondary traumatization, and secondary traumatic stress disorder. In its psychoanalytic evolution, countertransference has emerged from its limited construction as a treatment obstacle and therapeutic contaminant into a resource for therapeutic understanding (Natterson, 1991)—an instrument for gathering data and illuminating ongoing intrapsychic and interpersonal relationships (Boyer, 1979). It has come to embody the totality of the therapist's emotional reactions and to stand for their utility for understanding the patient in ongoing treatment and for formulating interventions (Kernberg, 1976; Searles, 1959; Gorkin, 1987). A heightened interest in the patient-therapist relationship as a forum for the reenactment of past experience (Aron, 1996; Ehrenberg, 1992; Gabbard, 1993) has accompanied the postclassical vision of countertransference.

Immersion in the transference/countertransference matrix when the psychic material of the patient is volatile and harsh places enormous strain on the therapist. To understand and empathically resonate with many posttraumatic psychic orientations, therapists must give up their usual hold on reality in favor of a kind of permeability that disrupts their own personalities when they open up areas they would rather keep dormant (Giovacchini, 1989). Genuine emotional release is essential—the willingness to have some defenses and the safety of the witnessing/observational distance broken down and broken through—so that a traumatized patient who has never been able to make an impact on anyone and fears that s/he would be destructive, seductive, or poisonous, can be encouraged to test new assumptions.

Giovacchini (1989) describes engulfment in the inner life of a disturbed patient as the psychic equivalent of invasion by a "foreign body . . . an unformed psychic amoeba" (p.178). McCann and Pearlman (1990) define the same experience of countertransference as vicarious traumatization—the cumulative transformative effect on the therapist of working with survivors of severe trauma—also construing it as a process rather than an event. The inevitable intimate internal changes, including lasting alterations in their cognitive schemas and representational systems, constitute an occupational hazard whose individual cost, if unaddressed, can metastasize into cynicism and despair: the therapist's inner experience of other people as trustworthy and benevolent may be disrupted, his/her sense of personal safety and power profoundly threatened; the collective cost can be a real risk to the profession.

Treating such a population challenges defenses that may never have been tampered with, forcing the therapist to examine his/her own emotional vulnerability as well as personal and philosophical issues with scrupulous honesty (Rivera, 1996); otherwise, s/he may have to leave the field to rebuild his/her defense system. Putnam (1989) discusses how extended encounters with severely dissociative patients produce feelings of intimidation and ineptitude. Herman (1992) cites the unbearable sense of helplessness that can lead a therapist to assume the role of rescuer. Kinzie and Boehnlein (1993) distinguish the problem of excessive identification with victimized patients and intolerance of patients whose suffering is less extreme; they also mention depression, anger, irritability, hyperarousal, and heightened vulnerability outside the office.

The literature also defines biopsychological effects: powerful visceral reactions like nausea, diarrhea, headaches (McCann and Colletti, 1994), along with disturbed sleep, loss of appetite, increased anxiety, increased fear, hostility, and distrust of others (Youngson, 1994). Davies and Frawley (1994) report feelings of numbness in an extremity, tingly skin, vaginal pain or contractions, dizziness, alterations in perception of one's body size, and disorienting sexual arousal, as well as difficulties in partnerships and family relationships; they go on to say that therapists are besieged by frightening and formless countertransference feelings and experiences far beyond anything their training has prepared them for, and that those psychic and somatic invasions challenge the integrity of their functioning. So even though some of the aspects of secondary traumatization can contribute to an experience-near understanding of the patient's childhood colonization by the perpetrator/caretaker, the impact of the process on the therapist can be so alarming as to actually compromise his/her capacity for empathic immersion.

And then there are the direct attacks on therapists engaged in clinical work with severely dissociative patients. Aside from physical and verbal assaults, their range encompasses: leaving dead animals on the therapist's porch, poisoning or releasing the therapist's pets, vandalizing the therapist's possessions, filing frivolous or malicious lawsuits or mailing letters of complaint to supervisors or ethics boards, making harassing phone calls, bringing guns and knives to the office, seeking information and gossiping about the therapist with others, making damaging or untrue remarks to friends or other patients or to the therapist's friends and family or both, refusing to leave the therapist's office, refusing to pay for treatment (Comstock, 1992); also undressing in the therapist's office, breaking into the therapist's office, stalking the therapist and the therapist's friends and family members, becoming interpersonally or sexually involved with the therapist's professional colleagues and/or relatives (Davies and Frawley, 1994).

Even the most fundamental rules of human relatedness can be broken in clinical work with MPD/DID individuals. Therapists may come to question what seems like an absence of coherent motivation or a "faulty work ethic" (Kluft, 1994c, p. 134) in the highly dissociative, severely traumatized patient population. Kluft describes how DID patients can lead the therapist to feel fooled, misled, and betrayed. Sometimes, when the therapist confronts the patient, Kluft says, the patient often

> responds either by self-attack (designed to propitiate the therapist by forestalling an anticipated attack), by attempts to represent the misrepresentation as essential and even wise in view of some other consideration, by further evasions, by counterattacks on what is perceived as the therapist's attack, or by

portrayals of himself or herself as so piteous (usually accompanied by a switch to a terrified and/or weeping child alter) that only a sadist would press the confrontation. (p. 134)

Reeling from a bewildering array of reactions provoked by (among other things) reversals run amok, the therapist can find it difficult to remain focused on the therapeutic task.

Davies and Frawley (1994) describe the strain on the therapist from exposure to trauma survivors' entrenched and bizarre forms of reenactment, difficulty with judgment, diminished capacity for reality testing, problems in learning from experience, pathological doubting, confusion about responsibility, blaming the therapist and playing victim, unresolved issues around honesty, integrity, and truthfulness—all of which collide with a therapist's expectations of treatment alliance and a secure therapeutic frame. The result is a sense of entrapment that parallels the patient's torturous core life-experience of a world with no relief, no redemption, and no exit. Eigen (1991), speaking of difficult countertransference pressure, asks if flexible benevolence on the part of someone under attack is possible, suggesting that there may be a limit to how much exposure the therapist can bear.

Russell (1998a) comments that the most powerful source of resistance in psychotherapy is the therapist's resistance to what the patient feels. Describing the essence of transformation and the blocks to it

> We resist feeling ourselves what things were really like for the patient. We tell ourselves we know their history, but it is not possible to do this work without resistance against feeling the pain. And it's no mystery that what we do not want to feel with our patients bears directly on what we resist in ourselves. What we have to ask of ourselves is nothing other than what we hope the treatment process may make possible for the patient, namely that urgencies be used, not in the service of repeating, but as a way of feeling what could not be felt before. (p. 18)

Predictable responses to treating dissociative survivors of severe trauma take shape as behavioral permutations of either denial/withdrawal or over-involvement/hyperarousal—and they in turn will impact on and interact with the patient's independent dynamics (Wilson and Lindy, 1994). The therapist is at high risk of enacting one or both patterns—that is, of getting rid of the patient directly (terminating or transferring the case, refusing to treat any such cases at all) or indirectly (rejecting the diagnosis, refusing the reality of the patient's experience, shutting down, medicating), or of psychologically adopting the patient (overidentifying, rescuing, reparenting, merging, taking responsibility for the patient's life).

The therapist must understand the need to create the most facilitative relational conditions for the patient's relinquishment of dissociative isolation, and that presupposes understanding the patient's imperative to preserve the illusion that s/he can "stay the same while changing" (Bromberg, 1993, p. 151), can maintain the dissociative structure while surrendering it (Bromberg, 1996a). The therapist must recognize the perceived threat embodied by the goings-on in the transference/countertransference matrix: the patient comes to feel that, by asking that s/he assimilate so much newness, the therapist is destroying his/her world.

A major force in disrupting the patient's dissociative modes of relatedness is the therapist's creative use of self and self-disclosure (both of which remain highly controversial topics within psychoanalysis and across all psychotherapy disciplines). Personal clinical experience with severely dissociative trauma survivors supports Maroda's (1999) recommended emphasis on the (potential) curative effects of the therapist's use of his/her emotional availability and vulnerability with patients (sometimes by sharing aspects of his/her experience) for breaking through stalemates and in facilitating personality transformation. Within a process of mutual emotional engagement between therapist and patient as a vehicle of therapeutic change, Maroda describes how many patients need to feel that they have emotionally impacted the therapist in some significant way and/or that the therapist has given over something in order for the patient to release him/herself into a new relational experience. Maroda notes, however, that some patients who cannot bear to receive any emotional input from the therapist (at all, or just at a given point in time), may need to flee or punish the therapist for violating him/her.

The need of severely dissociative trauma survivors, especially early in the process, to feel they are making an impact on the therapist and the often distorted experience of this impact as evidence of betrayal, seduction, or abuse by the therapist appear simultaneously. Therefore, the process of mutual emotional engagement with severely traumatized individuals can offer contradictory outcomes. A patient may open up or seem to be moved and then cancel sessions or drop out of treatment, or simply move on to other topics acting as if nothing important whatsoever has taken place, failing to integrate the experience within the lived history of the therapy relationship. Or, conversely, a patient may initially block or distort disclosure by the therapist, seeing it as potentially dangerous, and through dialogue, where distrust and ambiguity are tolerated, shift gears into a more emotionally vulnerable state. Sometimes too much of the therapist's aliveness can be threatening and overwhelming for the severely dissociative patient to bear. Sometimes emotional distance is what is needed by both patient and therapist.

It is however essential for the therapist to remain aware of what s/he feels and when s/he has lost connection with feeling altogether. While a therapist's ability to empathize with suffering and loss and create or develop affective bridges to (and within) severely traumatized patients is considered essential to treatment, humility about what we can and cannot feel or know is as important in honoring the level of violation many of these individuals have experienced.

> Some experiences are so scorching, some feelings are so frightening or painful, that, at whatever cost, the patient will know far more about them than we do. They do not need us to know immediately. But they do need us to know that we do not know. (Russell, 1998a, pp. 18–19)

THE THERAPIST'S PSYCHOLOGICAL AND PROFESSIONAL SURVIVAL

Cultural and external professional pressures also impinge. The increasing incursion by managed-care systems has impacted the quality, duration, and economics of long-term treatment. In the current litigious climate therapists work under the potential threat of legal prosecution (Davies, 1997), and there are ever more legal demands on therapists—to monitor patients' suicidality and dangerousness to others as well as the ongoing or potential abuse of children—and ever more legal restrictions on the freedom to work with and take traumatic memories seriously. Patients, their families, or even spouses and friends of patients can and do misrepresent therapists for all kinds of secondary gain including revenge, financial rewards, unification around a common enemy, or simply reenactment of complex group interpersonal betrayal and sacrifice dynamics; being unprepared for how severely traumatized, dissociative people (and their social systems) relate means being unprepared for the battles that may result.

It is unwise for clinicians treating trauma, especially those who believe in raising consciousness about abuse and women's oppression, to lose sight of the fact that every victim is also in some ways a perpetrator—toward him/herself and toward others. Therapists must get beyond the myth of the noble trauma survivor to avoid splitting this core paradox of victim-perpetrator and to hold the tension between the two; they must, without judging or moralizing, come to accept the fundamental power-based nature of relational trauma, which produces enormous identification with the aggressor and huge quantities of unmetabolized, raw destructiveness in personalities with limited and/or shattered capacities to assimilate, process, and sublimate them. Victims of organized child abuse and mind control often have completely split-off centers of agency that operate outside of their own will and conscious control and serve the will and ideology of their perpetrators regardless of whether or not they are still associated with them.

Trauma therapists are positioned between an extremely challenging patient population that exudes toxins and massive social and professional forces that diminish their capacity to heal. For clinicians treating DID and other severe dissociative disorders at this juncture in the history of both psychotherapy and Western society as a whole, there is essentially no secure professional and cultural "holding environment" (Saakvitne, 1995). The therapist must come to know with whom to undertake treatment and with whom doing so would exhaust his/her reserves of energy, goodwill, and tolerance for pain. S/he must know how and when to be aggressive in holding and supporting him/herself in terms of respecting limits, boundaries, and beliefs in what makes therapy effective. S/he must leave behind the polarizing questions from without (e.g., did this trauma happen?) to engage with what Davies (1996a) calls traumatic relationship dynamics, not in a hunt for traumatic memory.

The therapist's survival of the patient's dissociative camouflage and relational espionage depends in part on the therapist's ability to connect with his/her own inner ruthlessness (Pizer, 1998). If a therapist can be coerced, corrupted, intimidated, manipulated, or rendered ineffective by a traumatized patient, then not only is the therapeutic potential foreclosed but also the patient can become terrified and begin to act out (Ehrenberg, 1992); defeating, destroying, or duping the therapist can confirm a patient's worst fears about abandonment, rejection, lack of protection, and his/her own omnipotent destructiveness. In the end, the only movement possible is from the contest for domination (you or me) to mutual survival: either we both sink or we both swim. Surviving the emotional collisions—tolerating the tension, trusting in the process, sustaining faith in not knowing—and being able to reflect together on their meanings will unite the psychotherapy pair, except of course where the need to traumatize the therapist and communicate by means of reenactments is unnegotiable, rendering the patient unavailable for reflection and unable to mobilize the emotional generosity requisite to forming an alliance.

Some patients find trying to harm, deceive, or reject the therapist the only way they can be known and manage their suffering (*I have to hurt and destroy something or someone. It's the only thing that keeps me from losing my mind*). Interpretation in such cases may be too distant from the operant self-state to bridge the disparate aspects of the severely dissociative patient's personality. Sometimes empathic inquiry into the motivational system of the destructive alter is the most promising route to mutative dialogue. When a personality is organized significantly by dissociation the therapist must be able to "relate to several selves simultaneously while maintaining an authentic dialogue with each" (Bromberg, 1994, p. 534)—to hold concurrent citizenship in several domains of reality "with passports to multiple self-states of the patient" (Bromberg, 1991, p. 410).

With the intersubjective space dominated by duplicity, dissimulation, and selective amnesia, therapists may lose their bearings and begin compulsively to doubt themselves and their competence and come to feel outmaneuvered, manipulated, or betrayed—much as the vulnerable child the patient felt when s/he was at the mercy of cunning perpetrators who assaulted his/her sense of functional integrity along with his/her sense of reality. Chronic, pathological self-doubting by either member of the therapy dyad can be consensually validated in the treatment relationship, fueling ever shifting power dynamics as patient and therapist play the roles of believer, denier, doubter, and revealer.

Davies and Frawley (1994) describe the "game of turnabout" (p. 111) whereby a patient, identifying with the perpetrator, relentlessly attacks the therapist's sense of reality (e.g., denying, distorting, disremembering events and conversations that took place in treatment, fostering confusion and compulsive self-doubting; acknowledging traumatic memories replete with displays of affect and somatic pain followed by recantation then followed by de-recantation, etc.); when the patient does not acknowledge participating in such an enactment, the therapist feels marooned, viscerally ripped-off. The therapist's healthy aggression is required to confront dissociative strategies, however, and to disrupt traumatic fixity and steward mutuality, lest the treatment dissolve into a quagmire of double binds. Too many therapists end up intimidated—afraid their patients will leave treatment, kill themselves, act out against the therapist's property or family, or initiate malicious lawsuits.

At the root of the patient's chicanery, of course, are the evasion of pain, the maintenance of attachment to childhood abusers and malevolent introjects, and the warding off of annihilation anxieties. But since the treatment alliance is built on candor, truth, and identification with the therapist, the patient's relentless reenactments of betrayal and deception assault the therapist's capacity to generate the goodwill and benevolence essential to attaching to the patient altogether. An inexperienced therapist who does not understand the psychic milieu of a severe trauma survivor may feel unnecessarily guilty for mistrusting and resenting the patient; the insidious reversal whereby a beleaguered therapist is essentially persuaded to sacrifice his/her sanity for the hope of a patient's improvement is a predictable MPD/DID power play, however. Most severely dissociative trauma survivors will also unconsciously toy with a therapist's intuitive resources in an effort to insinuate doubt, distrust, and fear where therapists are most used to accessing reliable impressions and information about the world. Dialogues must replace enactments of sabotage in all its forms in order that the therapist's failing voice be restored and the patient's observation of his/her dissociation-driven self-sabotage begin. Psychological terrorism should not be tolerated for long.

The dissociative web redistributes traumatic anxieties, annihilation anxiety, and unbearable meanings to the point of containing that which might otherwise have led to a breakdown or the cultivation of a more psychotic or paranoid delusional system. If the patient's house of cards is exposed as such before enough wherewithal is developed to handle the psychic earthquakes attendant on the deconstruction process, the patient will likely take flight, generate innumerable crises, or find other ways to stalemate the treatment. Yet as the therapist is drawn deeper and deeper into an unreal world of disabling relational patterns, s/he will be seduced to act on the wish or to act on the wish to "cure" the patient of his unrelatedness as quickly as possible (Bromberg, 1995b, p. 177). Retaliating by foisting too much reality on the patient too soon is, in fact, a survival strategy for therapists who feel they are losing their own minds in the swirling and fragmented treatment process.

The DID patient's continuous shifts between revealing and concealing, capacity to sustain plausible denial about everything and anything, chronic forgetfulness, injections of confusion, and proneness to concretization, etc., disorient the therapist and render some of his/her usual regulatory and reality-testing tools unworkable. The ubiquity of reversals, a sense of underlying suspense and urgency, elements of terror and dread, the patient's overreliance on magical thinking, trance logic, and omnipotent fantasies, the frequent blank stares, interpersonal voids, states of psychic emptiness or numbness, the patient's tendency to bargain with unpleasant realities (past and present), the collapse of the utility and meaning of language—all create an interpersonal atmosphere that violates the mind of the therapist.

The countertransferential reluctance to confront the patient for fear of being considered an abuser or of letting him/her down or of seeming unempathic or of driving the patient to leave treatment, have a breakdown, or attempt suicide paralyzes the therapist when s/he needs to pull him/herself and the patient out of the destructive quagmire of relatedness-by-reenactment. By so assiduously trying to avoid recapitulating betrayal, the therapist may unwittingly participate in cocreating the conditions for a painful therapy failure that the patient will construe as betrayal in another form. The patient can be given so much rope that s/he hangs him/herself, the therapist, or both of them.

We as therapists need to acknowledge our limitations to ourselves and our patients, along with the inevitability of some failures. By colluding with patients to believe that we are absolutely devoted, completely tolerant, infinitely patient, and unceasingly generous we are only setting ourselves and our patients up for disappointment. (Personal consultation experience suggests that most therapists who end up transferring or otherwise abandoning their patients have made errors of this kind, often in quite concrete ways.) Placating traumatized patients in a desperate effort to reparent them or escape their unbridled sadism and retaliation (or our own) and/or avoiding confrontation with their many varieties of self- and other-destructive behaviors is not doing them any favor. A therapist treating severe trauma survivors must use his/her own protective aggressive responses early in treatment and set the stage for disrupting all forms of domination, collusion, and exploitation. We do not lose compassion, power, or authority when we negotiate the patient's needs and limits and our own along the way. We are not only thus modeling essential forms of mutuality from the start, but also we are preempting avoidable disasters.

UNDERSTANDING LIMITATIONS

There is no guarantee that the patient, the therapist, the therapy relation-ship, and as of recently, the institution of psychotherapy will survive the multiple assaults and complex systems of denial, dissociation, and reenact-ment within the therapy relationship and within the culture. Surviving de-struction (Winnicott, 1971) as a central metaphor and practical reality in the treatment of severely dissociative trauma survivors always involves the ba-sics of sustaining transformational space, that is, resisting the lures of with-drawal and/or retaliation (and identifying and often acknowledging their emergence to the patient). Surviving destruction also means tolerating the fallout from the deconstruction and reconstruction processes inherent in both psychological and cultural transformation of trauma. Patient and ther-apist must be allowed to explore multiple narratives, multiple subjectivities, multiple transference/countertransference paradigms, and multiple mean-ings in a prolonged and uninterrupted dialogue of mutual respect without interference from outside forces, and the potential/transformational therapy space must be able to survive a historic period when such liberatory psy-chological and political spaces are fast disappearing, regularly misrepre-sented, and under systematic attack.

Although the success rate with severely traumatized and dissociative pa-tients has improved in the past two decades with heightened professional awareness, an ever increasing body of research, and revised clinical ap-proaches, the reality is that we cannot successfully treat everyone. As Bloom (1997) points out, sometimes we fail with traumatized patients because the trauma has done overwhelming developmental damage to the physical and psychological systems necessary to engage reparative and recovery processes; sometimes we lack the power or knowledge to reverse this dam-age. Although many severely dissociative patients do make progress in treatment they remain so vulnerable to stress that their wounds are continu-ally reopened and inflamed whenever they come near situations that are similar in ways to the original traumas. Sometimes we fail to reach many pa-tients or to hold them in treatment long enough for significant change to take place because there are not sufficient economic, social, cultural, or pro-fessional resources available. Sometimes therapists fail because a dissocia-tive patient has extensive sociopathic features, ongoing involvement with destructive families or criminal groups, or an impenetrable and spiteful commitment to self-destruction. Sometimes therapists fail because they are not aware or educated enough, not honest and direct enough, not sensitive and empathic enough, not aggressive enough, not cunning enough, or not emotionally available enough.

JOHN

Like many high-functioning DID patients who go to great lengths to mask their pathological multiplicity, John was more invested in sustaining his persona and functionality than in self-knowledge, truth, or depth. But after five years, during which we had to fight to survive an interpersonal field charged with destruction, threat, intimidation, and torture, John broke through his terrors to come face to face with what he called the "abyss" at the core of his being—only to conclude that the consequences of exploring it could be so hazardous that he probably could never "go there." He was too damaged.

Brilliant and cunningly avoidant, terribly afraid of regression, dependency, and healthy forms of human love, John camouflaged his inordinate need to be in control at all times beneath a veil of apparent compliance; he could fill his therapy hours with details of his daily life events that completely obscured any feelings or meanings. He would turn out to be one of the most profoundly fragmented, high-functioning DID patients I would ever meet, and his personality contained some of the most extreme polarizations I have ever seen in one individual— among them, innocence and diabolism, compliance and dominance, permeability and impenetrability, precise recall and recurrent amnesias, lovability and hatefulness, knowing and unknowing, doing and undoing, cleverness and denseness, dependency and refusal to need or be vulnerable, hyper-responsibility and externalization of blame.

Background: John was a 41-year-old gay physician who entered therapy several months after moving to California, where the symptoms for which he had been in traditional psychoanalytic psychotherapy for about ten years did not, as he had hoped, magically disappear. A new acquaintance who had been a patient of mine (though not himself treated for trauma or dissociation and unaware of my specialization in the area) was the source of John's self-referral to address his familiar and mounting "adjustment disorder" problems, which included depression, anxiety, recurrent nightmares from which he awoke screaming so loudly that he roused the neighbors, panic attacks when alone, somatic preoccupations, chronic self-loathing, compulsive high-risk sexual behavior, dependency on marijuana and sometimes also Valium, inability to tolerate conflict with colleagues and peers, sociopathic entanglements, unusual fears of unknown origin triggered by innocuous stimuli, and out-of-the-ordinary concerns about death and dying.

Among the salient memories that emerged before any direct traumatic material was revealed were his diagnosis with anal fissures at age three, his virtual decompensation on seeing *The Exorcist*, and severe anxiety attacks and the press of irrational fears throughout his youth. John had had what he termed a "nervous breakdown" on discovering his first significant lover's infidelities at the end of their relationship, whereupon his parents, to whom he was not at all close at the time, came to live with him (allegedly, since other narratives later emerged) to prevent further collapse. He reported consistently extreme reactions (obsession, fascination, revulsion) to any material having to do with the Holocaust or other gruesome crimes against humanity, but had absolutely no associations to those patterns.

Early Treatment: John said his former therapist used to tell him that he "had the word 'trauma' written all over his forehead," adding that he never really knew what the therapist meant but acted as though he did so that the matter would be dropped—as it always was until the next time, when it would be dropped again. John acknowledged manipulating that therapist by means of distraction, evasion, and playing dumb, seeming entirely unaware of his own intentions or their possible implications. When I expressed curiosity as to how that pattern might play itself out between us if I said something that threatened him, he showed both fear and relief.

Once, during the early months of therapy, as John was describing the "craziness" and cruelty of many of his family members, he began to talk about their large summer gatherings at his grandparents' house. I casually asked about the sleeping arrangements, and John nearly fell off of his seat. He froze for some minutes, then shifted into a hostile stance I had never seen before, and asked me contemptuously why I wanted to know. My original question went unanswered; in fact, it remained unanswered for the next four or five years. Finally, John asked, puzzled, "If I have no memory for any of this, why is this such a big deal for me?" We reflected on the possibilities that he had experienced my question as intrusive or suggestive or that it had stirred something he was

unable or unready to deal with. Later in therapy, on more than one occasion, John forgot that this conversation ever took place.

I treated John during the early to mid-1990s when scarcely a day
passed without media mention of something related to the false memory syndrome (FMS) controversy, which was to play an extraordinary
role in the dynamics of his therapy. He would begin, in a fragmented
and highly dissociated manner, to switch self-states and spew out numerous stories of mostly extrafamilial (neighbors, teachers, family
friends) and some intrafamilial (aunt, grandfather) sexual abuse—only
to have some of his alters revise the material to conform to the therapist
memory-implantation theory, specifically to the assertions of the voices
in his head that told him that I was a trickster who used techniques he
had not yet heard of to, variously, input the memories or somehow
make him invent his alters because I only wanted to work with dissociative patients. Not only some parts of John but also some parts of his
social circle were focused on false memory rhetoric as the anti-MPD
campaign was reaching its zenith.

The idea that he was "crazy," losing his mind, served to deflect his
MPD identification for a couple of years. Such deflection is one of the
most common tactics among severely dissociative trauma survivors
(and a commonly used programmed message from perpetrators) in
search of some frame or meaning when they are inundated by memories, affects, or flashbacks. Some can actually use repetitive statements
about being crazy to contain and stop the flow. John didn't subjectively
feel he was crazy, but the voices in his head said he was, so frequently
and so adamantly that the distinction had no meaning and he became
thoroughly anxious about going mad, and would plead for help in differentiating clinical psychosis from dissociation. John often forgot this
particular therapy dance and wanted me to repeat and repeat it, in spite
of the fact that we came up with the same conclusion time and time
again in our respectful collegial reviews: his symptom profile matched
severe dissociative disorder, probably DID.

Middle Phase: John's repetitive cycles eventually became a source of
humor and playfulness in the therapy. Beyond analyzing their multiple
possible meanings (my corruption, his dissociative processes, his deception, media and family influences, etc.), John began to be able to
laugh at his own state-changes and his methods of managing and controlling the treatment. That freed up a new arena for engagement and

conflict about the truth/falsity of his memories, breaking out of the binary or otherwise rigid thought-loops (I'm crazy; it can't be real because it doesn't feel real) that precluded the establishment of a consistent observing ego and a real treatment alliance.

John was one of the few patients for whom the "conflict" about whether he was dissociative and a trauma survivor dominated the treatment for several years. He was also one of the few who exhibit all the classical MPD/DID symptoms but could not comprehend even the idea of being dissociative or traumatized. He had what I would call radical dissociation of meaning, dissociation for his impact on others, and unusual dissociation for his own dissociation. So brilliant (and professionally successful) in so many ways, he was unable to think certain thoughts, hold inconsistency in his mind without dissociating, or put two potentially meaningful clues together when they concerned himself; he was actually incapable of grasping how he could have part-selves with diverse opinions, attitudes, and modus operandi.

Meanwhile, regardless of whatever other meanings we generated together, some of John's voices kept insisting that he was "just acting." John knew as well as I did that he had a compliant side, so we examined his notions of my exploiting it as he used his acting talents to mutate into my alleged favorite diagnostic type. (I did not, after some time, hide from John the fact that I was actively engaged in the clinical specialty of trauma and dissociation.) In fact, however, John would have been a terrible actor at anything aside from passing as normal: he had extremely limited fantasy abilities and rarely elaborated or even finished any memory material once he reached a certain level of anxiety.

John's functional selves were quite porous to internal voices and yet quite impervious to the voices of other people—particularly voices of love, compassion, and respect, or voices that could potentially validate his trauma history and dissociative organization. At the beginning of treatment John seemed unclear even about whether or not someone in his life was insulting or manipulating him. His putative compliance was more apparent than real; actually, beyond coming across as the nice guy likable by all, John mostly did just as he pleased.

Internally, he lived as though in a world of one-way mirrors where some parts of him could be seen and influenced while other parts would remain oblivious. It was difficult for John to sustain observing ego and critical thinking capacities about his own complex, polarized, internal, and interpersonal process. We spent a good deal of time hypothesizing as to the mechanics of the collusion, suggestion, and influence alleged by some of his voices to be the real issue between us and also as to how his protector personalities might be using the others' allegations for avoidant or nefarious purposes. Sometimes our discussions had a collaborative tone; at other times, the derision coming from him was difficult to bear. Because his hate was so split off, the energy behind it was particularly foul, and his contempt could take on such a haughty, demonic cruelty that I had to struggle to keep the rest of him in my mind.

In spite of the fact that I leaned in the direction of feeling that John had DID and was probably a survivor of multiple-perpetrator sexual abuse, I tried to keep our dialogues about influence as open as I could while being quite frank about what I tended to believe and why. Who was suggesting what to whom, who was submitting to whom and/or what or for what purposes became important issues. Was John compliant with his own highly developed dissimulation practices, compliant with his family—its myths and relational practices—or dominated by the biases and interpretations of his therapist? All points of view were looked at simultaneously. Nothing was ruled out or decided upon. Multiple realities were held simultaneously in the potential space of the therapy relationship, and, in some cases, much was left unresolved. However, John's recurring amnesia for therapy sessions did frequently interfere with discussing the psychotherapy relationship. When John forgot what took place in sessions, he simply changed the focus to work-related problems.

He was afraid to have any strong feelings toward me or toward anyone else for that matter; merely speaking of (or reporting the comments of the voices in his head about) his aggressive, sexual, or cruel feelings or impulses was threatening for John and made him feel like he was losing control. Yet the more John revealed pieces of his sexual-abuse history, the more his overall psychological, interpersonal, and professional functioning seemed to improve. In fact, he actually developed more of a capacity for emotional presence, interpersonal conflict, and affectivity—when he wasn't denying, disavowing, and recanting.

A Game of Cat and Mouse: John couldn't help complying with and believing whatever his internal antitherapy voices were telling him—for example, about the perpetrator's presence in the room and influence on our relationship—but at the same time, he felt continually assaulted and demoralized when the voices that told him awful things about me (to whom parts of him had become quite attached) and about himself. Over time, however, his tolerance for conflict steadily increased as he was able to eventually see the issue not as two separate positions that had nothing to do with one another, but rather as a dramatic manifestation of an intense inner ambivalence about being known, about having feelings, vulnerabilities, and attachments, about experiencing family members in an unfavorable light, and about risking retraumatization in his relationship with me. Because John used FMS ideologies to regulate our exchanges and his access to painful material, the therapeutic movement into more symbolic, dialogical, and potential space took a couple of years.

Although eventually John said he didn't believe what his inner voices were telling him, they continued to distort his perceptions and distract his attention; they almost always automatically entranced him. Devaluation and overvaluation were enacted in the most extreme form using the FMS template as theatrical set to the therapy dialogues. John's distrustful and dissimulating alter personalities developed an unusual attachment to me. Occasionally, when caught and confronted in the act of subverting the therapy through false memory syndrome antics, these mischievous and sometimes malevolent and arrogantly hostile part-selves would act like they were enjoying toying with me in an elaborate chess game that I was reminded I was good at but would never win.

John described his subjective experience of alters taking over or influencing him in terms that paralleled "possession"[1] experiences reported in the anthropological literature. That is, in spite of his intelligence and his increasing familiarity understanding dissociative processes, John's subjective experience was that these voices from inside his head were totally "not me." However, John was too terrified to associate to who else or what else they might be, and in fact the mere request to look into it or to let whatever comes up come could trigger heart palpitations and mini-anxiety attacks.

To say that this patient lived in a house divided is an understatement. When out from under the spell of his hostile/blocker personalities, John's other part-selves could see the absurdity and illogical nature of most of what was being proposed, but a week later when under the spell again, John would act as if the conversation never took place. With

John anything could become unreal or be recategorized at any given point in time, including his own or our mutual history. Most therapies with severely dissociative trauma survivors involve continuous reinvention of the proverbial wheel, but this one often felt like it was regressing instead of progressing, and like we were endlessly caught in quicksand: I felt at times like he was pulling me in as I was trying to pull him out; at other times I felt like letting him drown in his own machinations and misery.

How a highly functional medical professional responsible for life-and-death decisions on a daily basis could show the kinds of memory deficits I witnessed often shocked and baffled me. Whenever we discussed it, John dipped into the litany of confabulated answers he had been using for years—"Oh, I'm just crazy," said dismissively, or cavalier versions of "I don't know," meaning "I'm not interested in knowing." Equally confounding was his indifference to the glaring inconsistencies in his life and his unusual thoughts and behaviors, and his utter lack of curiosity to explore them.

Eventually it was revealed that John's DID system had a very well-developed and highly protected functional set of self-states that could perform professionally without interference from any feelings, fears, or doubts—an essential adaptation. The host personality in his case was a dominant cluster of self-states responsible for work and functionality that weren't, in the words of some other parts, "designed for critical thinking." Of course, the meaning of the word "design" was not open to mutual reflection. This kind of thing was never negotiable. I eventually learned to accept and respect it as a form of containment.

A Deepening Bond or Bondage: It was difficult to know how John saw my use of power in our relationship. He would sometimes thank me for being confrontative enough to break through his façades and his duplicity, liberating him to experience honesty and intimacy for the first time, and advancing his treatment and his life. At other times, John would tell me that I was mean, harsh, impatient, and "over the top" with some of my formulations. The more evasive and distrustful parts of him would claim that I was being abusive—the same parts that denied that anything abusive had ever taken place in his early life.

John's feedback was probably on target some of the time, insofar as my frustration and irritation with the process would often be visible, becoming fodder for our discussions of the transference and countertransference whenever possible. (Like most of the DID patients I have treated, John never used that kind of sharing to subvert trust.) In any case, John benefited from the opportunity to give me feedback and I valued his regulating our relationship by telling me how I was affecting him. This was a totally new aspect of human relating to which John had never been exposed. Discussing power seemed to neutralize some of the underlying hostility, but never all of it.

John's systematic avoidance of traumatic affects and memories defined much of his waking life. As we became closer, he alluded to horrific fantasies of sexualized violence that his voices were imagining enacting toward me; he was terrified and unwilling to articulate them, fearing that the words or ideas alone could destroy our relationship. For a long time, no analysis, interpretation, or reassurance helped John risk revealing those fantasies; what freed him somewhat was my gradual acceptance of his governing subjective reality. Clearly, John was afraid of facing either the perpetrators of his past or the perpetrator(s) within, although by keeping me in the role of perpetrator much of the time per the FMS paradigm, he was able to ward off partially his feared encounter with himself and his history.

John and His Family: John declared, then disowned, memories of childhood promises that adult affection would be forthcoming— promises that turned into forced sexual liaisons with relatives, neighbors, or friends of the family. From his descriptions of childhood, John appeared to be quite vulnerable (almost to the point of having a neon sign on his forehead announcing his availability for abuse) to any disturbed adult's interest in him; at the same time, and for reasons that never became completely clear, John's early life brought him into an unusual amount of contact with numerous perpetrators. John was completely unable to feel any anger at any of those authority figures, even the ones whose specific betrayals he remembered. He was admittedly reluctant to learn anything about his past that would disturb the positive connection he had lately cultivated with his family, and emphatically invested in what he called his "Disneyland" relationship with his parents. Although he eventually described their hateful treatment and rejection of him, he maintained a superficial congeniality with them; as soon as some of John's alters made reference to the sexual abuse perpetrated by both of them, other alters immediately refuted it and recanted. Absolutely anything I said to slightly challenge or question his defen-

sively protective attachment to his parents was met with a total emo-
tional-cognitive shutdown. John recognized the way he automatically
activated such a powerful force-field but reported feeling helpless to
delve into it.

John had no difficulty remembering his parents' sadistic emotional
abuse, however. In fact, that was his presenting narrative of his life history, according to which a highly attractive couple gave birth to a less-
than-perfect child who became the object of constant scorn and ridicule
in scenes of humiliation intermingled with neglect. What with his father's pornography addiction (the extensive collections outstripping
available space in his bedroom), derisive behavior toward John, and seductiveness toward his sister, and his mother's addiction to tranquilizers and other mood-altering prescription drugs, they sounded like two
disturbed people who were "passing" as ordinary suburbanites. John
would also occasionally mention but never fully examine the extensive
psychological disabilities of his two younger siblings.

John had always longed for—no, craved—parental approval. He finally had achieved some version of it with his professional success and
corresponding financial resources. His parents were sometimes actually
deferential to him and strove to stay in his good graces. (They often convinced him to buy them expensive gifts or to give them large sums of
money.) The idea that therapists force patients to abandon their families
struck me as hilarious at many points in John's treatment, not only because it was elevated to the center of the professional and cultural debates at that time. Dissociative subterfuge was so intense where John's
family was concerned that an army of therapists could not have pried
John (or, for that matter, so many other dissociative trauma survivors)
loose from his convoluted involvement with them.

John felt helpless to do anything for his young nephews and nieces,
all of whom were showing signs of bizarre behavior and disturbed adjustment. Eventually able to recognize that they may have been exposed
to some serious abuse, he compared what he was in a position to offer
them to "what a German could do by passing a potato to a Jewish captive through the barbed wire of a concentration camp." Since he was not
willing to remember certain things about his relatives as he knew he
would have to were he to report on the risk to the children, he decided
simply to stop thinking about them, which he was quite able to do.
When upon termination John asked that I write up his case so that oth-

ers might benefit from what I was learning from working with him (even where he could not), I understood his request as an effort to pass a potato to someone else on the other end of some kind of intrapsychic barbed wire. The idea that anyone might gain from his struggles, suffering, and psychotherapy moved him deeply and surfaced a kind of hope that doomed people show when they realize that it is too late for them, but not for everyone.

John could dissociate his concerns about his nephews and nieces. I, however, could not. Here was the quintessential transference/countertransference enactment in our relationship, which is a part of most trauma therapies at one point or another—the patient's depositing of trauma, danger, suspense into the therapist's mind and then taking dissociative flight. This particular minefield was unusually complex because John knew that if he had ever clearly revealed sexual or physical abuse memories about his father I might have to report him to the child-abuse authorities in the state where they lived. He never dissociated his awareness of the potential for legal intervention, and I believe that, together with the rest of his perpetrator-protecting pattern, it accounts for why he always skirted details about his father's culpability even while revealing memories of abuse by several other relatives.

John made sure I was never in a strong enough position to file a child-abuse report while keeping me on the edge of my seat with respect to the children who might be subject to harm. There was nothing either of us could do about it. Like John in his own early life and even in his current family experience, I was now a silenced collaborator, bound and gagged in the face of possible abuse. The combination of legal, ethical, clinical, and moral stresses in treating John sometimes felt like a form of torture—and that, too, seemed to be communicating something to me about John's internal world that he could not otherwise express.

The Therapeutic Use of "False Memory" Rhetoric: John himself acknowledged that, as a professional physician, if he had been diagnosed with any medical condition other than MPD/DID, he would have been in the library poring over every reference he could locate. Of course, his ability to reflect upon or to connect any meaning to this inconsistency was limited. Several alter personalities pointed out that reading would have been useless anyway because his hostile blocker/protectors would distract his attention and "drain" from him any of the memory of what he read. Any discussion of how such an elaborate intrapsychic suction-

ing mechanism could have developed or still be so powerfully operative was met with a wall of confusion and superficial dismissiveness.
He was, however, on top of the "false memory" controversy as it was
depicted on television and in newspaper articles, and he felt compelled
to bring all of this material into our dialogues. After a year or so, the
compulsion was driven by paradoxical intentions, embodying not only
defensive and sadistic impulses but also an effort to minimize secrets
between us as we analyzed the media reports together. This was
progress for John: he was letting me in on how he was trying to defeat
me and destroy our relationship (as he had done with so many others)
instead of just playing it out. After a lifetime of keeping secrets, the idea
of revealing the very material he could and did use internally to advance his system of opposition to the therapy represented a level of intimacy he had never ventured into before.

One of John's many enactments of his inner dividedness and reenactments of his family dynamics was to speak to numerous people in his
life about his therapy and to provoke splits in opinion about it. The romantic partner whom he met about a year into our work together as
well as his most intimate friends saw evidence of his multiplicity and
heard his screams at night; they aggressively supported the therapy,
whereas others, who were influenced by the waves of FMS material hit-
ting the media (and some of whom John believed to be survivors themselves) would organize interventions to try and get him to leave his
therapy. Although John could see that what was in his head mirrored to
some degree the schisms represented in his circles of friends, he had
trouble perceiving his role in creating them. He upped the ante every
time his own ambivalence about therapy provoked another friend to
make vague threats (which he told me about) of reporting me to the
"authorities" for doing "false memory therapy" with him. We could
never mutually reflect on the sadism John thus enacted as a reenactment from his childhood since he either couldn't remember or refused
to believe the horrific tales of sexual abuse and betrayal his alters had
told me. Escalations of this rhetoric sometimes kept John's core issues of
dependency and sadistic aggression in dissociated compartmentalization and at other times completely shut down the flow of traumatic material within the therapy hour and in John's outside life.

John's self-states and alters were the most sociopathic and perpetra-
tor-like I have ever seen in an MPD/DID patient (identifying reflexively

with the intuited pain of child molesters interviewed on television; taking the name and playing the part of the Devil; maintaining the haughtiest, most contemptuous attitudes imaginable). At the same time John was gentle and in some respects very easily hurt—yet he had no real empathy for others and little capacity for true remorse. Although mildly aware of his propensity for surprising people with unexpected shifts into cruelty and exploitativeness, John's only concern seemed to be restoring their trust and affection toward him. As he began to see some of the effects of his behavior on me—someone he was growing to love as much as he was trying to hate and destroy—during the course of the therapy relationship, some authentic, healthy guilt emerged for the first time in his life.

John read Lenore Terr's popular books on memory and nonfiction accounts of the now-famous Eileen Franklin case, and I encouraged him also to consult Ofshe and Loftus's work along with classic material on trauma and MPD. He was able to apply his sophisticated intelligence to deconstruct some of the FMS perspectives, but only vis-à-vis others. He could not extrapolate to himself, and in fact reported having extreme difficulty understanding one section in a popular book about trauma—the chapter on MPD, about which there was absolutely nothing complicated. Written material about MPD actually exacerbated John's confusion and memory problems.

We finally did come to a point in our discourse where we could explore different possible meanings of his behavior and diverse narratives and recantations about his traumatic history without eliminating any and without his forgetting any. He learned to reflect on my thoughts without dissociating, without derisive hostile alters taking over, and without shutting down the dialogue. It was almost as if a new personality was formed—a self that could do the therapy, remember, feel, observe, link, and critically think about himself. After about three years, John accepted the obvious evidence of the DID diagnosis.

He remained unconvinced that he had experienced any childhood trauma, however, and when he did begin to integrate traumatic material and its implications, he continued to claim that he had not been severely effected, focusing consistently on his professional achievements as a way of demonstrating that the damage was minimal. He became able to think inquiringly about the inconsistencies in his life and his therapy without the cavalier dismissals that foreclose rather than promote dialogue. As exhausting reenactments gave way to reflection, we could examine everything in a spirit well beyond accusations or confrontations. John felt secure that he could disagree radically and irritatingly with me without being abandoned, punished, or withdrawn from.

And we could collaborate, knowing that agreement wasn't simply compliance. I recall one session in which I described in detail how critics like Loftus and Ofshe would probably conceptualize an important piece of trauma work we had just done together. This was part of how we manipulated the FMS, betrayal, and distrust themes—evaluating the same interpersonal process from a variety of perspectives, increasingly with humor: John's hostile alters usually played the parts of the FMS Foundation and I played the various protherapy roles. As John began to work through his defenses against acknowledging his pathological multiplicity and some of his traumatic history, we began to be able to define our therapy relationship and our conclusions from either side of the memory and MPD debates. Instead of the obstacle it was initially, FMS rhetoric became part of the play of therapy.[2]

A Tentative Breakthrough: Usually, following a productive therapy session with John some form of backlash, amnesia, or sabotage could be expected. However, during this time it was I, in the context of playing with different points of view, who generated the reversal fantasies of who was doing what to whom. It was I, not John's hostile blockers, who raised doubts about how the week's therapy might be projected from the FMS/anti-MPD postures. My creative portrayal of our recent piece of work as a dance of my coercion and John's compliance was very convincing—both a serious and humorous moment because we had visited so many times the landscape of absolute paranoia and confusion over who was doing what to whom. Usually some form of backlash, amnesia, or sabotage could be expected following a productive session with John—but by literally beating him to the punch, I somehow upset his dissociative apple cart enough to trigger a different reaction to our traumatic-memory work.

The hostile/blocker part-selves who had orchestrated the bulk of the "false memory enactments" were shocked and impressed that I was giving them so much ammunition with which to fight the therapy. I replied that, if after all we had been through, John were to take the FMS route once again in the same old way, I would recognize that something had disrupted our trust or that I had made some kind of error—or else

I would understand the regression to be a statement that John didn't think he could go into the depth of his pain. My flexible take on the meanings of any resumption of false memory rhetoric undermined some of John's cognitive rigidity and subtly eroded some of his dissociative barriers; it advanced us further toward disarmament, enhanced our trust, and allowed John some space to depolarize internally. As a consequence of that playful session, John asserted in an uncharacteristically somber tone, "You know I could go down that path [FMS] and avoid all of this pain; it would be so much easier." Then, after a pause, "And, I am not going to do that. "

A new sense of will, agency, and ownership of self set in at that moment. An almost four-year siege against the therapy gave way to a new level of depth and a wider window on his complex multiplicity. John began exploring more troublesome traumatic memories and developed a stronger capacity for staying with feelings and gruesome images without retreating to dissociative flight. For an uninterrupted period of time, he was able to make and sustain links between different states of mind and to wonder about their relationship with one another; no longer was every attempt at bridge building followed by demolition. Soon, very disturbing memories of sadistic abuse, ritual abuse, and group perpetration began to surface, and John focused on them for a couple of months before he shut down in a combination of terror, incredulity, and stubborn refusal to go further.

By then, our joint history of surviving his extended nay-saying and our working through of new ways to say yes without compliance and new ways to say no without sabotage and dissimulation had engendered considerable changes in his interpersonal life. John had been able to deepen outside relationships and also to handle increasing administrative challenges at work. The subsequent increase in responsibilities and acceleration of his professional ambition were among several factors that ultimately discouraged him from wanting to face and follow any more traumatic material wherever it might lead. During a kind of breakthrough session, some very deeply buried alter personalities emerged to say, "I don't want to be helped, I don't want to be loved, I am too damaged." John began to sob deeply, which is something he had rarely done in his life and something he had never allowed himself to do with me. After his years of psychic deadness, endless doubting, and his brilliant avoidance of vulnerability, I was profoundly moved to witness this opening.

John's resistance to feeling any pain or loss of control was enormous. He could, however, experience real intrapsychic conflicts about wanting to be known, recognized, and loved. They no longer had to be externalized and enacted, concretized by DID and by FMS ideologies. Once these core conflicts finally found their way into the therapy discourse, core issues—attachment, dependency, fears of retraumatization—could be accessed and discussed. John's defenses yielded to more emotionally vulnerable dialogues that led again to the ritual-abuse memories. It was they that elicited a level of anxiety that remobilized some of his more rigid dissociative defenses.

The Beginning of the End: Following major events in his professional and private lives—a big promotion at work that would mean greater demands on his time, his lover's unexpected HIV diagnosis—and several months after he reported a series of memories involving animal torture and killing and the abuse by a group of perpetrators of several children at once, John told me that the voices in his head wanted him to stop therapy. One of his alters identified those recollections of animal sacrifices as screen memories for human sacrifices; another began to allude to the possibility that John had committed some form of sexual abuse on his younger sister. Those revelations would prove to be John's last: analysis of his dependency, erotic, and sadistic issues was difficult enough, but he could not tolerate exploring the perpetrator within.

What was different from John's familiar one-step-forward/two-steps-backward pattern was that for the first time what he called a "majority" opinion was presented. John moved through a variety of enactments and excuses to conclude, honestly, that he believed there was "an abyss" at the base of his being that was so dark and so deep that he needed to take time to think about whether or not he could take on the dangerous journey. In that moment I realized that John might be terrified for good reasons: not all traumatized, dissociative patients can integrate. Sometimes trauma has outstripped the capacities for repair in what is left of the shattered self. Sometimes it is simply better not to know. Sometimes the decision to not go forward in treatment is an issue of faith—in the self, in the therapist, in the process, in a benevolent universe, in a benevolent deity—and sometimes it is the only way to keep on living.

Termination: By the end of the twice-weekly therapy, John was in a stable long-term relationship. He had resolved most of his fears and anxieties about being alone and was able to buy a house for the first time in his life. His sexual addiction and dangerous acting out had completely subsided; his reliance on chemicals for anxiety-reduction had significantly diminished. He had relatively few nightmares, was no longer anxious and depressed, and had begun tentatively exploring a spiritual life. In spite of those remarkable improvements, John was never able to consolidate and integrate trauma/memory material in any consistent, enduring fashion. And while he could now acknowledge his extreme pathological multiplicity, he remained primarily organized by dissociation and was unmotivated to change that. His capacities for intimacy and self-observation were still quite limited. The level of fear, hate, malevolence, and spite he carried within his psyche was reduced but not significantly diffused.

Our work, therefore, was successful, but incomplete. John spoke of his opposing hopes and dreads that leaving treatment would dislodge something fixed and rigid in him so that he could resume therapy with access to deeper places in himself; enable him to return to a less complicated, less conflictual life where he could be satisfied with what changes he had made; and allow him to be completely left alone and not bothered in any deep or meaningful way by anyone, providing a final reprieve from the pressures of intimacy. He expressed feelings of love and gratitude toward me along with fears and sadness over terminating—yet at the same time his hostile alters snickered about the money he would save and about their victory in preventing John from delving too deeply into his memories; having spent long periods of time locked in and retreating to small, dark, enclosed spaces during childhood, these alters longed to go back to that impersonal world. My own feelings mirrored John's. I was sad, relieved, disappointed that so much effort could not take him to another level of trust, faith, and integrity, and hopeful about moving on at some point in the future.

Within every trauma survivor there is the ongoing debate about preserving functionality versus the digging into posttraumatic material and characterological patterns so freighted with pain, grief, and rage that it inevitably disrupts functioning, at least temporarily. Some severely dissociative patients, in spite of extreme trauma, can generate enormous faith in the process of deconstruction and reconstruction and some cannot. Some have the capacities for the process and some do not regardless of issues of faith. Similarly, some therapy dyads are able to

generate hope and a capacity for faith that can see them through extremely difficult times and some can do so only in a limited way. The
analytic process is sometimes conceptualized as a duet of two voices,
interweaving tonalities and lyrics of resonance and difference (Pizer,
1996a).

Whether a different therapist might have taken the treatment further
is a question that both patient and therapist should always explore, and
John and I did. I pressed John to make his termination-decision as consciously as possible, so that it would be uncontaminated by old patterns
of self-deception or compliance and defiance. I shared my complex ambivalence with him. John and I had gone either as far as he could go or
as far as he could go with me, at least at the time. In spite of his gains in
internal and external adjustment, the relentless reinvention of the wheel
with respect to certain parts of the therapy, the continuous disruption of
attachment, and the continuous problems with amnesia and purposeful
forgetting left me feeling exhausted and sometimes exploited. John was
quite afraid of finding out who he might be. Any further therapy, it
seemed, would be motivated more by his fear of not being in treatment
than by his commitment to investigate his traumatic material and the
abusive relational paradigms cocreated in the treatment process. At the
end, John could be honest about his lack of interest and motivation to
know about himself in all of these ways. He would take refuge in his
work, his friendships, and his relationship with his lover. Something inside of him, inside of me, or between us could not be stretched any further.

Epilogue: I saw John on three separate occasions for two or three sessions each in the first few years after his termination. He would call me
in the midst of an overwhelming life crisis that precipitated massive
posttraumatic responses (e.g., nightmares of violence and abuse, return
to sexual compulsivity), suggesting, among other things, that deeper
material (from the abyss) might be trying to surface once again. Just
reaching out and being in the presence of my capacity to hold and remind him of the whole of him seemed to alleviate those transient de-
compensations. Although we revisited the possibility of our doing
supportive therapy only or of his working with another therapist each
time he renewed his attachment to me and the same set of conflicts
about going deeper presented itself, we would always come to the same
conclusion: John could not or would not engage in a more intensive

therapy dialogue. He never fully left the concentration camp of his own mind—but I am sure that because of our experience together, he worked out an interesting and more spacious compromise with the internal perpetrators and demons that plagued and controlled him. Some corner of hope inside him had become ignited and if now there was only a candle in the dark, someday, I thought, somewhere and with someone else it might catch fire.

Khan's (1978) and Winnicott's (1967) comments on the limits of the therapy contract have permeated my reflections on the way John ended our work together. As they point out, sometimes it is more important for a therapist to sustain a person in living than to rid him/her of his illness. The "absence of psychoneurotic illness may be health, but it is not life" (Winnicott, 1967, p. 100). As Khan (1978, p. 259) elegantly articulates:

> The demand for life, and if that is not possible, for not living, is made upon us by the patient and is not a bias of our restitutive omnipotence as therapists. When a patient makes this demand upon us, we have every right to refuse it, but not to confuse it. The patient is willing to stay ill and suffer its consequences so long as he or she is living or not living. If we try to subvert his life by a cure he either escapes us or gives up the right to be alive and ill and enters into a complicity with us which we mistake for "treatment alliance."

SURVIVING DISSOCIATION

The therapist treating severely dissociative patients must become, in a sense, "bilingual," able to shift frames of reference between unitary and multiple modes of relatedness and fluent at navigating violent internal and interpersonal politics. The therapist can succeed in forming a relationship with one aspect of the patient's personality system only to see that part ejected, covered over, or domineered out of the relationship by another, more aggressive or avoidant part. The normal clinical attachment process is subverted in relationships with severely dissociative patients.

There exists a unique cross-cultural difference (Kluft, 1989) between the therapist, whose own self-states are presumably organized predominantly by repression and other higher-order defenses and the MPD/DID patient who is in large measure dissociatively self-constructed. (However, since most human beings also deploy dissociation in various forms, long-term immersion in the transference/countertransference with severely dissociative trauma survivors is likely to bring most therapists into contact with their own dissociative self-experience; these experiences can be mild, moderate, or overwhelming for the clinician). Working with such a patient can feel like being on the receiving end of a series of repetitive abandonment, hit-and-run, bait-and-switch maneuvers, and the therapist's natural reactions to those feelings can impact the ability to trust the patient and cocreate an effective holding environment.

Of course it is not the therapist alone who creates a therapeutic holding environment. The patient contributes to the process if only insofar as a level of consistency and continuity of self comprises the basis for a treatment alliance—but that assumption, with the severely traumatized, dissociative population, cannot be counted on. The feeling of trying to create and maintain a holding environment on one's own is, as so many different therapists have commented, a symbolic replication of the traumatized child's abandonment to the desperate and lonely effort to restore him/herself without the assistance of a protective, soothing, and nonabusive significant other. The solitary construction of a holding environment by the therapist is so critical to treating dissociative individuals that the inability to make it happen will be a stumbling block to the healing process.

Modell (1990) comments on the precocious yet fragile patterns of maturational adaptation by children who experience early and massive losses of parents as protectors. In the face of such parental failure, which is one of the hallmarks of the severely dissociative patient's experience, the child can only sustain him/herself by relying upon his/her own constructed reality—a reality often largely composed of grandiose, omnipotent fantasies through which the unshielded child seeks safety and self-sufficiency. The life-preserving creation of an alternative inner world leads to resistance to taking things in from others because accepting the ideas of others confronts the individual with the limits of his/her omnipotence. Thus the severely traumatized, dissociative patient may consistently reduce the therapist to talking to him/herself while superficially offering a kind of affable compliance just sufficient to regulate the interpersonal field.

The abandonment of the therapist through relational retreat by the highly dissociative patient and the attitude of indifference on the part of an abruptly "absent" patient can leave the therapist with paralyzing anxiety and rage. The presence of this absence—the deadness and nonbeingness through which the dissociative patient passively allows certain internal and interpersonal enactments to occur without intervening, without applying critical thinking, and without grasping the destructive meanings and historical implications of the events—may be the single most difficult unconscious identification with the perpetrating/collusion system that blocks attachment to the therapist. Based on the internalization of the nonintervening, collaborating, collusive, and therefore ultimately abandoning parent, this identification also interferes with new learning and keeps the patient distracted, confused, and permeable to maladaptive forms of aggression from within and without.

Reversals and *polarizations* commonly take place during therapy (within the patient and between patient and therapist) between adult and child states, deadness and hyperarousal, clinging attachment and antibonding sentiment, impervious superficiality and depth of feeling, masculinity and femininity, belief and incredulity, rebelliousness and obedience, fragility and sturdiness, attentiveness and distraction, confidence and self-doubting, trust and distrust, collaborativeness and sabotage, loving and hating, arrogance and helplessness, remembering and forgetfulness, yearning for specialness and fear of any recognition whatsoever, attachment to life/hope and tenacious suicidality and clinging to death, anxiety or distress and numb or cavalier attitudes, and cooperativeness and abusiveness.

In particular, tentatively emerging healthy grandiosity can suddenly transmute into virulent self-denigration; other people may be simultaneously heralded and derided by different aspects of the self-system as the patient negotiates a safe intimacy/distance balance to avoid retraumatization; and, especially after the leakage of traumatic material, dependency needs (or unbridled sadism and vindictiveness) can abruptly resurface and totally overwhelm an individual's dissociative equilibrium. Meanwhile, independently, the therapist may be attempting to bond with and treat some fragment of the patient's self created to manage superficial functioning issues, erroneously thinking s/he is creating an alliance with a more important aspect of that self. In the extreme, a hostile adult alter may cancel an office visit while a pleading child-part phones the therapist, misinterpreting (perhaps through the passive influence of more dominant personalities) the missed appointment as therapist-initiated and evidence that the therapist no longer likes the him/her.

Indeed, some of the most disconcerting and troubling facets of the switching and reversing process transpire around being in and out of treatment— forgetting to show up for appointments, canceling sessions, threatening to end the therapy, arguing over paying for it, making special requests, and generally bouncing around the most elemental commitment to treatment (or, in analogous cases, to sobriety or recovery from other addictions). Some patients are so overstimulated and overwrought by the therapy process that they manage their anxiety by starting and stopping several times a year, never getting beyond the initial stages or past specific power struggles. In the multidimensional world of a severely dissociated individual, each interruption in treatment may be experienced as wiping the slate clean and in no way connected to previous interruptions or to any ambivalence/enactment pattern—which, not incidentally, portends a particularly poor prognosis. Surviving destruction in those instances consists in the therapist's ability to tolerate repeated comings and goings without giving up on the patient and in the patient's gradual ability to tolerate increasing tension-states before taking flight the next time.

At a certain point in the process, however, if the therapist is not willing to lose the patient altogether by taking a stand that the patient agree to an uninterrupted treatment, then the therapist will have failed to engage the patient in a deeper mutual survival of destruction. In the treatment of torture survivors (for whom the blocking of avoidance, escape, and dissociative defenses was pivotal to the traumatization) more flexibility may be called for, and many therapists working with individuals who have suffered either containment traumas—being buried, locked in closets, put into cages and trunks of cars—or other absolute forms of loss of control allow extra leeway to approach and avoid. Overall, the therapist's most important tool for disrupting this form of chronic switching is the eventual sharing of his/her experience of the patient and of the therapy. Such modeling of emotional availability and directness can access the patient's underlying terrors in a way that encourages their interpersonal negotiation (in contrast to the nonrelating, defensively autonomous way most trauma survivors have learned to manage fears and anxieties).

At the most basic level, as Ross (1997) explains, the therapist must be prepared to let the patient die, otherwise he/she can't help the patient. When a therapist is continuously frightened and worried or desperate to "save" the patient, neither of them will develop the necessary capacities to tolerate the work of integrating traumatic memories and affects or dissociated identities. More than likely, in fact, the therapist will become uncomfortably entrenched in the rescuer position and the patient will become infantilized and never integrate his/her aggression; s/he will either remain chronically regressed, embark on sprees of destructive acting out, or drop out of treatment entirely.

The inevitable chronic suicide threats and attempts and other, less lethal flirtations with danger that trauma survivors compulsively repeat are particular sources of stress for the clinician. The patient performs an elaborate dance whose postures alternate between clinging to life, damning the world, feeling condemned, courting death, and begging for rescue. The therapist is always both witness and participant and also is expected to continuously, simultaneously, and undauntedly hold all the hope while the patient enacts the dance. In terms of "proving" to the patient that s/he is capable of the level of devotion and caring tragically missing from the abusive family, the therapist is thrust into a role that somewhat resembles that of a child-victim living on the brink of disaster and doom, never empowered to make a difference in the course of events.

GINA

A therapist senses a spike in the curve of what has come to be "normal" suicidality in Gina, who insists however that nothing unusual is going on.

So the therapist questions her intuition: is she projecting her own destructive wishes—or is she picking up on something real? Or is the patient baiting and switching?

Later, one of Gina's child-alters leaves a message on the therapist's answering machine spelling out a detailed suicide plan. The therapist calls back, but the primary adult-alter who answers (persona-restoring, functional type) cavalierly claims to know nothing about it. Is her innocence denial? dissociation? conscious manipulation? all of the above?

The next morning Gina herself, shocked and distraught, leaves the therapist a message saying she awoke from a trance to find that she had turned on all the gas appliances and sealed all the doors and windows. Who's trying to kill whom? Is this suicide or homicide?

The therapist feels she's holding a life in her hands. Should she call the police and, if so, when? Gina will hate her if she does—and also if she doesn't. Professional ethics demand evaluation of the suicide risk but evaluating risk in DID patients is difficult to do and difficult to document. The whole situation turns into a forced choice about which hate and betrayal the therapist is ready to cope with on this particular day.

And, of course, that which is being avoided either within the patient or between patient and therapist—at the very least a direct encounter with aggressive feelings—will easily get lost in the management crisis.

When the patient attempts to pass on core responsibility for life itself, the therapist can be kept spinning between legal dilemmas, professional obligations, and personal attachment to the patient and their joint history—often while holding alone the identification with redemption and healing. S/he is apt to feel either the urge to implore the patient to sit still and give him/her a break or the impulse to say "go ahead and drop out of treatment, or kill yourself already, I'm sick of the back and forth of it all." Therapists will certainly bounce rapidly between optimism and hopelessness, between supporting and devaluing the patient—who will assuredly pick up on the ambivalence, accelerating a downward acting-out spiral.

By continually reversing directions, the severely dissociative individual avoids bringing polarized beliefs out of the realm of sequestered trance logic into a reflective consciousness. Until a certain point in the treatment, often far into the middle phases, the severely dissociative patient cannot help but keep things whirring to avoid stepping on any trauma land mines. For the therapist, the result may be a kind of motion sickness that generates chronic and disorienting disequilibrium.

JIM

Even though Jim is onto the shenanigans of his tricksterlike voices that consistently block emerging feelings, memories, or attachment longings, and even though he sees through their attempt to disrupt his struggle to go deeper in therapy, when they insist that there's nothing to go deeper about ("You're making things up just to please the shrink"), he's thrown off course by the same internal reversal he experiences in intimate relations as the voices remind him not to get close to anyone. They let him reveal alters and parts of traumatic memories in therapy, but only as long as he subsequently negates them.

Jim's brutal, cunning perpetrators manipulated both his attachment system and his neurochemistry to train him not to trust anyone but themselves. In one scenario, after they drug, multiply abuse, and momentarily abandon the boy, the father who brought him to the group and who has been raping him since age three (as a training exercise rather than solely for personal gratification) reaches out to him. The almost-embrace lasts one second before Jim is turned around and raped yet again. The group laughs derisively as he's humiliated and emotionally tormented for daring to hope and daring to believe in rescue.

This is just one of Jim's experiences of coerced bonding, "lessons" in the futility of hope. Yet for years this man has been unable to locate his compulsive distrust in his treatment by his perpetrators. He feels no anger toward them; in fact, the very thought of it agitates and terrifies him. He describes his alters "hard-wired to deflect closeness of any kind"—that is, to reverse direction in the face of any intimate encounter—but to pursue connections with a high potential for abuse, like promiscuous sex in public places and/or with strangers.

In patients with histories like Jim's, the therapist's empathy, compassion, or love triggers reminders of the early direct and indirect assaults on hope, setting back their intimacy projects by catalyzing new rounds of acting out. Such patterns can bury patients for years in the mental health system where their cycles of provocative and self-destructive behavior are never fully understood. In some very disturbing cases, where the therapist is made into an enemy for a long time, certain of the patient's parts (sometimes in conjunction with the abusive family or perpetrator group if it's still in the picture) will actually institute dangerous threats, blackmail, or even malicious lawsuits against him/her.

As dissociative reversals interact with projection, projective-identification, and denial and combine into multiple levels of transference, almost everything the therapist says and does—move a clock in his office, take a vacation—can be portrayed as dangerous by subcomponents of the DID patient's system. Still, however, the patient often cannot experience his/her actual abusers as dangerous, and the reversals around siting danger, particularly in the therapist and in the childhood perpetrator, will continue throughout much of the treatment process. The therapist's tolerance for being perceived as dangerous, along with willingness to confront the patient's manipulation and avoidance and to honor the patient's anger by negotiating its possible meanings, creates a climate in which the trauma survivor may find his/her protest-voice as well as the courage to challenge real and internalized perpetrating systems.

SANDRA

In the space of one month, Sandra's pet dies, Sandra's friend dies (HIV), and a celebrity dies. Feeling that she was the cause in all cases, Sandra tells the therapist she's too dangerous to come in for treatment for a while lest she bring harm to him. She adamantly refuses his invitation to discuss and actually test out her belief. It's unclear to the therapist what parts of Sandra's stance connect to treatment dynamics and his letting her down, and what parts are rooted in triggers or surfacing memories or fears of retraumatization.

Sandra is always conflating safety and danger. By producing an excuse for interrupting therapy, she's choosing to stick with her familiar omnipotent fantasies and delaying collisions with the therapist that might undermine the dissociative rigidity of her beliefs. By reversing her state from relation to isolation, she keeps herself safe from stimulating any overwhelming traumatic affects and safe from the risk of retraumatization; she also forestalls the abandonment she predicts will result from the impact of her destructive influence on the therapist.

Interpretation is rarely what gets a therapy dyad through impasses born of entrenched reversals of cause and effect. Sandra was impelled to take a brief hiatus from therapy, and in this case the therapist's empathic understanding and tolerance of a decision the patient had feared would result in his withdrawal or retaliation, together with his sharing of his sorrow and frustration at being kept out and prohibited from working in partnership with the patient at such a crucial time, is what seemed to break through the otherwise impenetrable wall Sandra had built around herself.

FORGETTING TO REMEMBER AND REMEMBERING TO FORGET.[3]

We all hover at different distances between knowing and not knowing about trauma, caught between the compulsion to complete the process of knowing and the inability or fear of doing so. . . . The knowledge of trauma is fiercely defended against, for it can be a momentous, threatening, cognitive and affective task, involving an unjaundiced appraisal of events and our own injuries, failures, conflicts, and losses. During massive trauma, fiction, fantasy, and demonic art can become historical fact; this blurring of boundaries between reality and fantasy conjures up affect so violent that it exceeds the ego's capacity for regulation. To protect ourselves from affect, we must, at times, avoid knowledge. (Laub and Auerhahn, 1993, p. 288)

Therapists treating severely dissociative trauma survivors must not only grapple with the posttraumatic vicissitudes of memory as it plays out in the therapy relationship, but they must also struggle with aftershocks of recent cultural civil wars about the veracity of delayed (or traumatic) memory and the potentially contaminating effects of psychotherapy. In many cases therapists and patients alike must find a way to pursue treatment for posttraumatic issues while maintaining their equilibrium and integrity during a period of cultural ambivalence, incredulity, and disparagement toward (interpersonal) trauma survivors and psychotherapy.

Trauma distorts the memories of its victims; no one disputes that. What is disputed, and disputed widely and often bitterly, are the cognitive and dynamic mechanisms underlying traumatic forgetting, memory recovery, and the motives and contexts that enhance both processes. Memory is a tricky business and the politics of memory is even trickier. The ownership of memory is inextricably related to the ownership of history, and the ownership of history (including personal history) is largely a function of power. Refuting the capacity or reality of someone's memory is, correspondingly, disempowering—an act of subjugation and remarginalization.

On the one hand we must acknowledge the limitations of memory and of our ability to arrive at objective interpretations or reality, and on the other hand we must acknowledge that memory preserves in the internal world important interactions with external reality that would otherwise be lost (MacVicar, 1997). Memory involves pruning, selecting, registering, and retaining, linking and delinking. As soon as events occur we begin forgetting them, altering them, making them better or worse (or in the case of DID, possibly both at once), changing the characters, making myths about them, and attempting to fit them in with what we already know (Schacter, 1996). The accrual of a clinical base of knowledge to guide the assessment of memory and other psychic material that emerges during psychotherapy needs to be informed by cognitive research—but not dominated, subverted, or marginalized by it.

Many people's memories have been systematically manipulated (usually by perpetrators and collaborators). Some people flee from their histories and others desperately search for lost memories. Some are haunted and chased by memories and others willfully avoid and manipulate their memories or their access to them. Some believe their fantasies and cannot integrate their actual memories, some use fantasy to cover actual memories. Some DID patients maintain false memories of nonabuse, affirming how wonderful their families really were; others enlist actual pleasant or innocuous memories to defuse emerging traumatic narratives. And some finally come to believe their often brutal or bizarre memories, only to experience the reignition of their chronic self-doubting in the reigning culture of skepticism.

All kinds of dichotomous characterizations of memory—implicit and explicit, traumatic and nontraumatic, semantic and iconic—coexist in the same individual. The fanatical focus on veridicality by extremists on all sides has supported simplistic conceptions of psychopathology and psychotherapy (Berger, 1996). A preferable epistemology tolerates complexity and ambiguity; Frawley-O'Dea (1997) enjoins preservation of the dialectical tension between narrative and historical truth. "The aim of analysis is not to recover the past, but to make recovery of the past possible, the past that is frozen in repetition" (Phillips, 1994, p. 69).

Remembering can be healing but is not necessarily healing in and of itself; similarly, not remembering and not knowing can serve *or* subvert the process of healing. By bearing witness to the patient's suffering, the therapist can ameliorate some of the essential isolation of the trauma and neglect experience and support the reestablishment of healthy attachment bonds and soothing introjects (Laub and Auerhahn, 1989); still, however, whatever traumatic material is uncovered needs to be integrated in terms of its impact on and for the patient's developmental tasks (Barach, 1999c).

Since reinstating development and fostering personality growth and integration is what is essentially healing about memory work, Kepner (1995) believes that the goals and purpose of working with a patient's memories necessarily vary with the stage of development of both the patient and therapy relationship, and he describes the most common course of emergence and assimilation of traumatic memories. Initially, memory fragments often do not emerge in recognizable form unless some degree of support is available; also, they often do not appear in logical or linear fashion but are, rather, disconnected. The patient is apt to move from a state of shock to one of self-doubt and then to cycle back and forth between them for some time; eventually, s/he can begin to affirm that what has emerged has at least some kind of truth in it and to start the difficult work of integrating new meaning structures and reorganizing identity.

Accordingly, therapists may need to provide the initial ego resources for severely traumatized patients who are learning to trust their basic perceptions and may also need to validate some of those perceptions (Steele, 1999). Until patients begin to develop a modicum of trust in their sense of reality, however, Steele cautions that this process is better undertaken with current and daily issues than with history and memories. In that connection, it may sometimes become necessary for the therapist to acknowledge the essential truth of the patient's experience or to challenge what appears to be unlikely.

In a relational perspective, the focus of treatment is on the impediments that interfere with a free commerce between various "layers" or "levels" of the patient's mind (Pizer, 1998), rather than on its repressed contents or on gaps in the patient's history. Close attention to process elements and to the intrapsychic realities observable on-the-scene replaces the collection of historical vignettes; the therapist can concentrate on "removing obstacles to intrapsychic freedom" (Berger, 1996, p. 171).

The actual complexities of clinical work are often bypassed, however, by memory researchers consumed with true/false dichotomies, by clinicians who believe that rapid collection of trauma narratives can actually lead to a realistic and lasting cure, and by those who refuse to accept the real possibilities of extreme violation reflected in some patients' memories. In all such limited conceptual frameworks "one does not have to tolerate the anxiety aroused by extended uncertainty, by working within a complex, subtle, uncertain clinical, and epistemological framework, and by accompanying a patient in an unpredictable, complex, frightening therapeutic journey" (p. 174); and in the matching treatment approaches, the psyche will not be liberated from patterns of internalized domination and colonization.

In the final analysis, as Davies (1996b) indicates, the truths we come to accept and ultimately to own during psychotherapy are those that improve clinical symptomatology—those memories whose processing ameliorates or even reverses posttraumatic, addictive, and self-destructive patterns. While it can certainly be argued that mutative elements of the attachment and relationship dynamics between therapist and patient, and perhaps the symbolic reparation involved in discussing and grieving over retrieved material (accurate or inaccurate), are the operative variables in generating positive changes from memory work in psychoanalytic psychotherapy, the reality probably fluctuates between and incorporates both possibilities. Portraying any form of memory work as an isolated project of its own stripped of the dialogical give-and-take of any well-conducted psychotherapy would be to misrepresent the process therapists and patients actually engage in.

Brenneis (1994) recognizes the double bind whereby the therapist's belief in the possibility of the existence, recoverability, and reconstructability of repressed or dissociated abuse may constitute a necessary precondition for the emergence of valid memories on the one hand, and fertile ground for overt and covert suggestion that could lead (in combination with the patient's quest for approval and affiliation), to the production of false memories on the other. "At some points, we may find ourselves forced to choose between bearing false witness or failing to bear true witness without knowing with any certainty which we are doing. Neither of these alternatives is without clinical consequences" (p. 1050).

In the American trauma drama there may be false accusers, false innocents, and false recanters, along with true victims, real innocents and legitimate recanters. And no one can ascertain the difference for certain in any of these conditions. False memories of abuse and false memories of nonabuse may actually coexist in the same person (and vice versa). The existence of one does not necessarily negate the existence or validity of the other. False memories of nonabuse, or minimization of abuse and omnipotent forms of disavowal, may even be the most prevalent form of "false memory" in human psychology. Whatever the situation, falsification of memory is most likely to take place under conditions of subtle or overt domination, whether it is a political or incestuous family system (Grand, 1995) or an unethical or clumsy clinician. This understanding must help us prevent overintrusive and dominating psychotherapy in terms of excessive suggestion, overidentification with victim roles, denying the patient's experience, or foreclosing on purely ideological grounds the exploration of possible trauma and dissociative self-organization.

Doubting is as infectious as credulity. Doubting is more hypnotic than credulity. We are all vulnerable, often in subliminal and subtle ways, to the forces of cultural and professional doubting, just as we are to those cultural and professional forces that would enlist our support. Doubt can itself become a phenomenon of paradoxical influence. A patient's doubting of him/herself can make a clinician doubt the patient. A clinician's doubting can make the patient doubt him/herself. The culture's doubting can make either or both of them doubt the veracity of the patient's material.

Too much emphasis on memory recovery at the expense of characterological work can imbalance a treatment, while the avoidance of memory work and accessing dissociative states can make a treatment overly intellectual and stale, reducing its transformative value. Therapists need to focus not just on the content of memories, but on the process of empowering patients in their relationships to their memories (Pye, 1995). That mandate encompasses the rehabilitation of imagination and restorative fantasy capacities, which when integrated and interacting with memory work, allow for a deeper integration of trauma and dissociative aspects of the personality.

Who's Influencing Whom?

> So the question is: given his or her training—whatever its theoretical allegiances—what is the repertoire of life-stories the analyst can allow, or allow himself to hear, and consider plausible? What are the acceptable shapes of a life that the analyst by virtue of his profession and his conscious and unconscious aesthetic preferences, find himself promoting? At what point, in listening to a life-story, does he call the police? Everybody sets a limit to the stories they can be told; and in that sense there is a repertoire of stories they are likely to hear. (Phillips, 1994, p. 70)

It is imperative that we take a very wide-angle view of the dynamics of influence in psychotherapy. Not all influence is coercive, nor are all attempts (conscious or otherwise) to influence equally effective: influence is fluid, and neither linear nor unidirectional. Indeed, much that is influential in psychotherapy (from the overarching interpersonal power dynamics to the particular offering of interpretations), can be made conscious and can be negotiated; influence is not inevitable and certainly is not automatically tantamount to indoctrination.[4] Indeed, relational psychoanalytic theories specifically emphasize the clinical utility of reciprocal influence.

Clinicians working within an intersubjective frame value difference, disagreement, and the exploration of paradoxes and alternative explanations. Patients are invited to disagree, to comment on the therapist's behavior, even to disclose suspicions of the therapist's motivations and to learn the workings of the therapist's mind, thus creating an atmosphere of mutual influence that promotes critical thinking and leaves possibilities of meaning open. The intersubjective vehicle is one in which the elements of influence are discussed and analyzed, and where there can be a recognition of mutuality of influence between therapist and patient while preserving an asymmetry of roles (Aron, 1992). In other words, relational and intersubjective theorists affirm or even at times take pride in the element of influence in their clinical work.

All therapy patients differ in the degree to which they are vulnerable to suggestion or hypnosis (Whalen and Nash, 1996). No trauma survivor is a sponge without some critical thinking ability and some defenses against impingement. Indeed, many of their life experiences have made them quite distrustful of authority and less receptive—and possibly less vulnerable— than others to influence and suggestion (Leavitt, 1997). The same dissociative strategies that may spare a patient psychic torment from abusers can also insulate him/her from assistance.

If the influence phenomenon in DID was a simple unidimensional construct as the critics and false memory syndrome proponents would have us believe, treatment would move along at a lot quicker pace. It is in the very nature of dissociation to encapsulate experience, affect, and belief systems in such a way as to make patients impermeable to influence except when brought into direct affective contact with, and direct perceptual awareness of, the therapist and the therapy relationship. If these patients were extremely suggestible, their self-hate could probably be dissolved with a year of sensitive, empathic, and supportive therapy. That isn't what happens.

Why is it that the media has chosen only to show the most primitive, bizarre, and exaggerated forms of treatment and mistreatment, instead of seizing the chance to educate the public about the complex nature of trauma, PTSD, dissociative adaptations, and child abuse? Why do television documentaries consistently pair MPD and trauma with past-life regression, UFOs, half-baked cathartic group-encounter sessions, and therapists who either are (or are edited to look) foolish and incompetent? Why does the media not seek out competent therapists to interview about sensitive MPD treatment (and then not manipulatively edit their testimony)? Are these influence phenomena not also essentially part of what we need to include in the current debates to attain a fully balanced perspective?

Clinicians will position themselves on different points along the skepticism-belief continuum in keeping with their own characters, histories, anxieties, and personal exposure to life's horrors. Their mental biases, including tendencies to overdiagnose or minimize the possibility of abuse, may play a role in the way in which patients come to understand and categorize their experience (Rogers, 1995). Those therapists familiar with the dynamics of sex offenders, sex rings, mind control, or perpetrator groups perceive and respond to patients' reports of such phenomena differently from those who are either new to such manifestations of human evil or afraid to listen.

Skill at handling prolonged ambiguity, informed conviction about the nature of memory and fantasy, willingness to agree and disagree with patients and to make and correct errors are what clinicians working with abuse victims should strive for, in contrast to the self-serving comfort of indefinite skepticism and ivory-tower neutrality. But the role and responsibilities of the therapist, wherever s/he is on the skepticism-belief continuum, should be distinguished from those of a judge or a lawyer in a courtroom. There must be room for "knowing" and "not knowing," for intersubjective knowing, and for consensual validation, all as part of an overall plan consistent with restoring lost connections in the patient's psyche.

The therapist's beliefs and expectancies may dovetail destructively with particular patient vulnerabilities. A patient with a pronounced need for closure to problems, or a need to find a single, comprehensive cause or explanation for his/her suffering, may embrace new information or interpretations without testing them. On the other hand, of course, patients determined to avoid emotional exposure may resist new information without testing out its possibilities.

According to contemporary relational theories, change does not come about because of the lifting of repression, nor insight through interpretation of conflicts: change occurs as a consequence of new experience and awareness of interpersonal entanglements (Levenson, 1972); and those—new representations of the self, others, and relationships—emerge as a result of new experiences in the therapy situation (Greenberg, 1986). This form of benevolent influence is rarely alluded to in the polarized discourse about memory and psychotherapy.

Consistent with the relational psychoanalytic conviction that neither patient nor therapist has sole access to reality, each partner influences, deflects, and changes the other. Building on the dynamics of that intersubjective truth, it is a relational ambience that can best moderate the destructive potential that inheres in inappropriate influence—an ambience where a willingness to believe the patient replaces either radical skepticism or unwavering belief; where a welcoming atmosphere of safety and validation makes way for expression of all the patient's protest responses and so-called resistances; and where the therapist is willing to repair disruptions, take responsibility for his/her effects, and simultaneously entertain multiple viewpoints without prematurely foreclosing any potential meaning.

The combined recommendations of most experienced clinicians regarding issues of influence and suggestion consistently lead back to the same focus on the patient as final arbiter of his/her own reality, as final authority on his/her own memories and history, as final determinant of his/her relationship with his/her family of origin (or cult, or perpetrator group), and to the central therapeutic goals of the patient's enhanced sense of agency, autonomy, relatedness, and critical thinking capacity.

BEYOND SURVIVAL

Only to the extent that we expose ourselves over and over to annihilation can that which is indestructible be found in us.

—Pema Chodron, quoting a well-known Buddhist saying

Therapy for trauma, like all depth therapy, involves an interplay of deconstruction and reconstruction; the core psychological structures, organizing principles, and beliefs of both members of the dyad will be challenged. To some extent, new identities must emerge for both or neither partner will feel an enduring sense of completion. As Russell (1998, p. 18) writes, "the difficult treatment forces us to widen our experience, to recognize that there are parts of ourselves, much more than the troublesome parts of our patients, that we do not yet understand."

From this perspective, survival of destruction involves more than just avoiding the inevitable impulse to retaliate or withdraw from the patient. Underlying that survival are the therapist's struggle to stay connected to his/her own feeling-states (and the shifts that take place during the clinical hour), and the therapist's ability to communicate about personal feelings and vulnerabilities to the patient in a way that breaks through the stalemates of dissociative retreat, the endless interlocking chains of double binds, and the persistent identification with the aggressor. It is both troubling and gratifying for a therapist to be so consistently challenged to face his/her own fears, anxieties, and limitations along with previously dissociated states of mind in the service of the therapy. The humility that comes from such courageous encounters with self and other bonds therapist and patient in a sacred process of mutual transformation that powerfully transcends many forms of internalized and institutionalized domination.

> The patient often harbors the fantasy which the therapist sometimes shares, that if the therapist can avoid the repetition, some kind of corrective emotional experience can occur. The thing that is in fact traumatizing is not the repetition, which has to happen in some measure, but the therapist's not being in touch with what he or she feels. The failure to feel on the part of the therapist does in fact recreate a context-specific loss of connectedness. (Russell, 1998, p. 17)

Sometimes fire can be fought only with fire. Sometimes the patient has to know that s/he has pushed the therapist to the absolute limit before something inside can give way. One subtext here is the trauma victim's quest for the *No* response that never came from his/her own lips because of terror and subjugation, nor from the mouth of any family member, nor from the community, nor from the whole society because of one or another level of collusion. Encountering the therapist's self-protective, limit-setting *No* in the context of compassion and empathy can be a central integrative experience.

And so can encountering a passionate other who will not settle for distancing intellectualization. Indeed, witnessing the therapist's struggle with his/her own vulnerabilities and limits can puncture the patient's dissociative armor. The essence of the therapist's struggle to survive is a kind of risk-taking—yielding his/her identity to be challenged and deconstructed—motivated by fierce protection of the treatment relationship and stewardship of its potential space. It is also the survival of the patient and the therapist's inevitable despair[5] and survival of the core assaults on hope, faith, and reality testing that carves a path from mutual survival to shared faith. Ultimately, the therapist survives destruction because something inside the patient—call it generosity, integrity, soul, the awakened capacity for love (or for achieving the depressive position)—interacts with the therapist's courage, compassion, humility, love, dedication . . . to constellate a new holding environment that transcends the isolation of the original trauma and the reenactments it generates.

When the core of a patient's traumatic experience has been an encounter with archetypal human malevolence or evil, only such a powerful communion can help the patient find the courage to remember, work through, and renegotiate this devastating experience. Only such communion of patient and therapist based on numerous experiences of survival and a growing mutual trust and respect can foster a belief in the power of human relationship and of psychotherapy dialogues to metabolize and transform pure destruction into developmental progress, creativity, and wisdom.

When therapist and dissociative patient survive destruction together, the shared experience is so profound that it not only counteracts the dehumanization of the trauma but also engenders something beyond the psychological—in the area we commonly refer to as faith. Eigen, rejecting mere mastery as the goal of therapy, refers to the area of faith as "a way of experiencing that is undertaken with all one's heart, with all one's soul, and with all one's might" (1981, p. 413). At times, Eigen points out, faith requires catastrophe to be met with catastrophe. "Certainty is beyond certain reach," he goes on, but anything less than the attempt to take up the journey "is self-crippling. The undertaking itself involves one in continuous re-creation."

In the cauldron of trauma therapy, catastrophe can be transformed into redemption. Underscoring the inevitability and importance of the therapist's secondary posttraumatic stress, the *Kaballah* tells us that the most powerful faith of all is faith that is lost and refound in the journey through the darkness—*the descent for the sake of the ascent* (Sholem, 1974).

CHAPTER 10

The Descent for the Sake of the Ascent: Revelation, Witnessing, and Reparation

The greatest sorrow is witnessing. . . . The greatest sorrow is to be a veteran, witness to the atrocities of humanity.
—Deng Ming Dao (Taoist Master)

There's a difference between knowing the facts and hearing the details.
—Anonymous torture survivor

There is a cultural gap between the inhabitants of the traumatized and non-traumatized worlds. Those of us relatively unscathed by interpersonal violence and domination often choose not to confront its consequences: it is simply "more orderly . . . to ignore the victim" (Nachmani, 1997, p. 203).

REPARATION AND RECONSTRUCTION

Victims of torture live in a different universe of discourse from the ones in which nonvictims live (Langer, 1996). Borrowing from Langer's attempt to articulate the value of narrative reconstruction with Holocaust survivors, we can probably agree that the developmental movement from victim to survivor entails finding one's voice, creating narrativity and historicity, and being witnessed by another in an empathic relationship—one in which the urgent mandate to tell and bear witness continually runs into the impossibility of telling (Laub, 1995).

Stern's (1997) relational perspective on healing trauma emphasizes the facts that the witness—in this case the therapist—is an active participant-observer in the conarration/identity- restructuring process, and that dissociative experience most often shows up indirectly in the organization of the patient's internal object relations. Hence, the heart of treating a patient whose current difficulties are rooted in dissociation of the past is articulating the shared experience of the therapy relationship as coconstructed via the transference/countertransference. "In the completeness of such narration, what was absent becomes present, what was silent enters speech, what was fragmented becomes linear, enactments, flashbacks, body memories find cure" (Grand, 1997, p. 212).

Van der Kolk and Van der Hart (1995), echoing Pierre Janet's (1889; 1986) clinical wisdom, refer to this process of witnessing and reconstruction as the reliving and integrating of trauma, making meaning by taming the transference experiences. The task is complicated by the severely dissociative patient's inconsistent memories, self-sabotage, alternating identifications, and unwillingness to resign him/herself to the realities of his/her subjection to horrific acts and the subjugation of his/her will and autonomy. In most victims' lives, observational, critical thinking abilities and reflective curiosity are supplanted by chronic self-doubting and incoherent narratives. Effective psychotherapy, then, must create dialogues where the isolation and confusion of the victim and the annihilation of history itself can be subverted by mutual reflection, collaborative reconstruction, and the generation of transformative protest responses.

Revisiting the traumatic experience in the transference links past and present, facilitating mutative process—by drawing from history without the compulsion to repeat it. The relational, cognitive, and witnessing process also inevitably involves disconfirming in the here-and-now of therapy the painful past traumatic interaction (Van der Kolk and Van der Hart, 1995), as per the trauma survivor's ongoing unconscious testing of the therapist.[1] Evidence of the weakening of the power of traumatic memory (with its attendant elaborated fantasies) and the trauma itself to dominate or contaminate current cases empowers the patient to remember and also to imagine alternative scenarios. A renewed capacity for narrative memory rooted in a recovered sense of agency requires that the patient develop a sense of self as separate from others, including the perpetrator(s) (Slavin, 1997)[2]. When the trauma patient is no longer at the mercy of the will of others, of the haunting absence or unwanted intrusions of memory or posttraumatic imperatives, s/he is free to experience a restoration of the dialectic between narrative and historic truth, free to discover him/herself (Frawley-O'Dea, 1997).

REPARATION AND CULTURAL INFLUENCES

A central problem in both clinical and cultural forms of reparation and witnessing of trauma is that prevailing images and definitions have been too narrow: the dominant group defines the discourse and writes the diagnostic manuals. The traumas that lead to the development of severe dissociative disorders are those private, often sexualized, and insidious abuses in which there are inherent gaps in shared reality, shared experiencing, and shared responsibility (Brown, 1995). And the posttraumatic syndromes are based not only on the events themselves but also on the psychosocial atmosphere of the cultural surround, which can variously support or hinder the process of coping with and integrating their effects (Kleber, Figley, and Gersons, 1996). Consequently, traumatic experiences—and what it takes to heal them—need to be conceptualized in terms of the dynamic interactions between the victimized individual and the surrounding society over time (Summerfield, 1996). Unlike adult war veterans and political prisoners who may have had the opportunity for identification with comrades (and for corroboration of the realities of traumatization), survivors of sadistic child abuse and torture have had only their perpetrators to identify with and no sense of community or alternative viewpoints—and certainly, no sense of shared or consensually validated history. In sum, *context* is critical to both interpreting and transcending traumatic events.

Keenan and Caruth (1995, p. 258) identify the "double trauma" whereby cataclysmic events that produce symptoms and calls for testimony are compounded by denial or devaluation and an absence of witnessing and testimony. Laub (1995) observes, "The loss of the capacity to be a witness to oneself . . . is perhaps the true meaning of annihilation, for when one's history is abolished one's identity ceases to exist as well" (p. 67). Indeed, a survivor who does not tell his/her story becomes a victim of distorted memory that contaminates his/her life; s/he begins to doubt the reality of the original events. The ultimate irony is the victim's coming to believe that it was s/he rather then the perpetrator(s) who is responsible for the atrocities s/he suffered. This displacement of responsibility occurs in an extreme form in almost every case of dissociative identity disorder. Concepts of reparation in therapy with child-abuse survivors must attend to both the internal (fantasy) and external (historical) worlds and recognize the effects of the "double trauma." Therapists must strive toward grasping elements of historical truth that persist within the labyrinth of the patient's narration, in spite of the fact that absolute knowing most often remains an impossibility (Grand, 2000). "We must persist in attempts to know historical truth because it is the truth of oppression" (p. 54).

BARRIERS TO REPARATIONS

One can be simultaneously victimized and responsible; neither negates the other. (Flax, 1993, p. 108)

The psychological damage from chronic child abuse does not easily lend itself to accurate recognition or simple reparation. Recognition and disavowal, believing and disbelieving, alternate like a metronome in human life and human history. Individual and/or collective readiness to accommodate or assimilate new, often terrible realities is as much a part of the actual discovery of the true nature of these traumatic realities as is the locating of actual evidence. (Sometimes monuments are built and public declarations or ritual processes conducted to commemorate the social maturation process.) The readiness factor applies as much to an individual's ability to access, believe, and tolerate his/her own traumatic past experience as it does to whole societies' capacities for locating, acknowledging, and expressing compassion toward victims of violent trauma, be it rape, incest, ritual abuse, political torture, or slavery.

The posttraumatic symptoms, the multiple self-states, and the suffering— the rage and pain forbidden explicitly by the perpetrator(s) and tacitly by social indifference and the victim's own sense of unworthiness—are legitimized and respected. That is not the same as "encouraging a culture of victimization" (Loftus, Milo, and Paddock, 1995, p. 307), however, and not the same as relieving individuals from responsibility for their actions and their consequences in the name of *empowerment*—which is not about abdicating responsibility any more than it is about endorsing retribution.

On the contrary, helping patients who are completely dissociated from the intrapsychic, interpersonal, and historical realities of their lives come to understand their experiences of victimization as *part* of the process of identity integration leads them to enhanced senses of agency and mastery. For many survivors of chronic childhood trauma, in fact, self-compassion, self-forgiveness, and even self-pity represent enormous developmental achievements, whose by-products may also include capacities for self-soothing that are not based on reenactments of destructive relationships with caretaker/abusers.

While some therapists are indeed prone to infantilizing their patients or overidentifying with their suffering, critics of trauma/dissociation theory seem inordinately worried that validating victimization will foster irresponsible, infantile, or entitled attitudes and behavior. Horevitz (1994), attempting to take a more moderate position, suggests that making past trauma the central treatment issue leads to inappropriate emphasis on retribution and litigation, and advocates focusing instead on the patient's pathological dissociative processes. But a few litigious patients and a few nationally popularized legal cases cannot and should not be used to define a complex and diverse victimized population. Supporting reclamation of previously disorganized protest responses is quite different from supporting retaliation, as critics like Paddock (1994) and Loftus, Milo, and Paddock (1995) suggest. Psychotherapy is not a search for unequivocal truth or some Holy Grail.

> Psychotherapy is not intended to help patients extract a pound of flesh from those they believed have wronged them, to blame others for past misdeeds, or to help them seek legal damages. Treatment endeavors to help people make sense of the incomprehensible, to relieve suffering, to modify pain of past hurts, to alter unwanted behaviors, and to function at a higher psychological level. (Althof, 1994, p. 249)

Relational theorists like Mitchell (1993) and Bromberg (1993), moving beyond concrete notions of fixed time, blame, and responsibility and favoring appreciation for the dialectical, the permeable, and the paradoxical, are concerned with linking- and meaning-making—returning narrativity and historicity to the patient, and with them ownership of his/her own identity construction, memory, and validation processes. (The clinical reality is that most severely dissociative patients are carrying the guilt and shame of the world in their minds, and their ideas of responsibility have been perverted in their psyches; the worry about creating a mass culture of victims out of a population of extreme self-loathing individuals is yet another reversal of truth, another variation on "blame the victim.")

Most victims of child-abuse trauma want and need a witness (a human heart and mind operating in harmony, that can listen and bear the effects of listening), an apology, someone to *not* look away in disgust, contempt, or incredulity when their story is told, adequate health care, and an opportunity to make sense out of the chaos and confusion of their life experience in order to move beyond being perpetually defined by the cascading effects of traumatization. The persistent portrayal of child-abuse victims as whining, self-pitying, welfare-chiseling sympathy seekers and "borderlines" can only be seen as part and parcel of the social problem of reparations for injustice and oppression that characterizes so much of American history, where perverse stereotyping of the disadvantaged and the disenfranchised, primarily women, African Americans, and Native Americans, "justified" their exploitation by the dominant culture and served to expiate guilt (Cushman, 1994a).

Although many people believe that Nazi Holocaust survivors have been treated with a level of recognition, compassion, and respect uncharacteristic of other oppressed and traumatized groups, this is not the case. When Danieli (1988) conducted open-ended interviews with psychotherapists working with Holocaust survivors, many therapists admitted to deploying a variety of denial, avoidance, and victim-blaming attitudes. For example, some therapists admitted to numbing themselves during sessions when Holocaust stories left them feeling overwhelmed; acknowledged not entirely believing their patients; accused patients of exaggeration; repeatedly forgot details of their patients' narratives and history; became impatient at hearing their patients repeating the same story; lectured and admonished patients for complaining; and insisted that the patients leave the Holocaust behind and talk only about here-and-now issues. Danieli summarized her findings stating that regardless of how compassionate or enlightened therapists believed themselves to be in their theoretical or political attitudes toward human cruelty, many interpreted the urgency of Holocaust survivors' needs to understand what happened as a lingering and unhealthy obsession and not as an entirely natural and appropriate response to their traumatic experiences.

In child-abuse territory, stereotypes sustain the appropriation of victims' psyches and self-respect. Caricatures of the oppressed discourage protest and function as obstacles to the empowerment necessary to break out of conditioned thought patterns and pathological attachments. The myths of false memory currently circulating ironically reinstitute the double binds to which abuse survivors had to accommodate as children (Hegeman, 1997). To the extent that trauma patients are portrayed as entitled, self-serving manipulators or as the compliant dupes of incompetent, exploitive therapists, the quest to expose intrafamilial and organized criminal child victimizers will end up in the same old cultural graveyard.

Throughout the history of psychotherapy, there has been unending debate regarding the reality of the pain and the credibility of the memories of victims of trauma—combat, incest, battery, rape, and childhood abuse. The consequences within the mental health professions of collective doubt include inadequate and inappropriate treatment and, in turn, retraumatization (Herman, 1992; Ross, 1989; Putnam, 1989). Freud's legacy has left us titillated by the unconscious fantasies and alleged sexual and aggressive desires of children—but without corresponding concern about the conscious, predatory sexual impulses of adults toward them. Why have the tastes of a considerable subset of adults for bizarre and brutal sex with children never become an object of study while the alleged perversions of children's imaginations have literally become embedded like granite in our psychological theories?[3] Moreover, since the same dysfunctional culture that permits the victimization of over one-fifth of its children also has the power to construct an understanding (and evaluation) of the abuse and its effects, we should not be surprised by the labeling of abuse victims as secretly desiring abuse (the Oedipal approach), or as manipulative and untrustworthy (the borderline approach), or as unwitting liars (the false memory approach) (Briere, 1996). We thus marginalize and revictimize "those who carry evidence of our own sins: our willingness to permit the wholesale sexual victimization of our children" (p. 50).[4]

How do we conduct psychotherapy with, and how does our society begin to make reparations to, children or adults who have been victimized by multiple perpetrators, tortured, gang raped, drugged, forced to hurt innocent others, and used in pornography and snuff films? Do we delay resolving this nightmare indefinitely because it is so unbearable and unfathomable, or because cognitive memory researchers have questioned the memory and therapy processes? Do we remain bogged down in debates targeting those who remember and those who speak out—survivors and therapists—so that we do not have to take the next step?

Posttraumatic Society

We are living in a traumatized environment, a traumatized culture, a traumatized society. Collective forms of PTSD—apocalyptic anxieties, breakdown of community, escalating polarization and violence, alternating hyperarousal and numbness—intersect with individual PTSD, whose sufferers constantly rename, recode, and otherwise revise their unusual and unvalidatable experience. Unaware of its traumatic roots and unable to make sense of their own intrapsychic assaults or the destructive interpersonal patterns that follow, survivors rely on disguise, distraction, and camouflage—sometimes called confabulation, dissimulation, denial, or hysteria.

The collective analog to the biphasic individual PTSD syndrome—the splits between believing and disbelieving, feeling (or remembering) too much or not at all, for example—probably accounts for the academic/professional, legal, and cultural schisms, where people overwhelmed by or overinvested in attention to violence in the world are locked in debate with people who enact denial, minimization, and numbing. Usually, there is a combination of both reactions in a given individual, with perhaps a predisposition to one of them; in many cases the response to trauma is linked to scope of imagination, such that if a person can't conceive that something so awful could happen, then it can't.

Also militating against recognition of extreme sadistic, sexual, and criminal abuse of children is the built-in organizing principle that people usually get what they deserve.

In preference to struggling with disorganizing information whose assimilation would shatter existing meaning structures, those professionals polarized into the disbelief camp adopt the anaesthesia of victim-bashing, therapist-bashing, and false memory propaganda. There is little middle ground left, since neutrality may be more of a fantasy posture than anything else. In Flax's (1993, p. 12) words: "Everyone might be better off if we acknowledge we are all operating on the terrain of power and not truth or objectivity." Our theoretical/ideological positions derive from a whole web of factors, ranging from idiosyncratic psychological desires, personal temperament, family dramas, and larger group loyalties and identities, to the contingencies of historical events and locations and the set of language games available at the time. One of the most important lessons for psychology from feminism and postmodernism, as Flax emphasizes, is that clinical treatment cannot be politically or socially neutral.

Whenever therapy liberates or recognizes the voice of the socially oppressed, or legitimates a marginalized discourse (Price, 1995), the institution of psychotherapy is bound to be targeted for a backlash by other forces with a vested interest in the cultural status quo. After doing almost nothing for the past century to expose the predatory nature of pedophiles and other perpetrators of sexual abuse, the psychotherapy world has spawned some left-turning wings—triggering the coalescence of opposing forces like warriors on a battlefront protecting the status quo, chiefly in the name of "the family," through intimidation, scary projection and propagandizing, and creative, new forms of denial, all fueled by partial truths that promise an alternative to participating in suffering, bearing witness, and reparation.

In the North American trauma drama, the legal system has now begun to take a large role. Alleged survivors are suing alleged perpetrators; alleged perpetrators are suing the alleged survivors' therapists; recanting ex-patients are suing former therapists with the help of family with whom they've recently reconciled; factions are lobbying for legislation of clinical work with patients whose memories affect their perspectives on their families.

> You can be sued for failing to diagnose what is wrong with the patient, and you can be sued for diagnosing something the patient doesn't *want* to have. You can be sued for failing to warn somebody about your dangerous patient. You can be sued if your patient decides to attempt suicide but survives, and you can be sued by the patient's estate if the suicide is a success. You can be sued just because the patient doesn't feel like paying your bill. In fact, in many states you can be sued even if there is no evidence of wrongdoing just "because" the patient is angry at you and the patient's attorney expects a settlement offer from your malpractice insurance company. (Barach, 1999d, p. 1)

When the legitimacy of traumatic memory, diagnosis (MPD/DID), and a given treatment are questioned, "The authority of the therapist is in danger of being supplanted by the authority of the lawyer" (Hegeman, 1997, p. 155). And when the scourge of child abuse receives the media attention that has been showered on the False Memory Syndrome Foundation/Movement with a passion and a zeal unlike anything the profession has ever seen, recovery from the epidemic will be well on its way. For the present, the fact that journalists . . . should so unquestioningly peddle inflammatory . . . attacks on incest survivors is very disturbing. News reports echoing the Foundation's propaganda frequently mention aliens, witches, fairy tales, UFO's in the same breath as the agonizing memories of people who were raped in childhood. (Landsberg, 1996, p. 1)

Reparation and restitution are always stormy processes. Even in unambiguously traumatic accident/disaster situations, victims are quite quickly admonished to get over it or put it behind them (Gelinas, 1995), or to forgive the perpetrator(s). When that impatience is compounded by disbelief, restitution is that much less likely. And, as Gelinas points out, those who are the most seriously abused are the ones who are most apt to be disbelieved: they tell the most terrible stories, and they are the most symptomatic and the most dismissable. While overt contempt for victims and their supporters is ego-dystonic with the American national character, there does appear to be what Summit (1989) calls an "entrenched, religious ignoring" (p. 418). Herman (1992) cites a cultural form of dissociation on the part of a society that finds acknowledgment of the realities of child abuse too great a challenge to its belief in a just world. Society's dissociative silence cannot help but compound the victims' torment and experience of betrayal.

THE TRAUMATIZED SELF: VICTIM/PERPETRATOR PARADOX

All traumatized individuals must somehow integrate the internal splits that reflect their identifications with victim, colluder, and perpetrator psychologies, whether by maintaining lifestyles of reenactment and/or addiction, becoming disabled, becoming perpetrators themselves or other kinds of criminals, achieving worldly and professional success that excludes an inner or intimate life, managing the destructive effects of trauma creatively on their own, or undertaking psychotherapy to put the pieces back together.

Default Mechanisms of Survival to Chronic Traumatization

According to Briere (1996), because s/he is chronically deprived of any real sense of control or self-determination, the victimized child can sustain illusions of safety only by extreme denial, "other-directedness" (relying on the reactions of people outside him/herself as a basis for self-esteem, reality testing, and safety), strange, paradoxical alternations between hypervigilance to danger and complete unawareness of danger, conditional reality (i.e., reality viewed as a relative abstraction, "a construct that can be molded or altered according to external contingencies" [p. 58]), avoidance, and extreme forms of self-loathing and "negative specialness" (e.g., a magical sense of power deriving from the ability to do bad).

To make a lifestyle out of denying the reality of a traumatic childhood is to make full use of such defensive tactics as identifying with the aggressor (projecting the victimized self on to others); glorifying authority ("cleansing" the abusive parents); thinking rigidly (creating artificial boundaries of safety and containment); avoiding introspection (flattening the psyche); or cynically distrusting all others (controlling and distancing the projected bad object)—Godwin (1996). Making a personal and/or professional lifestyle out of radical denial, for example, a victim may identify with "toughing-it-out" approaches, denying personal vulnerability and choosing relationship and vocational contexts that mirror these choices. S/he may make a lifestyle out of "identification with the aggressor," and seek safety by joining various authoritarian groups, movements, and religions, or the military. Godwin (1996) sees this pattern of victim denial as a breeding ground for conservative and reactionary political values and positions. Terrorists from the political right and the left may originate from such self-organization and traumatic experience.

Alternatively or concurrently, the victim can organize perpetration against him/herself within an internal dissociative system that contains subjectively compelling representations of victims, perpetrators, and collaborators. S/he can transpose all hurt into self-hatred, self-defeat, self-sabotage, and worthlessness. S/he can develop a condition of extreme vulnerability to reenactment through repeated enmeshments with abusive or sociopathic individuals. This deficiency of will in the service of the self is sometimes juxtaposed, as Howell describes, by an active gratification of and devotional service to others. Having dissociated the unbearable pain to which s/he was exposed as a helpless victim, the survivor in masochistic mode is deprived of the pain cues and the signals and sources of aggression vital for self-protection and self-defense (Howell, 1996). In the extremes of "other-directedness" described by Briere (1996), victims of chronic childhood abuse demonstrate boundary problems, isolation and neediness in the absence of internal support, hypersensitivity and extreme emotional reactivity to others, and suggestibility or malleability when faced with expectations and demands of peers or authority figures, and an impoverished sense of entitlement that can lead to the extremes of subservience and arrogance.

A victimized individual can also become what Whitfield (1995, p. 118) calls a "co-abuser," variously colluding or collaborating with traumatizers in what may be among the most common adaptations to childhood trauma. Women abused as children may fail to protect their own children from abuse, perhaps by directly offering them up, perhaps by looking the other way; then they deny their roles in the arrangements. Such women are identifying with, or at least covering for, the abusers (their spouses, say), just as they did in the cases of their own abusing parent(s).

In other adaptations, survivors frustrate, tyrannize, and terrorize their therapists as well as significant others in their lives. Professionals must endure the stress of witnessing, containing, and finding meaning in extreme masochistic enactments (by their very nature sadistic vis-à-vis the helper). Victims can present as people without histories compliant with authority, as workaholic, as robotic-normotics, as drones, and can remain (willfully) confused about their backgrounds, identities, and circumstantial risks. They can become unable or unwilling to know their own minds, think their own thoughts, and speak with their own voices. They can echo internalized perpetrator messages, accepting them as the "real me." To maintain family ties and/or sustain their internalized domination-oriented object relations, they can trade in all possibilities of benevolent intimacy. To bind the processes of dissociation and disavowal, they can become addicted to anything, from sex, drugs, food, and work to extreme dogmatic, double-binding religions, extremist, righteous politics, skepticism, obsessive coveting or collecting, prostituting, and enslaving relationships. Victims can become expert in all forms of collusion and complicity in exploiting themselves or others. Taken together, these adaptations to extreme and chronic traumatization and neglect create extreme attachments to perpetrators and profound confusion over core issues of identity, responsibility, worth, and personal potential.

Complex attachments to perpetrators are some of the most insidious side effects of chronic child-abuse trauma and some of the most difficult to resolve (see Chapter 7). Van der Kolk's (1987b) review of studies of traumatic bonding reveals that children, like animals, cling more persistently when their caretakers are abusive. Fraiberg's (1982) work shows that infants exposed to unpredictable eruptions from caretakers and prolonged experiences of helplessness were able to obliterate pain from consciousness and participate in sadomasochistic play with their parents. Freyd (1994; 1996) and Ross (1997) emphasize the centrality of attachment to the perpetrator as an issue in the treatment of victims of (particularly intrafamilial) violence. Indeed, according to Salter (1995), there are usually three people in the therapist's office—the patient, the therapist, and the perpetrator. "Underneath the gentle tones of therapy, there is always a fight going on" (p. 281). The conflict has to do with the patient's struggle between sustaining bonds with perpetrators and entering into other, more mutuality-based relationships, including the one with the therapist.

One of the most prevalent clinician errors is to assume that trauma survivors can be cured with kindness alone (Blizard and Bluhn, 1994). When the victim's primary attachment has involved traumatic bonding with a perpetrator, all moves are suspect and subject to interpretation as approaches toward abuse. Specifically, benevolence on the part of the therapist can so threaten the patient with the loss of the abusive internal representation (around which the self has become organized and identified) as to precipitate severe abandonment depression, flight-fight responses, and suicidal acting out.

In chronically traumatic relationships, abused children learn both victim and perpetrator roles and re-create the whole traumatic attachment dynamic in other circumstances (Sroufe and Fleeson, 1986). They do not actually have different working models for the roles of terrorized victim and gleeful sadist, however; they have only one model, of which the apparently polarized positions are flip sides, compelling them to identify with and enact abuser and victim roles simultaneously (Prior, 1996). Identifying four primary patterns through which the abused child constantly rotates—seesawing between victim and victimizer roles, identifying with the perpetrator, tormenting him/herself with blame and guilt, and seeking object contact through perverse or violent means—Prior (1996) captures the dilemmas that organize his/her psyche and future relationships.

> It is intolerable to live life as a victim: one is weak and powerless. But it is equally intolerable to live life as a perpetrator, for then one deserves all manner of punishment. It is intolerable to be completely alone and unconnected. But it is equally intolerable to seek relationship through perversion or violence. It is intolerable to be a passive and helpless victim. But it is painful to escape from this helplessness by believing that you caused and deserved abuse. The escape from passivity is achieved by feeling inescapably bad. (p. 75)

Clearly, there are infinite variations on maintaining the effects of trauma, passing it on, and organizing around identification with power, perpetration, and righteous disregard for the vulnerability of others. Most abused individuals do not go on to abuse others (but many go on to co-abuse). Severely traumatized individuals have to find some way to balance the victim-perpetrator dialectic within their own psyches.

FUSION AND CONFUSION OF
VICTIM-PERPETRATOR-COLLABORATOR POSITIONS

Perhaps the most insidious complex of victim-perpetrator dynamics occurs when the child is coerced into complicity. Encountered in almost every case of ritual abuse, pseudoreligious cult abuse, and organized crime, forced perpetration subverts the will of the child for the group's malignant ends, yet it is almost always experienced as "choice." When a dissociative individual (often through a child-alter) remembers hurting or having to have sex with other children, or luring or kidnapping them to be victimized and sometimes killed, or defecating on a Bible and "spitting in the face of God," or torturing and dismembering animals, s/he is guiltily locked even as an adult into his/her "voluntary" participation as a traumatized, entranced child with no other way to understand its cunning orchestration by the perpetrators. The manipulation of the psychic wounds of the child to solidify his/her identification with evil, generated dissociative splits organized around a perception of self as omnipotently dangerous and entombed him/her in secrecy, silence, and devastating shame.

Needless to say, forced complicity and the resulting amalgam of victim-perpetrator roles are among the more difficult aspects of severe trauma and dissociation to treat clinically. The real perpetrators and their intentions, directions, and coercion will be buried in some dissociated state beyond the possible reach of any reflectivity or critical thinking. Van der Kolk (1995; 1996) stresses that traumatic memories barred from consciousness and hence unavailable for the kinds of cognitive operations that create change over time are impervious to language and perceived experience. The corrupted sense of agency associated with forced perpetration will crystallize convictions about the self as unredeemable and unsalvageable, *making prideful identifications with malevolence a seductive alternative identity to unmitigated helplessness and exploitation.* Some dissociative patients' unyielding attachments to and identification with such unredeemability can either slow an integration process down for an extended period, or, worse, stand permanently in the way of complete healing in an otherwise successful treatment.

Confounding the clinical picture with many severely abused dissociative patients is the fact that they often possess many persecutor and perpetrator alter personalities—some of whom believe that they chose to commit acts of violence and some of whom claim to really enjoy hurting others. Some patients have committed actions against innocents over whom they had authority during childhood even outside of the primary abusive context. A few have committed abusive or murderous acts in the context of child care during their teenage years or in adulthood. A few have harmed their own children (or the children of friends or relatives) in mild or severe ways. Others have committed acts of violence only when involved as children with perpetrator groups but live in the dissociative world as if these events are still taking place in present time. Some are easily connected to guilt and shame; others, through complex dissociative processes largely shaped by the perpetrating group, are adept at keeping guilt and shame split into more distant part-selves while many of the rest highly and proudly identify with evil. Some internal persecutor alter personalities become perpetrators because they were trained to, and some commit acts of violence or sexual abuse whenever stimulated by specific triggers (e.g., a naked small child) and have little impulse control in the areas of sexuality and aggression.

Perpetrator-identified self-states and alters are probably more common in severely dissociative patients than has previously been appreciated and therapists are likely to encounter the most intractable forms of avoidance, distraction, and counterattack when trying to get near them—and likely to provoke a systemic uproar if they succeed.[5] The challenge is to find ways to empathize with and confront them, or at least move them to think critically and feel pain by linking them with other parts of the patient's system; the problem is that the sadistic parts are desperate to keep themselves and their massively dissociated vulnerability, dependency, and shame isolated from the rest.

Of course, like all other parts of the personality system, these self-states are part of an elaborate protective system. They deflect the locus of blame from the perpetrators onto the victim—some of whose host-personalities even believe that these parts *are* the real perpetrators—and perpetrator-alters may even be "best friends" of the actual perpetrator(s), in which role they provide excellent camouflage from legal and criminal investigation. They free functional alters from exposure to sadistic, rageful, and brutal feel-

ings and fantasies, defend against the enormous shame associated with coerced complicity, perpetration, and the inability to protect the self from psychic breakdown and takeover, and they keep the core vulnerability safely
hidden. Not all perpetrator-identified parts are equally responsive to treatment; indeed, where the internal splits are enormous, treatment is sabotaged
at every opportunity as the dynamics of evil and betrayal are relentlessly
reenacted, especially when the patient is revealing forbidden secrets or beginning to make a significant developmental leap by reclaiming aggression
or forging a deeper bond with a therapist.

There is a small minority of highly dissociative patients whose omnipotent perpetrator-alters/self-states refuse direct involvement in treatment or
cannot resist continuously sadistically undermining the therapy relationship, even given optimally balanced empathy, inquiry, interpretation, and
confrontation of abusive ideologies on the part of the clinician. Whether or
not the patients are still somehow involved with their abusive groups or
families, these part-selves cannot disengage for long enough to work
through any issue or conflict from the compulsion to wreak havoc with the
therapy and the addictive pleasure of making the therapist writhe helplessly. Direct dialogue is limited to those times when they are caught red-
handed in the enactment, which incidents they perversely enjoy. (Thus
pressed, one perpetrator-alter in a male DID patient whose outer presentation was quite gentle, affable, and compliant described his fantasies of inflicting harm on me and watching me suffer while I become confused as to
the location, origin, and reality of the experience; actually able to articulate
his recurrent need to be the cause of others' suffering without their being
able to identify him as such, this alter had absolutely no capacity to reflect
on the origins of that need—nor, of course, did the host personality.) The key
in some cases is to work around such alters to strengthen the rest of the personality system so that their internal and interpersonal power is disrupted
and then depleted from within. Helping patients differentiate *being* evil from
imitating evil in order to survive encounters with evil is a labor-intensive
process.

THE OBFUSCATION OF THE VICTIM AND
PERPETRATOR POSITIONS

If the victimization of children is the number one blind spot, number two is
what sexual offenders get away with (Salter, 1995)—the compulsive, repeti-

titive, chilling invisibility of their acts. The average person (who is the average juror) does not know enough about sexual assault to avoid being conned—and clinicians treating survivors need to be well-versed in the dynamics of offender psychology, not least because the internalizations of perpetrator consciousness can be the most intractable obstacles encountered in therapy.

> Sexual abuse is not an accident. It does not "just happen." It is not typically an impulsive act. It is a series of interlinking thoughts, feelings, and behaviors that are highly compulsive. It will not go away on its own. It is not easy to change, and it can never be cured, only controlled. (Salter, 1995, p. 103)

There is in fact a "syntactical process, grammatical structure, and violent semantic failure by which a person is rendered a thing" (Nachmani, 1997, p. 204). The relational processes that facilitate multiple and ongoing traumatic events involve systematic planning as well exploitation of power dynamics vis-à-vis the victims and propaganda-like effects on victims and bystanders alike.

It is not only perpetrators who go to extremes. Self-hating victims further empower them by losing sight of their own external oppression, identifying with their abusers consciously or not, and splitting off their inevitable aggression and their self-valuation; the result is the collapse of their protest and escape responses into collusive patterns, which enable the abusing system to perpetuate itself. Thus, the victim/perpetrator dichotomy is simplistic and false—yet many clinicians

> have fallen for the sentimental fallacy that dissociative adults are basically wounded children needing only parenting-like love and soothing to heal. . . . Although there are certainly aspects of these patients that experience themselves as childlike victims, our *adult* patients are *adults*. They can do everything that other adults can, including severe harm to others. (Barach, 1999b, p. 1)

Highly dissociative people can and do harm others. Many patients who have been involved in ritual and organized child abuse have reported committing murders (Barach, 1999b), and kidnapping, torturing, and training other children to become prostitutes and perpetrators. Some survivors continue to struggle with sexual attraction toward children and may talk about having molested children at some points in their lives; some may still struggle with urges to abuse their own children or children in their care. Because dissociative, traumatized patients are prone to reenact traumatic relational paradigms, emotional assaults on the therapist's sense of hope, faith, goodwill, and core emotional vulnerabilities can be anticipated during therapy. Treating these patients' perpetrative tendencies may force clinicians to "confront moral repugnance that goes well beyond the realm of countertransference" (Barach, 1999b, p. 1).

There is also the reality that some dissociative patients have also perpetrated against their current or former therapists—knowingly and intentionally spread rumors about them on the Internet and elsewhere, filed complaints with licensing boards or initiated civil or criminal suits fabricating claims of sexual molestation (or other violations) by the therapist and that misrepresent their own histories and treatment experiences. A small number of dissociative patients have threatened therapists' persons, therapists' property, and therapists' families. And this far-from-exhaustive list does mention damage from the severely disturbed families or criminal/perpetrator groups by which some dissociative patients remain controlled.

On the other hand, some dissociative trauma survivors hold in their psyches and spirits an extreme level of pain, terror, and knowledge of human evil, unburdening the rest of us from witnessing atrocity, often going to their graves at an early age, and often dying without recognition, treatment, valuation, or respect.

The victim-perpetrator dialectic is complex, involving reality, fantasy, projection, dissociation, and incomprehensible inconsistencies. No perpetrator is without his/her weakness and pain. No victim is without his/her cruel, sadistic, and aggressive side. No perpetrator commits acts of harm and atrocity twenty-four hours a day (viz., the Nazi war criminals who demonstrated adoration, concern, and generosity toward their own family members [Lifton, 1986]). Some perpetrators are dissociatively disordered and enact abuse on their victims for which they are completely amnestic the rest of the time; others commit their offenses while intoxicated and their memories for the events are clouded and vague.

Evil is mixed into the stuff of ordinary living, defying expectations, which is one reason it can be so elusive. One man, nothing short of a serial child rapist, murderer, and trafficker in child pornography and snuff films, tended a garden, raised pigeons, and occasionally went to church. The perpetrator who suffocates or drowns a child for his/her own sadistic gratification is the same one who "rescues" the child (albeit for his/her own aggrandizement, as a prelude to programming based on traumatic bonding, and of course also to keep the victim alive for future abuse) and to whom the child then clings for dear life. Sometimes the person who abuses a child is the one who protects him/her from the rest of the family. Or the day father may be entirely different from the night father.

BEN

Ben's father took him on a camping trip for his tenth birthday. Before and after the rape that came late at night (upon the father's usual signal, which by that point was a conditioned stimulus for a dissociative switch in the child-victim), the camping trip was like any ordinary father-son event—dinner followed by card games, then each to his own separate tent. There was a strange and strained silence right before and for some time after the rape, but when breakfast was served the next morning, it was back to the birthday camping trip complete with laughter, good cheer, and no sign that anything unusual had taken place during the night. Such juxtapositions, unimaginable to most people, were normal.

Psychotherapy with criminal perpetrators and pedophiles often involves accessing the hidden, split-off victimized child self. Psychotherapy with victims often involves accessing the hidden, split-off sadistic self. But to describe the victim-perpetrator paradox is not to define them as moral equivalents. In fact, although sadistic-trauma survivors can bring incredible pain and suffering to those who get close to them, their dynamics are not predominantly predatory. Rather, most of their enactments, outbursts, manipulations, and chicanery are best understood as desperate efforts either to attain safety and relief from pain (Salter, 1995) or to communicate in the only way they can about the abuses of power in their families of origin or the social systems that allowed them. Sometimes their relentless self-defeating and self-destructive behaviors are the results of deeply implanted or unconsciously internalized messages or injunctions from the perpetrators that have not yet been recognized and deconstructed.

Once a victim has become a perpetrator as an adult, however, and entered the often addictive cycle of regulating affect through acts of physical and sexual abuse, a shift takes place in his/her consciousness such that pain, vulnerability, and access to the original traumas are vehemently sequestered. The lifestyle of perpetration, with its layers of deceit, distortion, and manipulation, makes most of its adherents inaccessible to treatment. Solzhenitsyn (1974) invokes a psychic threshold of evil doing, and holds that some people can cross a boundary of identification with fellow humans that admits no possibility of return. Unfortunately, some survivors of sadistic and ritual abuse who were forced to perpetrate violence upon others believe they have crossed this boundary and have been repeatedly told as much by their perpetrators—but in fact they have not: their own intentions were completely supplanted by the will and agenda of the perpetrators.

Most patient-survivors in the beginning of their recovery have little connection to identities of self-as-victim or self-as-perpetrator. Often a mixture of confusion and vague self-loathing masks the complex web of victim, perpetrator, and collaborator self-states. Davies and Frawley (1994) suggest that for a traumatized patient to become fully healed, and especially for him/her to claim and internalize an appropriate sense of empowerment, s/he may need to try on the mantle of the abuser as well as the victim.[6] S/he will have to recognize and relinquish his/her own patterns of dissociation and rigid identification with both victim and perpetrator elements of the psyche (which entails self-forgiveness); s/he will have to reenact both parts, witness his/her systematic denial of both parts, and eventually integrate victim and perpetrator identification to bring the polarities into a new and different, conscious relationship. Most difficult of all to locate and work through are the levels of collaborationist/complicitous self-states modeled after negligent and collusive parental, political, religious, and social systems. These part-selves may be even more intractable than persecutory alters.

Transcending Victim, Perpetrator, and Collaborator Identifications

A final option for the victimized individual is to confront the emotional devastation hidden behind the mask of calcified normality. This choice will inevitably involve facing internalized and interpersonally enacted elements of many or all of the destructive patterns of relatedness just outlined. Eventually, the decision to seek healing will involve relinquishing the comforts provided by the elaborate systems of dissociative defense, pretense, and the omnipotent solutions of childhood: idealization and mystification of irrational authority and of violence will be replaced by a capacity for vulnerability and a tolerance for helplessness; domination and submission shift into the background while mutuality, equality, and reciprocity become increasingly prominent features of intrapsychic and interpersonal life.

The liberation and development of a trusted internal authority can challenge and then supplant submission to the internal persecutors and perpetrators that have been governing the self. Ownership of that self and its life experience is permanently registered and openly expressed. Internalized messages from the perpetrator(s) are recognized, deconstructed, disidentified with, and assertively mastered. Betrayal of self and other, as a way of life, is worked through as the confusion between loyalty and betrayal is examined. Subjugated proclivities for aggression and protest are realigned into productive achievement and empowering interpersonal communication. Capacities to feel pain, sorrow, grief, and despair, all lost in the compulsive use of dissociation, are redeveloped, and so is the aptitude for symbolizing, creating, and maneuvering intrapsychic representations and fantasies. Real empathy for the self (and all of its parts) and for others is nurtured. Most of all, conflict, emotion, and self-reflection are tolerated, even enjoyed, and no longer systematically avoided.

Survivors of tortured childhoods must integrate and deconstruct the particularly insidious forms of shame and guilt that have lodged in the spaces among their part-selves. Victims of encounters with human evil often bear the burden of that evil as though they had committed evil themselves, believing that they "allowed" it to happen to them. As patients, they must work through the self-protective omnipotent illusions ranging from "not-me" (*It didn't really happen; I wasn't there, she was*) to "all-me" formulations (*I made it happen, I liked it, I'm one of them*). The true desolation of the chronic trauma survivor is the reality that s/he was betrayed and violated by those whom s/he most trusted and needed, and was powerless to do anything other than capitulate and at some level join the perpetrator; will and sense of agency were completely undermined and assaulted. The victim's coerced moral transgressions represent "the marriage between ethical collapse and primitive desire; they precipitate guilt and reparative hunger. And they compel the survivor to want death for wanting life" (Grand, 2000, p. 93).

For many survivors of chronic childhood trauma, the grueling task of recovery is overwhelming. Relinquishing all forms of self-deception, omnipotence, and dissociation is more difficult than climbing the highest mountain with inadequate gear. Separating from entrenched attachments to perpetrators can leave the victim with a disorganized sense of self to which almost anything seems preferable. Thus, some may only get part of the way toward wholeness and healing. Some jump off the path when what has to be faced—or relinquished—seems too much to bear; some get pushed off by traumatic therapies or abusive relationships. Some choose a life of workaholism, numbing, and psychic deadness. Some rejoin abusive families or criminal cults. A small number commit suicide. A few become permanently physically disabled from the cumulative effects of childhood trauma. Some become chronic mental patients bouncing in and out of hospitals, day treatment programs, and brief interludes of work, and live on disability for the bulk of their lives. Many reach a compromise between the demands of full recovery and the limitations of their psychological capacities and other resources. Amazingly, some traumatized individuals do fully recover—but not without many scars. Some have such enormous wherewithal in spite of massive traumatization that they show their therapists the extremes of shadow and light—catastrophe and faith—in human life.

PSYCHOTHERAPY IN THE WAKE OF TRAUMA

People organize their lives to avoid the imagined catastrophe of certain conversations; and they come to analysis, however fluent they may be, because they are unable to speak. But some people, of course, have had unspeakable experiences, or experiences that have been made unspeakable by the absence of a listener. (Phillips, 1994, p. 84)

Trauma continues to build until its cascading after-effects are restrained and diffused by a more powerful (and benevolent) obstacle. Psychotherapy must become that obstacle. Nachmani (1995) says that what makes an event traumatic is the failure or the absence of a compassionate disruption. Moreover, he says, "Actions that traumatize are not restrained or inhibited or considerate. They are inflicted because a compassionate morality is absent, or because a cunning, perverse morality is cultivated" (p. 427).

A therapeutic relationship of reciprocal influence and emotional attunement, where coconstructed meanings and multiple narratives (and the feelings and fantasies they generate) can evolve over time without the limitation of dogma, theory, or incredulity is one possible transformative disruption. In this relational view of psychotherapy, an asymmetrical relationship continues to exist where hierarchy is not collapsed altogether; it reflects commitment to mutual exploration of therapist's and patient's participation and assumptions, including their use/misuse of power (Shapiro, 1997). When a trauma survivor's experience of authority has been deformed by exposure to torture (as is most often the case in DID), treatment must address the authority dynamic within the treatment relationship (Eckhardt, 1987; Brown, 1994) in an ongoing way.

What actually constitutes trauma is highly personal and contingent on preexisting mental schemata, cultural norms, personal history, and age at the time of the events (Van der Kolk, Van der Hart, and Marmer, 1996), yet almost all theorists across diverse schools of thought now emphasize that it is the *meaning* attributed to the event rather than the event itself that actually determines the intensity of the emotional reaction and eventually accounts for the resulting psychopathology. In patients with complex dissociative disorders, it is often those meanings—increasingly disturbing, unassimilable, and often intolerable—of events and relationship dynamics that fuel and trigger dissociative defenses. It appears to be easier for the severely dissociative patient to reexperience the somatic and sensory aspects of a physical or sexual violation than to confront the intentionality, planning, betrayal, and systemic collusion of the adults in the abuse scenarios. The realization and remembering of malevolent relational dynamics, the reassociation of meaning and context, can only take place after prolonged immersion in a nondominating, noncomplicitous therapy relationship.

Interpersonal trauma takes place in relationship, and it is spread through the medium of relationship. Its reality is denied and disavowed in relationship, so the sequelae of trauma must be met and contained, the contagion disrupted and healed, in an alternative model of relationship. Psychoanalytically informed, relationally focused psychotherapy gives rise to a relationship that recognizes, wrestles with, and survives the intrinsic traumatic feelings and the penetrating reenactments of exploitative and malevolent dynamics often played out by adult survivors of severe and chronic child abuse. Child-abuse trauma, like so many violent events, dehumanizes the individual; psychotherapy, when it works, humanizes the individual and reorients him/her at least to the world of mutual, reciprocal, and benevolent relationships.

The psychotherapy relationship is key to developing a facilitative level of awareness that can both access and penetrate dissociative states and the fears, beliefs, and identifications that hold them together. A relationally oriented therapy consists of an incisive intersubjective discourse and a refined mutuality. Such mutuality evolves out of an interplay of symmetry and asymmetry and the field of intersection between two different subjectivities

(Benjamin, 1995; Aron, 1996). In fact it is the patient's continual surprise and wonder at the therapist's failure to (completely) confirm traumatic expectancies and relational paradigms of domination, betrayal, sacrifice, and subjugation that so powerfully disarms compulsively deployed dissociative defenses. This encounter leads to recognition and working through of the entrenched, internalized after-effects of interpersonal trauma—especially distorted belief systems—that are often buried beneath, and camouflaged by dissociative structures and symptomatology. The therapist's noncompliance with the patient's traumatic expectations has this affirmative impact only where mistrust is overcome and safety guaranteed (Nachmani, 1997). The patient's expectations will not be disconfirmed without the therapist's reliability being assailed at every turn, without the therapist's making a few errors along the way, and without the therapist's encountering his/her own sadism, despair, futility, and rage.

Within a relational therapy process, interpretations and interventions must be grounded in the experiential interactive field occurring between therapist and patient, rather than exclusively oriented toward the inner life of the patient, as in classical psychoanalysis. In the treatment of DID, interpretations must move back and forth between descriptions of the patient's internal world and the interpersonal dynamics produced by the collision between the worlds of patient and therapist. Severely dissociative patients often use distraction (sometimes diversions toward the interpersonal) to deflect attention from their inner worlds and traumatic pasts; likewise, they sometimes focus on their internal worlds (or crises) and their pasts to deflect interpersonal tensions arising in the treatment. Relational and emotional collisions, traumatic reenactments, confusion over who did what to whom, and painful alterations in worldviews are some of the inevitabilities inherent in the treatment process for therapist and patient alike.

TRAUMA, PSYCHOTHERAPY, AND REPARATION

Whenever chronic brutalization and betrayal have been part of an individual's early life, psychic dismemberment will find its way into the therapy relationship. And, even if most of it originates in the patient, the therapist's own lived experiences plus his/her defenses against primitive anxieties never concretized in lived experience will be stirred. Hence, the psychotherapy relationship with severely traumatized patients necessarily involves the traumatization of the therapist and, to some degree, the retraumatization of the patient. According to contemporary psychoanalytic paradigms, therapists necessarily enter the relational worlds of their patients, and they get to know the essence of their patients by what is lived out between them (Hirsch, 1994). From the relational perspective, these working-through processes involving the therapist as participant-observer create a new object relationship for the patient, one that substantially changes what the patient comes to expect from significant others (Davies, 1997). However, as Davies states, for the therapist, living within the patient's internal object world is no easy task for those internal objects of the patient's will invariably collide with the therapist's own internal objects and self-representations. "We must expect, in the course of treating adult survivors, to experience the most ravaging self-doubts, to be subjected via projective forces of transference-countertransference reenactment to the same forms of coercive mind control that once seized control of the patient's reality" (p. 69).

When an individual who bears the burden of psychological trauma (especially chronic childhood sexual and physical abuse) and a psychotherapist willing to recognize the damage and participate in the healing come together, they will inevitably collide, destabilize each other's worlds, and be forever changed by the encounter. Traumatized patients may alternatingly or simultaneously experience themselves as destructive, dangerous, or punitive agents of control in all their relationships, as the denying Other(s) who minimize their own suffering and pain, and/or as passive victims of the therapist's and others' betrayals; they may perceive the therapist as helpless, naïve, uncaring, vulnerable, seductive, and/or malevolent (Neumann and Gamble, 1995). Apprehending the therapist's innocence—or their own—is among the encounters most vehemently resisted by dissociative survivors of sadistic abuse and coerced perpetration: in its presence, their core structures of identification with perpetration, malevolence, or evil collapse, evoking enormous vulnerability. Invariably, the patient also regards the therapist as savior and redeemer.

As for the therapist: clinical work with survivors of chronic child abuse inevitably challenges his/her helper identities (Neumann and Gamble, 1995); s/he feels as though s/he has "been thrown into a maelstrom with no lifeline" (p. 342). Clinical experience shows that dissociative survivors will do almost anything to avoid reexperiencing their own pain, grief, and suffering. They will also resist all efforts to support their relinquishing attachment and intrapsychic bonds with their childhood caretakers/perpetrators, as annihilation-panic (often articulated directly as fear of falling apart) surfaces with the destabilizing of their elaborately constructed identities and the dreaded rupture of their dissociative barriers. Treating trauma often demands that therapists tolerate prolonged periods of helplessness, inadequacy, attack, shame, and abandonment.

Of course, much in the way of therapeutic intervention consists precisely of efforts to carve a path for affective expression of extraordinarily painful, traumatic feelings, and for the questioning of identifications with significant others of childhood. This makes therapy a dangerous enterprise for the patient, who at once reaches for it with primal, elemental longings, and compulsively seeks to circumvent and sabotage it. When his/her own disavowed and forgotten voices are discovered, the severely dissociative patient often simultaneously loves and resents the therapist—for the recognition and for the persistence and respect that follows it. Then, however, the patient may unravel as warring intrapsychic factions identify the therapist as most hated, most feared, and most revered and desired object. The ensuing transferential enactments reflect the traumatized patient's embedded expectations that power in the therapy relationship will be misused by the authority/parental figure. "This dynamic leads to a replaying in all forms, in the analytic arena suspended in time and space, of some of the nastiest behaviors of the species" (Hegeman, 1995). But if the therapist's becoming swept up into relational reenactments is "the source of the greatest turmoil in therapy, [it is also] the best single pathway to growth—finding and directly engaging the patient's dissociated voices as discontinuous but individually authentic . . . expression of selfhood" (Bromberg, 1995a, p. 521).

In these moments, the real conflicts and multiplicity of the patient crash into the conflicts and multiplicity of the therapist. That is, there are inevitable conflicts between their multiple identities and multiple needs that cannot be reduced to the "phantasms projected into the therapist" (Slavin, 1996) by the patient. The renegotiation and reintegration of identity and conflict on the patient's part can only take place when the patient taps into the therapist's conflicts and identity struggles in a way that takes us

someplace that is obviously hard for us to go. We go there and we often change in the process, because to some degree, having a relationship with this patient requires it. Our patients are, all the time, provoking in us (and reading) the quality of our inner dialectic between multiplicity and integration. And they are assessing its implications for renegotiating or reintegrating their selves in the context of inducing us to adapt to them and them to us. (Slavin, 1996, p. 623)

In profound statements about mutuality in psychotherapy, both Slavin and Bromberg speak to the states of being alone in the presence of the other, and together in collision with the other, to the value of the processes of mutual deconstruction—witnessing the other's struggle with disintegration dynamics, multiple identities, and conflicting loyalties—*and* to the negotiation of new meanings, identities, and relational paradigms out of that shared experience. Even in the absence of dangerous concretizations and the acting out of traumatic patterns of relating, the treatment of severe trauma survivors always involves gut-wrenching anxieties that tear at the very fabric of psychological cohesion and integration.

In other words, the process of mutual deconstruction is not without its consequences for therapists.

The therapist's private experience becomes the channel through which the patient's full range of dissociated self-experiences can first achieve linguistic expression, but optimal use of this channel depends on the analyst's ability to allow a transitional reality to be consensually constructed between himself and his patient. (Bromberg, 1995a, p. 521)

In the transitional zone, the severely dissociative patient's internal characters and less-well-organized self-states appear and disappear and they change and evolve with humanizing contact from relationship itself, from interacting with "otherness." But the battles in this zone unlike the original traumatic contexts are waged in fair and clear terms, and their resolutions are negotiated, not established through domination and terror. The therapist treating trauma and dissociation from a participant-observation perspective is continually challenged to respond, immerse, adjust, negotiate, and to change (Pizer, 1996; Bromberg, 1996b; Davies, 1996a; Slavin, 1996), and s/he does not emerge from this sort of experience unscathed (Eigen, 1992; Goldberg, 1990): s/he cannot conduct an effective treatment of severe trauma without risking being known, being touched, and, at some moments being just as terrified as the patient. The therapist must reach the patient and allow him/herself to be reached without the protection of psychological rubber gloves (Ehrenberg, 1996). "Our very vulnerability often becomes our most sensitive instrument, and paradoxically thereby, a source of analytic power and strength" (Ehrenberg, 1996, p. 281).

Therapist and patient will destroy each other's mythologies, worldviews, and identifications. If all goes relatively well, they can eventually move through and out of the series of traumatically defined, painful reenactment and merger states into a different kind of unity. This unification or integration is defined by a sense of having survived—actually and symbolically, of having weathered the stormy treatment, of having "come through the whirlwind" (Eigen, 1992). Ehrenberg (1996) views this emotional joining as emerging not so much out of the linear, intellectual part of the work as from the sharing of emotional availability and the affective experiences of the moment. Goldberg (1990) refers to the process as a "fusion of horizons" (p. 148, citing Gadamer, 1975), whereby therapist and patient are two persons on the road to discover" the necessary use of others as the building blocks of our self" (p. 148): a synthesis representing a previously unthought view of self and world can evolve. Goldberg's relational perspective proposes that truth is never final and exhaustive, and that meaning is in a constant state of creation and revision. Individuation (the development of an autonomous, interdependent self), respect (the capacity to value, honor, and hold in regard), and mutuality (the capacity for reciprocity, paradox, recognition, inclusivity, and empathy) are just some of the fruits of this new, differentiated union. Integration, maturation, and wholeness are some of the terms applied to the optimal or successful negotiation of such a psychotherapy process.

The patient's use of the therapist's self as a medium for accessing the communications of his/her own sequestered voices requires the therapist to balance and project openness and permeability with solidity, consistency, and distinctness. This is no easy task when the therapist's psyche is assaulted by the multiple challenges engendered by the therapy material and traumatic reenactments; it is further complicated by the media's persistent portrayal of therapists as dangerous and incompetent memory-implanting fanatics. The treatment of severely traumatized people—the *Kabbalah*'s "descent for the sake of ascent" (Sholem, 1974)—is redemptive for therapist and patient alike, but traumatization or retraumatization is always unavoidable in the process. If, accordingly, it can be said that the path to Heaven goes through Hell, that the greatest light emerges out of the most abysmal forms of darkness as the *Kabbalah* counsels, then the wise therapist will try to make space for the spiritual questions that inevitably enter the treatment and struggle along with the patient to come to terms with the spiritual implications of what has taken place in the patient's life.

MARJORIE

Marjorie is a high-functioning woman in her midforties whose subtle but complex disorder falls into the diagnostic category known as DDNOS (dissociative disorder not otherwise specified) because of the high degree of coconsciousness and cooperation among her various self-states and her only mild to moderate memory loss; she has never elaborately personified her dissociative self-system into the full MPD/DID symptom picture. Marjorie has always remembered some of her sexual abuse in the basement at the hands of her father. Therapy provides a safety net for remembering—and revealing, and integrating—the rest. She maintains a strong treatment alliance and is highly motivated to fully recover.

Courageously moving in and through her traumatic material and integrating it rapidly, Marjorie spends minimal time debating the reality of the events she recalls. Her major debate revolves around how deeply her extremely disturbed parents got to and damaged her. Did they win? Are parts of her like them, or did she somehow mysteriously resist the identification with her aggressor? When she sacrificed herself to protect her siblings, was she successful in sparing them the abuse she suffered? How much did she comply with her abuser father and how much did she fight him and resist?

Part of Marjorie's dilemma as a child, and now as an adult reconstructing her past and her identity, was that her father was someone she could attach to in spite of his brutality and escalating sadism while her mother's callousness and inhumanity left no room for any real bonding. She tells me about the time, over fifteen years ago, that she told her mother that her father had abused her. Her mother's one-sentence reply echoes in her mind to this day. "I thought he was doing your sister." So for Marjorie to remember her father's absolute sadism without diluting and deflecting it with her own self-hate is to lose, once again, the only parental bond that got her through.

One day, Marjorie was reviewing her initial trip down to the basement with her father, some persistent dreams making her think there was more in that episode to be looked at. For the first time in her life he had been playing a children's game with her in the living room. He had also been drinking, as usual. When he casually invited her to accompany him to the basement, Marjorie welcomed the rare moment of special attention—something she always craved since neither parent could ordinarily be counted on to be emotionally available.

Several memories blended together and Marjorie reconnected with fragmented images of a knife or weapon that had been plaguing her in dreams and in other intrusive images over the years but had never before surfaced into consciousness. The particular event she began to recall involved not just the sexual abuse that had become chronic by that time, but specifically sexualized punishment, imposed by way of retaliation for her interference with her father's efforts to abuse one of her siblings.

One of the triggers for this set of memories was a widely publicized case of child sexual abuse and murder by parents in the basement of their house. The child was found by the police tied up and with duct tape on her mouth. Marjorie's natural empathy, outrage, and identification with the child-victim were compounded by her increasing agitation and obsessive focus on the duct tape and the binding of the victim's hands. While open to the possibility that these images were merely suggestive but not actually reflective of her own abuse, Marjorie was prompted by the waves of nausea and resistance, fear and dread that had in the past always signaled unprocessed traumatic memory to explore what about duct tape and ropes was so disturbing her affect.

When describing a moment when her father threatened her with a knife if she cried out or refused to take her clothes off, Marjorie stops her story abruptly. Her eyes go backward and I feel as if I have lost her to some awful fate. Her face contorts, her neck twists back, her mouth is open in haunted terror, her eyes get wide in fright, then they close altogether; she shifts, puts her hand tightly over her mouth, and starts softly whimpering. Every time Marjorie has gone in and out of such states, she seems to return more whole, more self-aware; is she building another bridge now—to herself, to me—with her mind and body? Can I trust her process, our process?

I find myself moving in and out of anger, nausea, and my familiar clinical interrogatives. Is this yet another violation like the ones she lived through? Am I putting her through this or seeing her through? Is my willingness to wait, watch, listen, another kind of violation? Am I forcing her to do this—perpetrating? Or am I just standing by—colluding? Is she forcing me—victim—to witness helplessly? Who is seducing whom? Or are we knowing and not knowing together, liberating frozen parts of her experience to be voiced, making meaning? Are all of these things happening at the same time? Is it all a matter of mutual suggestion as the critics would say or is that a distraction? Must I link these expressions immediately to other patterns and transference experiences, or should I give her space to lose and then reinvent herself? Is testifying with her full self healing or retraumatizing? Is witnessing building faith, trust, and tolerance for anxiety and ambiguity, or another form of collaboration?

No words pass between us. I think I know what I am seeing as Marjorie's movements suggest that her arms are tied and her head held back while she's being orally raped. Coming back, she begins to choke, then cough. "Can you connect with me here and now," I ask. "Tell me about this pain your are in." I wonder if I have spoken too soon—to reduce my own anxiety—or not soon enough. Can I trust my own instincts and sense of the rhythms of integration?

Rubbing her neck and shoulders while returning to her adult communicative state, Marjorie answers in a somber voice, "What did I do to make him hate me? He told me that it didn't hurt when I said to stop. Then he put duct tape on my mouth, called me a liar and a slut. . . . Why did he want to kill me. He always said I made him do this to me because of the way I looked at him upstairs. He said he knew what I wanted and he was going to give it to me. What did I want? Since I wanted his attention, maybe he was right. I hate myself for needing it, for believing he would be nice to me."

I remind Marjorie that she always turns her rage on herself—as if she should have known what was coming or could have prevented it. "The shame and humiliation are all tied up in why you didn't do something to stop him almost as if there was no one else in the event but you, and also as if you're forgetting that you were a child when all this took place."

"Why didn't I scream or shout or hit him?" she asks herself, me, and the universe.

"What happened when you did try and protect yourself?" I ask.

"It enraged him and things got worse. But I could have done something else couldn't I?"

THERAPIST: It has always been so much you and so little anyone else in this world of self-hate you have built to cope with all of this trauma.

PATIENT: It's like he's not even there anymore . . . just me by myself, feeling defeated, like the images of me alone and cold in the basement feeling awful and feeling like I had done something wrong or failed to do something important.

[Long silence] . . . When I can remember that he planned it and knew what he was doing, that feeling does shift, but I have to come out of the memory of it in order to see that. Some places in me can't see that part of it yet.

T: His planning and intentions are some of the hardest part of this to get, along with your helplessness, which is the very hardest part.

P: I am trying to see this from different sides, and now it's about why did he have to tie me up, what did I do to deserve that. I don't think he directly said things like about my deserving it, but that was implied. What he did say was that he could and would kill me. . . . It wasn't just to silence me, it was more than that.

T: What do you think?

P: I think he maybe got off on stuff like that sometimes.

T: You mean he liked making you afraid as part of the abuse?

P: I keep moving in and out of it, then and now. It's confusing.

T: Being inside of it and outside of it at the same time is what we're trying to help you be able to do. When it's not so fixed it's not so overwhelming. You can move around the event and the feelings and fantasies you had about what was going on instead of being frozen in one place.

Marjorie and I have processed many memories together and at the end of this session she asks me what it was like for me, as she occasionally does by way of bridging and reconnecting to a living witness and by way of grounding herself in here-and-now reality in preparation for leaving. She also does so as a means of reversing the absence of witnessing in her family and as a means of having some sense of agency in the therapy process. First, I ask her what she imagines.

P: I think it is hard for you to see me go through this and it probably makes you mad and sick.

T: Anger and nausea were two feelings that came and went at different times this session.

P: I have been feeling sick and nauseous on and off the whole session. But something about you sharing, no, your even having feelings about this brings me more in touch with that in me, now more than before.

T: My words about my feelings seem to link you to yours, or help you give them a name.

P: Or maybe just help me stay with it more knowing I am not so alone.

T: The words can bring together pieces that have been disconnected. And the anger?

P: Still far away, but I can imagine feeling it one day soon. Somehow seeing this in this way reminded me that I was a child. I always think of myself as an adult being abused. When I see my true size, then I can begin to get angry. [*Pause. Silence*] . . . I have mixed feelings about making you feel bad.

T: I think there is a desire on your part to protect me on the one hand and to want me to know it up close on the other, which is even harder to own.

P: In the old days I used to want to rub your face in it to make you know it and that way I would know you felt it, and I would completely split off in those days and not know I needed you to know, so I could make you know more by force like he did to me.

T: The sick feeling is some part of this we can share, so even though you have to go through this alone in a way, you are also not completely alone. You need to have this shared in some deep way, but without anyone making anyone else feel anything by force.

P: Part of me still feels alone in some of this, probably because there is more about this to remember, I think. It's not as hard as it used to be to stay with it. I am sad for me now, but I am sadder for that little girl who I know is me but who I can't quite connect with fully yet as me. I know it matters to you, I matter, that changes it. The nothingness isn't completely gone I know, but it's different, you're different, I am different—we are both changed a little bit by this. Somehow this mattering to you makes me matter to myself in a little different way. It helps me move past wishing or pretending it didn't happen to feeling a little different about what did happen, or maybe even seeing it in a real way for the first time.

We agree that the nausea is passing for each of us. Some of it seems to be related to feeling isolated or alone with the material. When we can share something about it together, then neither of us is so much assaulted by images or sensations, and we can begin to make some sense out of them.

The processing of this set of memories was not complete for some time. Another trauma within the series of traumas emerged. Marjorie alternated between remembering her father smashing her hands down on the table to be tied and revisiting an image of her broken self submitting by offering her hands ("willingly") to be tied upon his request. The foray into this zone was particularly conflicted because complete submission was abhorrent to her; her pride and dignity were invested in the idea (real and imagined) that she fought back.

As I was encouraging Marjorie to free-associate to what she saw or felt, there was a switch. One part of her asked me why I was "making the child go back to that man" in such a vivid way that it seemed for a moment to both of us that the remembering and witnessing process itself was completely equivalent to retraumatization—or to the initial traumatization—and that I was a collaborator and perpetrator in that moment.

When we agreed to completely stop the process and to explore what was happening in our relationship, there was great relief. It led to a series of discussions of transference fears of repetition of domination dynamics. Marjorie needed to recover her sense of her own power in relation to me in the here-and-now of therapy before going any further into memories that shattered her illusions about her own self as always capable and self-protective, and about her father as occasionally protective. And that led to a reworking of a previously traumatic therapy relationship.

Hypnosis had been used from the second session on in that therapy to make Marjorie revisit her childhood bedroom, where she would repeatedly relive terrifying and painful sensations but where even after many years no verbal or narrative memory ever could be integrated. The timing and pacing of this prior therapy were rooted in the clinician's own systems (and inexperience or naïveté) and not based on anything happening with Marjorie, who ended up losing quite a bit of functioning and integrating very little during that time. Clearly she now felt we were verging on repetition of that kind of domination paradigm; Marjorie decided to call a halt to "exploratory work for her own good" for several weeks.

Marjorie had what she called "an elaborate temper tantrum," which to me represented the emergence of a new level of aggression whereby she was playing with her own power in relation to me and, of course, to her perpetrator. This was the first of a number of episodes of Marjorie's expressing anger at me for real or imagined injuries or boundary violations (for example, sharing too much with her, raising her fee, forgetting something she had told me a week before, and so on). Each always presaged revelation of another layer of more brutal sadistic trauma: her father seemed to like most to beat her into unconsciousness and then orally rape her; he tormented her at any sign of resistance and frequently engaged in various forms of bondage, torture, and verbal death threats.

Finally, Marjorie spent several sessions just being angry and talking about it quite eloquently. Marjorie was angry that these terrible things had happened to her, angry that she had to spend time and money dealing with them when not everyone else in the world had to, angry that anyone could do them to a child, angry that she had submitted, angry that she had to know about such things in the first place, angry that she didn't or couldn't protect herself, angry at the prior therapist for reenacting and not giving any credence to her protest responses about their process together, angry at me for wanting more from her, angry at the world outside the basement window that was indifferent to her suffering.

For the first time Marjorie was able to get in touch with a level of hate toward her father—hate that he put his perversion in her, hate that he broke her, hate that she helped him hurt her. During this period her omnipotent defenses against helplessness collided with her anger, disappointment, and despair. By choosing not to delve further into her memories for awhile Marjorie was saying no to me, no to her father, no to her mother, and no to society's collaboration, no to her prior therapist's impingement, control, and suppression of her voice of protest— and she was also saying, no I don't want this to have happened, I don't want this to be true; I can still make it not true, I have the power now and I want to play with it.

In this case, witnessing Marjorie's anger, protests, distrust, and negation was almost more important to her integration process than the witnessing of the traumatic events themselves. Welcoming and validating Marjorie's "nos" instead of writing them off as resistance or defense was essential to her accumulating enough resilience to face the next layers and to reverse the legacy of submission into one of empowerment. Before recovering any more memories, Marjorie had to develop a stronger sense of agency in order to tolerate the impact of the material that was still to come.

Destruction of the core experience of agency is the crux of what happens to victims of sadistic sexual abuse and torture, according to Slavin (1997), and restoration of agency is the crux of healing trauma.

> In the confusion of motives, the obfuscation of reality, . . . the toying with meanings and events, the crazy-making redefinition of pleasure and pain—in the moment of experiencing one's self instantaneously as both the helpless victim and the omnipotent perpetrator—the child's maturing and differentiated sense of self, and of self as agent, is irrevocably damaged. (p. 227)

In the treatment of survivors of severe trauma, patients and therapists always struggle over who will be the agent of memory recovery. The recovery of memory must always yield to recovery of agency even when—most especially when—the patient refuses (temporarily) to reveal, to remember, or to bear witness. And while the recovery of agency does not substitute for the recovery of memory, taking charge of oneself within the transitional zone of the therapy relationship does indeed enhance the capacity for narrativity, for the retrieval of personal history, and for tolerating that which may never be fully knowable. Most important, it develops the capacity for protest, for healthy aggression, and for differentiating self and other in new ways.

ALEC

Now in his late thirties, Alec is an exceptionally intelligent and successful gay attorney who survived a complex intra/extrafamilial sex ring, torture, and ritual abuse. When he began treatment during his first year of law school, his presenting complaints included a history of extreme sexual compulsivity and promiscuity, depression, and the recollection that he had molested his brother, three years his junior, over a period of seven or eight years during childhood.

Alec had already undergone several prior therapies and just gained full control over his high-risk sexual acting out in a 12-Step group for sex addicts. As a result of dangerous dissociative reenactments of the gang rapes of his youth, Alec had become infected with HIV. So although a healthy long-term relationship was helping him to feel safe enough to go deeper into his therapy, the entire treatment was shadowed and fueled by a beat-the-clock urgency.

Alec was always quite open to looking at his part in the interpersonal process and exploring its meaning, and to being called on his manipulations and unconsciously brutal reenactments. He appreciated honesty, even confrontation, from me, including my acknowledgments of frustration with ways of toying with his own and my reality testing; he learned that such transitory frustration would not lead to disaster. For Alec, emerging memory was always preceded by enactment, and there was a recognizable rhythm to approaching and distancing himself from relationship to me and his part-selves. What Alec does not like to do, however—giving rise to our ongoing tug-of-war over issues of attachment and dependency—is to link his behaviors with their origins in his family and associated perpetrator group: his split-off beliefs in the goodness of the criminal offenders and especially his mother who had a major role in the group was juxtaposed with his terror and utter fragmentation on receiving a phone call even from relatives never involved.

Like many complex, fragmented but highly functional DID patients, Alec both revealed and denied his dissociatively organized self-system. After months of negotiation about tolerating his own feelings and voices versus acting out, shutting down, and withdrawing, Alec had finally agreed to let some of the vehemently suppressed voices in his head (mostly child alter personalities) reveal what was on his mind, which in his case meant letting all of his voices speak without deciding if what they said was absolute truth or not. This commitment gave Alec great relief, for he had never known any real freedom in relationship. Life was always about bargaining, scheming, and avoiding.

One of Alec's signs that traumatic material is close to the surface during clinical hours is the onset of miniconvulsions—like hiccups without the belching sound; at different times they emanate from different regions of his torso, anywhere from his groin to his throat. The convulsions have been manifesting since the day—three years earlier, one full year into treatment of his depression and narcissistic personality disorder—when he first mentioned the possibility that his father had incested him.

We variously considered them somatic reenactments of anal rapes by his father, his uncle, and other groups of multiple perpetrators (as his history was to reveal), Geiger counter–like warnings that other voices were trying to break through, seductions, and even something that I had somehow placed inside him. To the part-selves who supported this last possibility, the argument that if a therapist could implant false memories, he could implant strange body movements seemed compelling. And Alec's flirtation with the false memory movement—one of his many defensive strategies to sidestep critical thinking and, by extension, his traumatic material—made this otherwise extremely bright man so vulnerable to internally constructed recantation dialogues that he could have been a national poster child for the False Memory Syndrome Foundation.[7]

Alec spent so much of his childhood being deceived and brainwashed and dissociating and lying to himself that he often became more convinced about unrealities than realities. Indeed, he regulated his early encounter with his multiplicity and horrific multiple-perpetrator memories by subscribing tenaciously to the notion that I was an evil genius who had mysteriously made him think and feel things that had nothing whatsoever to do with him. The running commentary in his head could transpose any newly generated meanings—about his victimhood or his parents' abuse and complicity—into certain very rigid and repetitive viewpoints: he was stupid or a liar or attention-seeking, I was untrustworthy or diabolical, he was simply trying to give his life meaning and nothing traumatic had ever happened to him, his parents were benevolent narcissists, and I was the false memory therapist par excellence. We left all of these prospects open for a very long time in order for Alec to locate and make up his own mind.

At any rate, a strong wave of miniconvulsions started up on the day Alec had agreed to allow himself to invite other part-selves into dialogue instead of actively excluding them. When I saw his throat wrenching, I became aware that I had seen so much of Alec's convulsing over the years that I had actually stopped inquiring about it, stopped listening to it as a form of communication, perhaps. This time I pointedly asked Alec what he thought the convulsions were about just now and why they were so specifically centered on the throat. I also commented on how we never distinguished among the different gestures and treated them like they were all the same. The smirk that showed up on his face was by now a familiar warning sign that either a line into traumatic memory had been crossed or his blocker alters had been caught covering up. He replied that he hated when my questions landed on the mark—meaning that his dissociative default mode was threatened and he might have to feel something.

There was a long pause. He convulsed again and again. I had the spontaneous thought that I was going to hear another child shock-treatment torture narrative. (I later wondered if I had somehow magically made him say just that—the notion an index of the impact of the dynamics of mind control and their reenactment, as well as indicative of the extent to which the role of false memory rhetoric in our dialogues inspired all manner of illogical doubts, which would have been easier to bear than what was probably coming.) I fleetingly remembered the time when as a child I put a knife in the toaster, and my whole world stopped for a moment. And then I remembered three detailed electricity tortures that previous patients had described. (I have since heard many more such revelations about the use of electricity in mind-control programming from patients of my own, my colleagues, and my consultees.)

Faced with the possibility of a similar story from yet another patient, I wanted to know and I didn't want to know. I would have to shift gears completely. I felt some shame and guilt that I might have missed this for so many years. Or was this an example of unconscious influence? Were my associations accurate?

Almost immediately, Alec said that his convulsions could be electric shocks. Then, following a huge motor discharge, he almost came off the chair. I took a deep breath and asked again if he felt he could tell me anything about that or, if not, if he would let the parts who could tell. He asked aloud (something he had only just begun to do) for other parts of himself to feel free to speak. And then I asked if he was willing to remember what was said.

He seemed furious at me, almost as if I was the source of his shock treatment torture. "Isn't it enough that I am doing this, do I have to remember it too?"

I said, "Alec, because I know that facing sides of yourself that you'd rather not have or know about can be extremely uncomfortable, I want to tell you yet again that you don't have to go forward into any feelings, memories, or contact with other parts of you unless or until you are ready. Do you believe me?"

"Most of me knows you don't like to see me in pain or hear about this stuff, and most of me knows I still can't hate my perpetrators so I hate and accuse you instead, but still I cannot say all of me believes that somewhere you are not getting off on this in some way. I guess I don't trust anyone completely, never have."

Alec then spoke of deep shame about aspects of the abuse that he may have liked, confusion about being told he liked things he didn't, and a fleeting realization that he was never permitted to have the thought or feeling or memory of not wanting or not liking some sexual, sadistic, or complicitous act his perpetrators' forced him to experience. There followed a moment of vitality when he realized that he could now actually decide that he did not like or want something. For Alec— in spite of his brilliance—it was a revelation. He reflected on his appreciation for my permissiveness, particularly my willingness for him to hate and accuse me of various things.

The issue of liking it/not liking it so central to Alec's confusion about who was responsible for his abuse had always come before, during, and after each and every traumatic memory. His conception of himself as a horny, oversexual, nasty child who was a sex maniac by age five was one set of cognitions that would immediately motivate redissociation of newly articulated memories. "For now," I said, "all I am asking is that you make a decision to not redissociate what you are saying to me . . . and to deal with your ambivalence about remembering and feeling with me directly instead of after you leave the sessions."

What was to be revealed was that Alec had been trained to lose his voice. In one of many training sessions, he was strapped to a chair and told to pretend it was after school, that the woman before him was a teacher he could trust. ("Pretend" was a word frequently used by his offenders to confound his sense of reality.) He was seven years old, in second grade, and already a veteran of organized abuse and mind control. So even though Alec knew this "teacher" from group sexual encounters (i.e., knew her not to be a teacher, let alone his real teacher), he was so desperate and so dissociative that he remembers pretending to the point of believing that the fake teacher would actually help him.

There was one man working the shock machine and another giving that man directions. Alec said that his father and a group of others were behind a barrier watching the whole thing. Two patches of white tape attached a wire to his body, possibly to each of his forearms, possibly elsewhere, he was not completely sure. In the charade that followed, the director told Alec to tell the "teacher" about people who hurt him—and Alec, obeying hesitantly, said something about sexual touching. He was given a mild shock. He jolted. Next the director told him to tell the "teacher" about things that scared him most. Reluctantly playing along, he began to describe "a group of people who hurt children," and the shock came full blast.

Alec then stopped telling his story. He shifted states immediately. He became vaporous and transparent, weak, and his face, jaws clenched tightly, lost all color. The world went dead. I brought myself back by noticing his locked jaw and by asking him to reconnect with me. "What is the pain, Alec?" My voice brought him back. "Can you still feel your connection to me here in the room?"

There was a moment of confusion when a perpetrator-identified part of him told the narrator part that he was being abused now, and that I was the person shocking him, not the others. That seemed to be both an extension of the deliberate mix-up of past and present orchestrated by some of his part-selves and a function of the dynamics of treating this survivor of complex torture, whereby my pressure on his dissociative defenses invariably placed me in the role of the perpetrator. Alec and I started to talk about how my asking him to remember felt like my shocking him, my perpetrating on him, but by now he was so familiar with his own internal reversals and avoidance strategies that, for once, he declined to detour to make me the offender and stayed with the experience instead. (Sometimes a patient's making the therapist the perpetrator is a measure of progress; sometimes, as here, progress lies in a compulsive patient's capacity to cease doing that as a deflective tactic.)

Alec said his jaws were shut tight for a long time after that shock, and he said the rest of the shocks were moderate. "They didn't have to do the real bad one more than once." He described how he would do anything to avoid the severe shock again and he fully complied with the abusers after that point. "All it takes is one shock like that and you're gone—and though you want to be gone, you'd do anything not to be made gone like that ever again. These people know what they're doing."

An alter personality appeared in the following session to describe how Alec pretended the white patches of tape were a doorway he could enter to avoid the pain he knew was happening to somebody, but not to him; on the other side was an imaginary room in which he placed his fear, his hate, his rage, and the members of the offending group. In that room anything could happen and he could use his power to destroy the abusers or save it for years later when he could hunt them down—yet Alec was afraid to go there now in his own imagination. As I articulated the isolation and terror of his predicament and the number of splits his psyche had come up with to cope with it all, he seemed relieved, and we could begin to discuss the value of his dissociative solutions side by side with the ways in which they left him so divided and broken apart that he was his own worst enemy. And we could begin to discuss his entrenched patterns of sabotaging all loving and potential helpful relationships in his life.

When I asked him if he believed he was actually another somebody when the abuse was taking place, he deflated slightly and said, "not really." He told me he hated me for reminding him. He hated when I said things that made him feel anything. I said, "This is progress. The hate comes at me like a flash whenever I threaten your dissociative barriers, whenever something I say reveals the pretend part for what it might really be—but the hate is between us and not locked away in the room, not aimed at yourself in destructive enactments. Maybe we could talk about it. We could even go into the white room together if you want, when you want."

Of course he hated me: not only was I making him feel, but also I was making him tell, which was not unlike the perpetrators making him not tell; the hate in one sector of his personality was trying to counteract the growing trust and dependency in the others. But Alec was introduced to safe hating, and safe hating means no one dies, no one is raped, and no one is tortured when you express negative feelings. It was the beginning of his ability to do just that. Later, he thanked me for letting him hate me, which seemed almost more important at that point than positive attachment because it allowed disparate parts of himself to be brought into our relationship, each on its own terms.

Alec had been caught between speaking and losing his voice in peculiar ways that were atypical even of other torture survivors. One of the mysteries of his peculiar incapacity to release the part-selves with direct knowledge of traumatic events was resolved. Alec was finally one with himself. And now some of the mysteries over his unusual patterns of following healthy bonding with sudden reversals (predominantly toward me, his partner, and some close friends) also began to clear up

In the next couple of dialogues devoted to processing and digesting this disturbing set of memories, another alter personality entered the coconscious discussion to describe how special he had felt as the only child at the shock session because being the center of all the adults' attention enabled him to pretend that he was actually controlling all of their actions. In other words, this electricity-training event was a privilege, not a torture. He was the one in charge. Moving in and out of awareness that this was fantasy, Alec expressed irritation with my interjections about the need of the child in him to come up with the power scenario to make it all less awful and him less helpless. He went on to elaborate on how he made up a story about being the real leader of the group, which gave him so much power that the adult perpetrators didn't even know about how powerful he really was, "although one day they just might," he added.

Since this alter had split off from the pain itself and from identification with the victimized child self, his omnipotent illusions were well developed and his representation of the events almost lighthearted. My admiration for the creativity of his solutions combined with my challenge to the dissociative process seemed to make the conversation less overwhelming for this part of Alec, who slowly began to move closer to his own pain. My desire to "shock" him out of his omnipotent and self-negating illusions came and went; still, I had trouble juggling my reactions to match Alec's different states.

Sitting with the shattered one, the electrocuted one, was more difficult. "I was naked in the chair, I could feel my back against and my butt against the metal. I thought I was tied down but I wasn't because when the shock came my hands went up in the air. Everything went black, then white; I could feel my finger tips and toes tingling and my jaw tightening and my head hurt, I don't know why I felt it in my head if the wires were connected to my arms. I felt my butt go up and down just a little on the chair, and then I didn't feel anything anymore. I just dissolved into it, and then there was nothing. It stopped hurting after a while, I felt numb. Everything went from black to white. Then there was no pain."

When Alec told me this, I said nothing at first. We both wanted the memory over with in some ways, but to leave it too quickly would be to enact yet another abandonment on his entire self, specifically the part holding pain in isolation from other parts. I had mixed feelings about the pacing. On the one hand I didn't want Alec to become unglued; on the other, he seemed more authentic in sharing the details of the event and I didn't want him to lose these hard-won connections to himself. I felt that if I made the wrong move the whole session could be wasted.

For his part, Alec had been trained not to make any wrong moves himself, and never to trust any professional societal authority with revelations about his other life. (Years later Alec disclosed that he had been trained specifically to hate therapists for trying to thwart the beneficent goals of the group and to target them for violent actions. He came to realize that he had been systematically programmed to deflect and negate any mention of multiple personality disorder, child sexual abuse, and so on; not so the term *dissociation*, however, which we had enlisted as the word of choice for communication about his inner life.)

Alec had tried to train me over the years to stay away from traumatic material, repeatedly reenacting shifts from alliance making to alliance breaking, in keeping with his perpetrator group's reversals. Now, by focusing on and positioning himself between the survival and denial values of his fantasies and alter creations, Alec was trying to move closer to the pain of the actual trauma and to what it meant. For the first time the motivations to connect with other parts—unfamiliar, amnestic, and cult-identified parts—of himself came from him. This was progress and I hoped it wouldn't get disrupted.

A heavy sadness emerged in that session. Alec's torturers had permanently altered his personality. Their expert mind-control tactics had left Alec with blank spots in his memory and an inability to apply what critical thinking abilities he had developed to an analysis of his predicament. The implicit denial operative in his disturbed family every day of his life, the pervasive atmosphere of terror in the perpetrator group, and the culture of violation of the laws of society and basic human rights in which he was captive over a period of many years had left him with a chronic incapacity for testing reality and tolerating uncertainty.

Shocked into full submission—terrified, literally out of his mind to the point of creating many minds around a single traumatic event, Alec was left in a tomb of numbness. As he told his story, parts of him became aware for the first time that its events had actually happened to him, not to some other little boy. He also became aware that the part of him that had been paralyzed did not have to stay that way. The trauma could actually be over with forever. The witnessing and testimony were inextricably connected to the subjective experience of the trauma abating.

Now there was no more pretending. From Alec's despair came a chorus of denial and recantation followed by an integrated sense of knowing what he had always known, to echo his words. It was still too dangerous to make associations to his perpetrators and to their intentions; that would come later. Occasionally, Alec expressed deep gratitude for the chance to have someone listen to those parts of him which he felt no one would ever hear from, which he had been explicitly told no one would ever believe.

Still, he felt the need periodically to attack our connection and my goodwill toward him in order to regulate his own strange attachment compromises, ward off the interference of more memories, reenact the assault on relationship that would have to be revisited many times in the months ahead, and most of all sustain bonds with his parents and their imagined innocence. Witnessing the original trauma was a turning point, however: after those sessions, there was considerably less recanting and denying, and a deeper and more consistent commitment to listening to himself emerged.

A couple of weeks later, Alec completed a major element of his testimonial about shock treatment torture and training. He remembered in fragments that the perpetrators had sexualized it at the end when the leader instructed the adults to masturbate as Alec was being shocked. Whether this was part of the omnipotent fantasy he cultivated to temporarily master the events or whether the group actually climaxed to his pain remained unclear. He recalled being carried off and tenderly dressed by the leader who at that moment felt strong and protective. So his first human contact following torture created another layer of trauma bonding, and putting together that this man was the same man who had orchestrated the torture took some time, as Alec's attachment fears were more complex than any others. Finally, after weeks of work, Alec was able to identify both of his parents in the circle of adults, and that was the most devastating part of the memory. Behind it was another: Alec was able to evoke an earlier ritual of sorts in which his parents publicly turned him over to the group and officially ended their parental relationship with him.

Some renewed protest responses emerged spontaneously, and Alec decided on his own to go into the memory of the physical pain to completely unlock the part of himself frozen in the electrocution trauma. This new piece of internal theater had the earmarks of an adult's taking appropriate responsibility for a child, reversing some of the internalized relational paradigms where children service the adults while pretending they have good parents. By facing the most excruciating of the physical and attachment pains and betrayals, Alec was able consciously to work through the convulsing of the first few years of the therapy. In the end it was his healthy anger affirming that he no longer wanted to be stuck with that pain that motivated this piece of reclaiming himself. What Alec wanted was to put his own holding arms around his child self and remove the posttraumatized boy from the arms of the perpetrator. Alec's description embodied the restorative fantasy operations newly developed to alter the past in the present and to cultivate a new sense of agency.

As Slavin (1997) states, when agency is taken away or toyed with, memory becomes unstable. When impaired agency begins to heal from the damage of cumulative trauma, not only does memory return but the ability to synthesize and integrate memory—and the ability to deploy fantasy operations (instead of dissociative solutions) to rework helplessness—also return or are developed for the first time.

THE WITNESS AND THE WITNESSED

I think it is important to recognize how much we get from our patients. Our patients are holding environments for us, as well as we for them. We organize ourselves through their presence. We immerse ourselves in them on a daily basis, and this immersion restores and enriches (not only drains) us. They give us a chance to use our minds and feelings creatively and usefully. We come up against our (and their) walls and find ways to keep flowing. (Eigen, 1998, p. 42)

With all that has been written about working with traumatic reenactments and transference analysis, clinicians and theorists can forget that the act of listening and witnessing the testimony of survivors is most fundamental to the reparative process. As psychotherapists, we take it for granted that we know how to listen and hear people in their pain but we have much to learn, primarily from our patients. Both the suffering and the complex maneuvering to minimize suffering of the dissociative survivor, however fractured and internally inconsistent, need to be witnessed. An atmosphere of safety is a precondition for the testimony and for gently but continuously steering traumatized people toward their pain.

Through testimony, the narrator reverses the process of objectification and loss of identity: "to testify is to engage precisely in the process of re-finding one's own proper name, one's signature" (Felman, 1995, p. 53). Through testimony and witnessing, the legacy of annihilation inherent in trauma is subjected to the reparative processes of making an impact and making a difference on the other. The patient's awareness of his/her traumatization cannot be presupposed. In fact, knowledge about trauma "can only happen through testimony: it cannot be separated from it. It can only unfold itself in the process of testifying, but it can never become a substance that can be possessed by either speaker or listener outside of this dialogic process" (Felman, 1995, p. 53). This illuminates one of the many problems in translating that which takes place in the clinical hour to courtrooms and legal proceedings, and even to case presentation.

Testimony as a process refers to the healing and *empowerment* aspect of language itself and reverses the *obliteration* of language and connection that took place in trauma. Using language and informed silence to penetrate to the state of being wounded and helpless is to both enter the state of paralysis imposed by trauma and held in dissociative states, and to foster a re-emergence from that psychic paralysis. Testimony also provides a link between the psychological and the political, between the private and the public, and its power can help restore affective ties and integrate fragmented experience. Without denying the reality of the transference/countertransference, and without ignoring the issue of unconscious conflict, clinicians have to work from a nonneutral commitment to help patients convert a sociopolitical crime from an individual illness into something amenable to cultural elaboration (Becker, 1996).

Rape and child abuse take place in the universes of sexual, gender, family, and interpersonal politics; like political torture, they may be regarded as pathologies of power relationships. Consequently, the posture of "neutrality" for caregivers is a fallacy when it comes to torture, child abuse, and organized violence against innocents, a variety of denial (Simpson, 1996). It must be revised so that doing nothing, or behaving as if nothing has happened, or not analyzing the meaning of what has happened is not neutrality. Not only is it a pathological form of denial but also it is actually enabling to perpetrators.

It is impossible to treat survivors of severe childhood trauma and remain morally neutral about some of our societal norms. Quoting Montaigne who four hundred years ago wrote that "science without conscience is but the death of the soul," Simpson states: "No doctor feels bound to be neutral toward cancer. Why should we treat torture, the cancer of freedom, any differently?" (1995, p. 209). Becker's (1996) position supports Simpson's: apolitical treatment of trauma, including the use of some clinical language and attitudes that excessively pathologize and decontextualize victims' responses and posttraumatic symptoms can mirror the self-justifying attitudes of victimizers. Cautioning against converting ourselves into traumatizing agents in our roles as helping professionals, Becker reminds us that the recovery from trauma, particularly the restoration of dignity and self-respect, is catalyzed when trauma survivors are regarded less as individually disturbed and more as people suffering the consequences of a disturbed society. Unarguably, traumatic experience and the search for meaning it triggers must be understood in terms of the patient's relationship with both him/herself and his/her social surround, not least since outcomes are influenced by always evolving forces located both within the individual and in the larger interpersonal, cultural, and political domains (Summerfield, 1996). Understanding the suffering of victims who cope and transcend and of those who do not can only be achieved, according to Summerfield, when the mental health field makes common cause with other disciplines and with the testimonies of the survivor populations themselves.

Creamer (1996) expresses in cognitive terms what most traumatologist-clinicians from Janet and Freud to Herman (1992), Courtois (1988), Briere (1992b), Van der Kolk (1995; 1996), Bromberg (1994; 1996b), and Davies and

Frawley (1994) recommend: recovery from severe trauma requires two conditions. First, reminders of the experience must be made available in a manner that will activate the traumatic memory network (affects, sensations, relational configurations, and meanings), since the personality alterations that coalesced around traumatic experience cannot be modified if the network remains dormant or dissociatively out of consciousness. And second, again so that modification can occur, information inconsistent with what is contained in that network must be made available—Nachmani's (1995) benevolent or compassionate disruption.

Like Creamer, most clinicians, whether working from cognitive, hypnotic, or relational psychoanalytic approaches, seek to access the direct perceptual substrate of traumatic experience within the therapy dialogue often enough and for long enough and at a mutually regulated pace and intensity that modification can occur. "Moving on" must involve a new engagement with benevolent interpersonal reality. And this benevolence must demonstrate itself and include a sharing of horror, speechlessness, and powerlessness. "What inundates a traumatized life is, really, at once overwhelming, void of meaning, and unsayable. That is what people in pain are telling us, if only we will hear" (Egendorf, 1995, p. 20). Though trauma may remain incomprehensible, through testimony and through countertransference experience it becomes accessible.

Foa and Kozak (1986) suggest that PTSD, like other anxiety disorders, can be construed as reflecting a pathological fear structure. Pathological fear structures are hypothesized to contain excessive response elements resistant to modification and also to include unrealistic appraisals of nondangerous stimuli that produce avoidance. The fear structure must be activated with matching input on the one hand in order for it to be modified—yet the information to be processed in the course of therapy will, on the other hand, be incompatible with the structure's pathological elements. This essential cognitive model, like Creamer's proposal, fails to take into account the complexity of the testimonial and witnessing processes, nor does it reflect communication through enactment or the use of the transference/countertransference to access and then moderate dissociated traumatic experience. Indeed, many cognitive approaches downplay the importance of the relationship between therapist and patient in favor of the linear transformation that can take place through reeducation, interpretation, and the replacement of old thoughts with new ones. In practice, the treatment of severe trauma survivors does involve accessing fear structures, unrealistic appraisals, and avoidance strategies; however the working through is hardly a linear or simply didactic process. In order to uncover and witness traumatic memories, therapists must confront, and in some manner transcend, their own feelings of horror and the desire to look away as well as the their voyeurism. Hegeman (1997) compares cognitive and psychoanalytic approaches to trauma therapy and reconstruction, referring first to the former.

> There are many recommendations that the transference be diluted as much as possible by the use of treatment teams, and changes in therapist are often encouraged. The idea of rebuilding trust gradually through a deeply valued analytic relationship, or of the treatment room as a special place for trust and play, free enough of reality constraints for the self to be re-imagined, is nonexistent for the cognitive behavioral approach. (Hegeman, 1997, p. 151)

Perhaps Bromberg's (1980) dual emphasis on empathy and anxiety, and the negotiated dialectic between attunement and confrontation best mirrors the essential features of transformative and interactional witnessing. Bromberg (1996b) believes that there is no way for a patient's personal narrative to be truly transformed through a cognitive editing process alone. Rather, only a change in the perceptual reality—which arises out of witnessing and testifying from the direct experience of the dissociated self-states involved in the traumatic experience—can make mutative alterations in the cognitive reality that defines the patient's internal object world. Without direct access to the affect, memories, belief systems, and programming, a severely traumatized patient may remain fundamentally isolated, permanently subjugated to the tyrannizing systems of childhood.

Such a transformative dialogue differs radically from neutral narration and listening, and brings new meaning to the term witnessing. Now an interactive process, it introduces a new relationship, and a shared consciousness, into the dissociative psyche's splits, blank spots, and points of traumatic overwhelm. Based on mutuality and a sharing of power, and with a substantial power of its own (harboring no intention to harm), the new relationship constitutes a bridge to the terror, anxiety, and pain that have existed previously in isolation, a bridge that the patient can choose to use or not. The challenge for the interactive witness is to tolerate confusion, ambiguity, and contradictory realities without prematurely foreclosing meaning or attempting to resolve paradox. Its successful resolution reverses the original trauma-tizing domination, intrusion, and appropriation of the victim's psyche.

Witnessing from within the transference/countertransference matrix means that the therapist cannot listen without getting his/her hands, mind, self, and spirit dirty. The clinician's struggle with his/her own confusion and painful affective states is as much a part of the witnessing process as inquiry, empathy, or interpretation. In contrast to the contentions of some of the more concrete or cognitive or hypnotism-based approaches, the revisionist mes-sage here (Egendorf, 1995; Ehrenberg, 1992; Bromberg, 1996b) is that treat-ment cannot be completely or even mostly "managed" or orchestrated. The listening process is not an uncontaminating one. The traumatic reenactments must impact the listener for the underlying perceptual substrate of the narra-tive to be accessed and the story to be told transformatively. "Therapy may involve skill, but it is also a form of prayer" (Eigen, 1998, p. 43).

WITNESSING AND SURVIVAL

Clinician/theorists who have spent a great deal of time in the presence of enormous suffering have attempted to organize theoretical concepts around the processes of witnessing and testimonials. Laub (1995) distinguishes three levels—being a witness to oneself, being a witness to the testimony of others, and being a witness to the process of witnessing itself. Standing in all these places at once is a key to avoiding collapse into an anxiety-relieving comfort of either arrogant and premature knowing *or* incredulity .

Hearing people through their pain is described by Egendorf (1995) as con-sisting of four distinct but overlapping registers: *decoding* ordinary mean-ings, *resonating* with the significance for another's life, *awakening* to the reality of one's experience and identity in the presence of a witnessing other, and *communing* with the other through the dialogues that occur between the witness and the witnessed. Egendorf likens this form of hearing to medita-tion and mindfulness. The exacting process of attending thoughtfully man-dates us to rescue ourselves from distraction and preconception. "What hits in the moment of confronting trauma is ultimately nothing we can name. Literally nothing. Nor some speculative category in a philosophical system, but a life-sucking void that takes our breath away" (Egendorf, 1995, p. 20).

Egendorf encourages us to remain in a constant state of readiness to be sur-prised, to discover hidden meanings not immediately apparent, and also to realize—in another version of the redemptive paradigm whereby Heaven is reached via Hell—that pain and illumination are so intricately intertwined that we must direct the search for understanding into the heart of human agony. This is at the core of the reparative process of psychotherapy. When patients are ready, healing dialogues can lead them through the confrontations with death, symbolic death, threatened death, near death, intentional evil, or capricious destructiveness to accept what is given and what is taken away,

> by inviting them to speak into being the great absence in their lives. And as they do, and grow willing to turn from their reflexive turning away, we may guide them further—to verify for themselves that they, as the ones who are raised up in wakefulness to meet trauma's demand, do not perish, not even in the face of nothingness. (p. 21)

DID AND WITNESSING

The processes of witnessing and testifying are different with severely dissociative patients from those same kinds of processes with survivors of collectively experienced adult trauma (e.g., the Holocaust). During DID psychotherapy, witnessing itself is fragmented, sporadic, and often interspersed with reenactments and alternate versions of events. The narrative process may be the nonlinear outgrowth of screen memories made up of fragmented images, themselves fragments of memories representing preliminary attempts to historicize (Kornfeld, 1996), all punctuated with revelations of omnipotent fantasies organized by a child-victim struggling to make a less disturbing, less overwhelming meaning of what s/he was experiencing.

The therapist often witnesses by direct experience through projective identification and through his/her participation in reenactments. Bodily sensations of nausea and pain may alternate with numbing and distraction. The therapist's rage at the patient's perpetrators may be difficult to contain while the patient—rarely even close to anger in his/her initial presentations—works at disentangling past from present and cutting loose from the frozen terror of reexperiencing for long enough to stay in affective contact with the therapist. Sometimes the therapist feels as though s/he is lowering the patient into a dark well and straining to prevent the connecting rope from breaking: when to tug the patient back into the present and when to allow the free fall into the traumatic material is the constant dilemma for clinicians trying to balance dosing, pacing, and containing with the ultimate goal of gently advancing toward the pain the patient has spent his/her entire life trying to avoid.

Sometimes, segments of traumatic experience appear as partial constructions of what may have happened, but the mechanisms adopted by the DID patient for sheer psychic survival may mask his/her recognition of them as elements of his/her experience. With the passage of time and the deepening of the therapy process, however, the reconstruction of gaps in the patient's own history is catalyzed (Kornfeld, 1995). The possession of the past by a self in dialogue with itself and a witnessing other supplants the possession (and fragmentation) of the self by the past (and the perpetrators). For DID patients no less than for other survivors of chronic interpersonal trauma, the witnessing process is still always a double-edged sword, as returning to the scenes and affects of the trauma produces losses as well as the hoped-for transformation.

REVERSING THE DAMAGE: "HEARING PEOPLE THROUGH THEIR PAIN"

Egendorf (1995) elegantly describes how hearing people through their pain is first and foremost a privilege, and how healing dialogues can raise communication to communion where two who remain distinct meet as one. Reminding us that hearing creatively and calling out to the survivor to enable him/her to voice the hitherto unmentionable is the most potent antidote to traumatic estrangement from the self and alienation from others, Egendorf believes that the patient learns through this kind of intense meeting and discourse that such speaking is indeed possible and worthwhile. "Hearing people through their pain therefore means . . . that we draw them out in the midst of what obscures them from themselves, and use talk creatively ourselves to show, rather than to tell them, that they not their hurt are foremost" (p. 18).

The witnessing, testimonial, and remembering processes in work with severely dissociative and other severely traumatized patients confirm that they have in reality survived (i.e., that the trauma is indeed over), and allow them to become full participants in their own suffering rather than dissociative managers committed to contain it and to avoid overwhelming trauma. Becoming a full participant in the presence of an empathic and benevolent other is a core and healthy reversal of the self-betrayal institutionalized in the trauma and posttraumatic symptomatology. To the degree that the therapist is impacted and uses the experience of impact in contactful dialogue toward a true "meeting of minds" (Aron, 1996) with the patient, a reparative and redemptive mutuality replaces the domination/submission paradigm emblematic of child-abuse trauma. By taking an active role in the reconstruction of narrative history and the reformulation of meanings, the therapist is assisting the patient to differentiate from the traumatic relational matrix—to think different thoughts from the victimizer or perpetrating system, and to have different feelings from those that governed the self-hatred that left the abusers out of the picture entirely, and thus to take steps toward reclaiming an identity independent of the ideologies and denial systems of the traumatizers of childhood.

Witnessing narrative testimony and witnessing through the countertransference facilitate the patient's assertion of autonomy and separation from the internalized (and actual past and present) abusive system(s) while simultaneously opening channels for new connections with the patient's self and benevolent others. "The individual not only has a history which an observer may unravel and describe, but he is history and makes his history by virtue of his memorial activity in which past-present-future are created as mutually interacting modes of time" (Leowald, 1972, p. 409). This transformational perspective—in stark contrast to the recommendations of Loftus and Ketcham (1994) and Ofshe and Watters (1994), who emphasize cognitive-behavioral treatment of the patient's here-and-now symptoms, behaviors, and circumstances to the exclusion of renegotiating his/her past and internal representations—fully respects the dialectical relationships among past, present, and future. "The modification of the past by the present does not change what objectively happened in the past, but it changes that past which the patient carries within him as his living history" (Leowald, 1980, p. 144).

For therapy to be truly transformative, it must engage in what Brown (1994) calls subversive dialogues. In this view, the patient begins to have access to the previously dissociated world of affective responses like rage, despair, sorrow, and compassion for the self. Such therapeutic conversations reinforce mutuality, deconstruct the power relationships in the patient's past and present (including the patient's experience with the therapist), and examine potent causal/collusive factors in the culture at large. Also paramount is the consistent return to the patient of the power to define meanings, by continually guiding him/her back and forth from the therapy dialogues to his/her internal authority in order to establish what ultimately feels valid. The patient's disagreements, protests, and accusations toward the therapist must be tolerated and explored to create a climate where trust and difference can coexist; this one element of the treatment disarms disso- ciative defenses for cult survivors in particular, and loosens their identifica- tions with the aggressor. The agency restored when authentic aspects of the self are freed from dissociated memories and omnipotent solutions to trauma confers the acquired power to search for and live one's own truth (Kafka, 1997). Psychotherapy's interpersonal reparations develop a self that will not be silenced or subordinated, a self that can subvert the dominant paradigms of social oppression rather than be subverted by them.

Notes

CHAPTER 1

1. Bremner and Brett (1997) found that dissociation in the face of trauma is a marker of long-term psychopathology; their results related to and supported Pierre Janet's (1889) turn-of-the century theories of dissociation.

2. The National Institute of Mental Health (NIMH) found that 97 percent of a sample of 100 MPD cases reported experiencing significant trauma in childhood; 83 percent reported being sexually abused, 75 percent reported being repeatedly physically abused, and 68 percent reported being both sexually and physically abused (Putnam, Guroff, Silberman, Braban, and Post, 1986). Other research findings (Bliss, 1984; Ross, Norton, and Wozney, 1989; Coons and Milsten, 1986; Ross et al., 1990), confirm sexual abuse—preponderantly incestuous and predominantly in tandem with extensive physical abuse—as the element most commonly reported by DID patients. Almost all abusive incidents examined by Putnam (1989) show extreme trauma involving sadism, torture, bondage, prostitution, isolation, severe punishment, and deprivation.

3. According to Kluft's (1996a) review of the DID literature, most child abuse is reported retrospectively in adulthood. Some studies, however, have been able either to document or corroborate independently a substantial number of reported abuse allegations (e.g., Coons, 1986; 1994; Hornstein and Putnam, 1992). These studies demonstrate that trauma can be documented in 95 percent of children and adolescents with DID and allied forms of DDNOS (dissociative disorder not otherwise specified). Ross's (1997) overview of the research across five major studies including over 700 patients, concludes that at least 88 percent of adult DID patients report childhood physical and/or sexual abuse at first assessment. (Most, incidentally, affirm continuous memory for some of the abuse throughout their lives, supporting Ross's contention that the stereotypical DID patient with no trauma memories at all before treatment reflects only a small minority of cases, and indeed may be a clue to iatrogenic, malingering, or factitious phenomena.) Ross's (1997) initial research on recantation reveals that most if not all DID patients in treatment (excepting those with either initial malingering, factitious, or iatrogenic presentations) toward integration do not recant their child abuse histories during or following therapy.

4. Secondarily, the individual can at once severely curtail and minimally preserve the capacity for reflectivity. Such depersonalized compromising (e.g., in observing self and other) has been noted to be among the major mechanisms of defense among survivors of Nazi concentration camps (Bluhm, 1999/1948).

5. Foote (1999) notes that the skeptical reaction to DID can largely be attributed to a specific set of transference/countertransference interactions that these patients tend to inspire in therapists. Comparing and contrasting the presentation, life histories, and underlying psychodynamics of DID and hysterical patients, Foote notes that it is the DID patient's experience of chronic interpersonal powerlessness that leads to presentation of symptoms in an unconvincing, "hysterical" manner: The "natural unconvincingness" of the DID patient is *not* the socially

adaptive interactional style of the high-functioning hysteric, says Foote, and, moreover, this style represents the DID individual's internalized expectation of agonizing impotence, often with associated rage and terror. He uses the term "pseudo-hysteria" to denote situations in which genuine psychiatric disorders such as PTSD or DID are perceived as hysterical productions.

6. See: Bremner et al. (1995; 1997); Southwick et al. (1993); Putnam (1999), Putnam and Trickett (1997), DeBellis et al. (1994a; 1994b; 1999); Charney et al. (1993); Krystal et al. (1996).

7. Personal clinical observation suggests that severe and chronic trauma (not unlike near-death experiences or chronic use of psychedelics) ruptures many kinds of psychological and neurophysiological thresholds and stimulus barriers, foreclosing some experiences and making way for others. The latter include subjectively compelling interface with "spirits" during and after specific traumas—sometimes the only sources of hope and help a patient has ever known. Whether such perceptions of benevolent "contacts" are construed as products of omnipotent fantasy, extensive hyperarousal and the vicissitudes of brain chemistry, and/or authentic mystical experience, working with severely dissociative patients requires open-mindedness and the willingness to temporarily suspend incredulity.

8. Braude (1995) has introduced terminology to categorize the enigmas of disordered awareness, disordered agency, epistemic barriers, and unusual self-ascription commonly found in the severe dissociative disorders. For example, a state is *indexical* when a person believes it to be his/her own (i.e., to be assignable to him/herself), *autobiographical* when a person experiences it as his/her own. Two or more self-states are *coreferential* when they may be ascribed to the same person, *cosensory* when they seem to be simultaneously aware of external events such as sights or sounds, *intraconscious* when they claim knowledge of the other's mental states such as feelings, memories, and/or beliefs; *coconsciousness* may reflect either cosensory and/or intraconscious features.

9. Hence, DID is predominantly a covert condition (Kluft, 1985). Its purest form is virtually isomorphic, occurring when a traumatized child creates another version of him/herself to hold traumatic or conflictual experience and/or to represent the wish to have been unaffected by it (Kluft, 1996a).

10. Rarely do single alter personalities operate without the copresence, support, or direction of others. What we call alters may actually be groups of parts operating in unison; some of our categories and labels for types still speak to the unitary conceptual approach to multiplicity inherent in our bias. In this connection, Putnam (1989) addresses the phenomenon of the "host," which is often equated with the presenting personality in treatment. An alter may actually be an alliance, a "social facade created by a more or less cooperative effort of several alters agreeing to pass as one" (p. 107). That alliance is easier to see in patients who do not dramatize their multiplicity and do not name and codify their alters; the pattern of blending and passing as one is more difficult to discern among those who have elaborated systems with large numbers of alters in complex relationships with one another, resembling three soap operas going on the same screen at once.

11. As Turner, McFarlane, and Van der Kolk (1996) have indicated, when shame of this kind dominates, avoidance reactions are pronounced and victims are likely to disclose their most traumatic experiences late in the course of treatment. Most DID patients will suffer in isolation for a long time even while firmly engaged in ongoing therapy.

12. Revisionist theorists like Haaken (1998) prefer to believe that oppressive cultural practices alone (i.e., independent of sexual violence) can evoke "storytelling" about incest, and that trauma/dissociation theorists in their quest to understand the literal are losing the symbolic. Although undoubtedly some public and private displays certainly fall into that category, *most* revelations about sexual abuse are hardly "storytelling" contrived for an audience—and severely dissociative individuals are not in the business of "concretizing cultural myths." On the contrary, the psyches of severely dissociative trauma survivors contain much of the culture's split-off knowledge of its own "sins" and crimes against humanity, making them exceedingly vulnerable scapegoats.

13. Discussing the suppression and censorship of the "Confusion of Tongues" paper, Rachman (1997) summarizes Ferenczi's brilliant early insights into sexual abuse: the robotlike obedience and emotional surrender of the child-victim in the face of domination and betrayal by the adult perpetrator; the development of adult characterological patterns from the child's use of dissociation to cope with severe early trauma; the child-victim's renunciation of his/her own reality testing to conform to the needs of caretakers/abusers; the presence of pervasive confusion in the mind of the victim as an overriding state, which results in the belief that the abuse was an act of love rather than exploitation for the adult's own gratification; and identification with the aggressor, leading to the shared pseudo-delusion that victim and perpetrator are in a mutually tender and beneficial relationship.

CHAPTER 2

1. The New Testament is more child-friendly. For example, Jesus preaches that "unless you change and become as little children, you shall never enter the Kingdom of Heaven" (Matthew 18:3); later when the apostles try to keep some children away from him, Jesus says: "Let the little children come to me" (Matthew 19:14). Paul (II Timothy 3:15) writes to Timothy (son of a Jewish mother and Greek father): "You have known the Holy Scriptures since your childhood," and so on.

2. The Society for the Prevention of Cruelty to Animals had intervened to stop the repeated physical abuse of a female child by her foster mother (Solnit, 1994; Weiner and Kurpius, 1995).

3. Fergusson and Mullen (1999), summarizing and integrating the results of a large number of child sexual-abuse prevalence studies, conclude that estimates suggest up to one-third of women may report exposure to unwanted sexual attention, with the majority of studies suggesting prevalence between 15 percent and 30 percent, with similar estimates reported for males (approximately 30 percent, estimates lying between 3 and 15 percent). According to Putnam (1999), the prevalence of child maltreatment in the United States has reached more than 1.6 million *confirmed* new cases per year. (Reports based on the annual survey by the National Committee to Prevent Child abuse [Wang and Daro, 1998] reveal that over 3 million allegations of child maltreatment were made to child-protective agencies nationwide.) Putnam's (1999) review of the breakdown of the confirmed cases reveals: 52 percent from neglect, 25 percent from physical abuse, 13 percent related to sexual abuse, and 10 percent from other sources. According to his review of the literature the number of children seriously injured due to abuse has quadrupled from 1986 to 1993. Briere (1992b) states that reported victimization rates jump to between 36 percent and 70 percent in clinical, hospital, and psychiatric settings, depending on the study.

4. According to a 1997 survey of adolescents conducted by the Commonwealth Fund (Schoen and Davis et al., 1998) one in eight (13 percent) high school boys had been physically or sexually abused or both. Two-thirds (66 percent) of boys who reported physical abuse said it occurred at home, and 68 percent reported that the abuser was a family member. Of those boys sexually abused, one-third (35 percent) said the abuse happened at home and less than half (45 percent) said the abuser was a family member. Approximately 21 percent (one in five) high school girls surveyed reported that she had been physically or sexually abused. The majority of the abuse occurred at home (53 percent) and more than once (65 percent). In their recent review of sexual abuse of male children and adolescents, Holmes and Slap (1998), like Fergusson and Mullen, conclude that such abuse of boys is common, but often goes undetected and untreated. Holmes and Slap found that although boys across the sociodemographic spectrum appear to be at risk for sexual abuse, the boys who were at highest risk were less than 13 years old, nonwhite, of low socioeconomic status, and living without their fathers. Typically, the abuse occurred outside of the home, was repeated, and involved penetration. Of particular concern was the finding that the number of children who report being exposed to acts of abuse that involve sexual penetration is as high as 13 percent for females and 11.3 percent for males, with the majority of studies reporting prevalence figures in the range of 5 percent to 10 percent. Although

females report an overall higher rate of sexual abuse compared to males, when it comes to the more severe forms of abuse involving penetration, the estimates do not vary widely between boys and girls (Fergusson and Mullen, 1999).

5. In one of his earlier comparative reviews of the research literature on child abuse, Finkelhor (1994) found that the studies were extremely variable in their scope and quality and that the variation in rates (found, for example between countries) probably does not accurately reflect variation in true prevalence as much as it reflects methodological limitations, sampling differences, and definition differences across studies. The influence of a society's overall consciousness about child abuse and dissociation issues on both the researcher's methods and interpretations and the response sets of the participants must be questioned consistently. (Prevalence rates range from a low of 2 percent reported in France, Great Britain, and Sweden to a high of 16 percent in the Netherlands, which is most comparable with the U.S. prevalence data. Countries in the middle prevalence range included Australia and New Zealand, Costa Rica, Canada, and Austria. Apparently the screening questions and interviewing sensitivity was most sophisticated in the Dutch study, where the highest rates were found.) According to most researchers (Briere, 1992a; Finkelhor, 1994; 1998; Enns et al., 1995; Oates, 1996; Fergusson and Mullen, 1999) the differences in findings from prevalence studies reflect some of the problems inherent in this research. These include heterogeneity among those who have been classified as sexually abused; indeterminacy in the criteria for defining abuse; the source of the sample (in terms of education, socioeconomic status, and ethnicity); the scope of the definition used in the survey; the upper age-limit of "child" (sometimes eighteen, sometimes fourteen); variations in the methods of questioning about abuse; sampling techniques (i.e., random sample, college students, community sample, sex of respondents); the response rate; and the accuracy of the respondents' memory. Oates (1996) notes the contrast between the high figures of prevalence studies with studies of reported incidence that tend to give lower figures. According to the reported incidence statistics, sexual abuse in the United States in 1993 was 5 cases per 1,000 children, with the incidence of *substantiated* cases revealing approximately 2 cases per 1,000 (Daro and McCurdy, 1993). In spite of the methodological flaws that might exist in prevalence studies or in the analysis of notification figures, Oates (1996) believes that the extreme difference between reported incidence and prevalence confirms the view that most child sexual abuse goes unreported. Fergusson and Mullen (1999) conclude that despite the debates about the true prevalence of abuse when less stringent definitions are applied, the prevalence of more *severe* forms of abuse involving penetration cannot be regarded as an inconsequential problem of childhood. These authors offer the example that if physically intrusive CSA only had a true prevalence rate of 3 percent, this would still mean that one child within each class of thirty schoolchildren in the U.S. would contain at least one child who was the victim of what is considered to be severe abuse.)

6. Especially since the failure of several important ritual-abuse day-care cases (e.g., in Manhattan Beach, California, and Jordan, Minnesota), articles condemning the reality or possibility of ritual abuse have appeared in magazines as varied as *The New Yorker, Harper's, Vanity Fair, National Review, Redbook, Mother Jones, Village Voice,* and *Playboy* (Jenkins, 1998). Further, a wave of debunking books (e.g., Jenkins, 1998; Hakken, 1998; Ofshe and Watters, 1994; Hacking, 1995; Kincaid, 1998) have been produced in recent years by academics (usually, but not always nonclinicians), all with rather acerbic and contemptuous approaches to the possibility of ritual abuse or other forms of organized perpetrator groups or networks of child exploitation.

7. This elevationist stance toward retractors often occurs without any consideration of the individual's complete psychiatric history complex overlapping dynamics of diagnostic comorbidity, factitious disorder, malingering, psychological and economic opportunism, not to mention the potentially powerful effects of posttherapy suggestive social influence (for example, from family members, lawyers, groups of false memory advocates or other recanters, and sensationalist media presentations). See Brown and Scheflin, 1999; Marmer, 1999; Brown, Frish-

holz, and Scheflin, 1999; Armstrong, 1999; Scheflin and Brown, 1999 for discussions of these issues.

8. Both cause and effect of the disinformation so destructive to patients and therapists alike are spurious generalizations based on a few poster-child cases, like this one from Jenkins (1998, p. 183): "Generally, a woman or teenage girl would consult a therapist for a personal problem like an eating disorder only to be convinced after some weeks or months that her real problem could be traced to an early history of ritual abuse in which her parents participated. The victim would sever connections with her family. . . ."

9. Former Representative Joseph P. Kennedy II claims that over 100,000 children are involved in child prostitution in the United States. "Frankly, most of my congressional colleagues have no idea that such an industry even exists. . . . We think of ourselves as civilized people living in modern times, yet child prostitution is a growing problem in both developing and developed countries" (1996, p. 2).

10. One of the biggest problems with child prostitution cases when they are prosecuted at all, according to Flores (1996), is that timely and efficient prosecution is rare; it typically takes months after an arrest for cases to get to trial. That means the pimp will be out on the streets almost immediately, and the child-victims are quite aware of this.

11. The Internet is, of course, an unsurpassed instrument for the distribution of kiddie porn ("chicken porn") (Muntarbhorn, 1996), which is generated both intra- and extrafamilially (Tyler and Stone, 1985). Until 1977, few states legally prohibited the use of children in obscene material or performances (Pierce, 1984). Back in the late 1980s, Crewdson (1988) wrote that the computer industry estimated that there were approximately 2,500 pedophile-related bulletin boards operating at any one time: "since they are mostly run from garages and spare bedrooms, it is impossible to keep an accurate account" (p. 104). In light of the incalculable increase in Internet–related child-abuse crime, a press release was recently issued by the Office of Justice Programs of the United States Attorney General's office announcing $2.5 million in grants would be given to help local law enforcement agencies combat Internet crimes against children (OJP, 2000).

12. Perhaps the most disturbing (and for many simply impossible to believe) part of child (and adult) pornography—the snuff-film industry—is still largely undocumented. According to some survivors' reports, a child can be kidnapped, tortured, raped, and murdered on videotape and the tape copied and distributed on the black market days or even weeks before his or her face even appears on a milk carton.

13. Approximately one-third of a national sample of psychologists reported that they had treated at least one case of ritual abuse (Jaroff, 1993). Braun and Grey (1987) estimate that about 28 percent of all patients with MPD have undergone ritual abuse; among inpatients the figure may go as high as 50 percent (Braun, 1989). In their national investigation of 270 cases of substantiated sexual abuse of 1,639 children in day care, Finkelhor, Williams, and Burns (1988) found that 13 percent of the cases involved allegations of ritual abuse.

14. Ritual abuse shares underlying dynamics with incestuous abuse (Russell, 1996; Herman, 1992), which also often involves torture and captivity. Indeed, Amnesty International's (1973) definition of political torture blurs the distinction between intra- and extrafamilial abuse—"the systematic and deliberate infliction of acute pain in any form by one person on another . . . in order to accomplish the purpose of the former against the will of the latter" (p. 31).

15. Numerous authors have described similar reports of other ritual actions including excreting on Bibles, defacing Christian images by raping children with crucifixes, publicly rejecting God and accepting Satan, engineering mock marriages to the devil or other malevolent deities, drinking blood, urine, feces, eating human flesh, being locked in cages or jails, being told that parents or siblings would be killed if they told anyone about the abuse, being held underwater, being threatened with guns and knives, being buried in the ground in coffins or "boxes," being injected with needles, bled, drugged, being photographed during the abuse, being tied upside down over a star or being hung from a pole or hook, being burned with candles,

being terrorized with snakes, spiders, or insects, having blood poured on their heads, hearing songs and chants, being forced to kidnap children from playgrounds, being given electric shocks, having observed animals being killed, having observed torture, mutilation, and murder of infants and children, being taken to churches, graveyards, other day-care centers, and other peoples' houses for sexual abuse and/or rituals, being threatened with supernatural powers (Noblitt and Perskin, 1995; Ross, 1995a; Ryder, 1994; Sinason, 1994; Smith, 1993; Young et al., 1991; Young, 1992; Faller, 1994; Waterman et al., 1993; Hudson, 1991; Bybee and Mowbray, 1993; Jonker and Jonker-Bakker, 1997).

16. Although some perpetrators operate out of pure malevolent instinct, others were trained in mind control in the course of their own abuse as children and/or systematically as apprentices to the abuse of others. Some patients have reported that their mind-control training was witnessed by groups of "doctors" with clipboards who were studying the methods of torture and brainwashing. During these training sessions these patients were trained to not see the "scientists" in the room or to see them as if they were behind a wall or a two-way mirror.

17. Smith (1993) presents data on 52 adults who claimed to be survivors of childhood ritual abuse and found that perpetrators were reportedly fathers (67 percent), mothers (42 percent), stepfathers (31 percent), stepmothers (23 percent), aunts (21 percent), uncles (27 percent), nonfamily member physicians (33 percent), nonfamily member clergy (17 percent), and nonfamily member teachers (17 percent). In her study of the occupations of family and nonfamily alleged perpetrators she found physicians (33 percent), teachers (25 percent), clergy (22 percent), police (15 percent). These findings were more or less consistent with an earlier study (Driscoll and Wright, 1991) that investigated the experience of 37 adult mental health patients who were alleged survivors of ritual abuse. In the latter study, perpetrators included fathers (63 percent), uncles (41 percent), mothers (38 percent), stepfathers (35 percent), stepmothers (22 percent). Other abusers included physicians (54 percent), neighbors (41 percent), friends and relatives (49 percent), church members (35 percent), police (27 percent), teachers (22 percent), morticians (19 percent).

18. Goodwin (1994) recounts the documented crimes of the Marquis de Sade to expose that plausibility: "What passions are detailed in story and deed? To mention a few: locking in cages, threatening with death, burying in coffins, holding under water, threatening with weapons, drugging and bleeding, tying upside down and burning, wearing of robes and costumes, staging of mock marriages, having victims witness torture, having them witness homicides, pouring or drinking of blood, and taking victims to churches and cemeteries. I mention these acts in particular among the 600 sadistic practices described in de Sade's book, because these are 15 of the 16 types of allegations found characteristically in children and adult psychiatric patients complaining of 'ritual abuse' in the 1980's and 1990's. The only one missing from de Sade's 1789 inventory is photography (not yet invented); its place is taken by use of peepholes and use of stages at the orgies, where each libertine could be seen to perform with his entourage of victims" (pp. 483–484).

19. According to Grand (2000), the perpetrator experiences his/her greatest triumph and concealment when the victim is coerced into perpetration and complicity. In such conditions, the real history of the perpetrator's culpability is occluded by the victim's/survivor's "shared monstrosity.... It is a tribute to the perpetrator's brilliance that the survivor's coerced transgressions obscure questions of agency, responsibility, guilt, and innocence. In the survivor's breach of his own moral integrity, the perpetrator locates a mirror for his own disavowed culpability" (p. 93). "The victim is haunted by her own moral failure, and the perpetrator is cleansed and obscured in the survivor's guilt" (pp. 94–95).

20. The most recent and conclusive review of victim-perpetrator relationships (Fergusson and Mullen, 1999), indicates that contrary to popular belief, the majority of episodes of child sexual abuse do not involve immediate family members (between approximately 6 percent and 32 percent of CSA incidents were committed by family members including parents, stepparents, and siblings; the weighted average estimate from the series of studies reviewed suggested

that overall 10.4 percent of CSA incidents involved close family members). Rather, most sexual abuse is committed by other acquaintances who are known to the victim (between 20 percent and 50 percent of CSA perpetrators are described in this category, with a weighted average estimate overall of 47.8 percent). These authors also found that when sexual abuse did involve family members it was more often of a *severe* and *recurrent* nature. (This fact may explain the popular belief that most common forms of CSA involve intrafamilial abuse because these incidents are more likely to come to attention in various ways.) This review also found stepparents to be at far higher risk (approximately ten times higher) of being perpetrators than biological parents.

21. Based on the estimated number of victims reported by state inmates in 1991, the more than 60,000 violent offenders who had child victims may have had as many as 95,000 victims. Three out of four child victims were female. More than 40 percent of child victims of incarcerated violent offenders suffered forcible rape, injury, or death as a result of the crime. About one in seven child victimizers reported that the victim died as a consequence of the violent crime; death was substantially more likely to be reported when the victim was an adult.

22. Two comprehensive studies (Abel et al., 1987; Becker and Quinsey, 1993) found extremely high rates of sexual offending. Of 561 perpetrators in Abel and colleagues' sample, there were a total of 291,737 paraphilic acts with a total of *195,407* victims. Of those, molesters of girls reported an average of 19.8 victims each; molesters of boys reported an average of 150.2 victims each. The numbers of victims per abuser documented by the legal system differ substantially from those acknowledged via anonymous self-reporting: for example, Groth, Longo, and Mc-Fadin (1982) found that incarcerated sex offenders admitted anonymously to two to five times more offenses than had come to the attention of the criminal justice system; Weinrott and Saylor (1991) found that a sample of 67 child molesters incarcerated for molesting 136 victims admitted to more than 8,000 sexual acts with 959 children.

23. "Distortions provide offenders with an interpretive framework that permits them to construe the behaviors and motives of their victims as sexual and allows them to justify and excuse to themselves (and others) their offending behavior" (Howitt, 1995, p. 93).

24. In these studies, researchers document that over one-half of the abusers had repeated early grades in school or been placed in special education classes, and about one-third suffered from documented neurocognitive impairment.

25. The diverse array of theories of pedophilia include: sexual learning theory, precondition models, cognitive distortion theory, psychodynamic (including Jungian) approaches, feminist theories of pedophilia as gender politics (including the role of pornography), theories of pedophilia as a biological quirk, and theories relating pedophilia to disturbances in fantasy including influences from pornography, cultural myths, and the media Howitt, 1995).

26. Estimates of the percentage of child sexual-abuse perpetrators who report being sexually abused in childhood typically range only from 20 percent to 30 percent (Freund, Watson, and Dickey; Murphy and Smith, 1996).

27. The abuser, having experienced the extremes of powerlessness, helplessness, lovelessness, and rage, at the hands of early caretakers, fantasizes the fetish as a weapon with which to beat the parent at his/her own game (Eigen, 1984).

28. In their review of eight major studies of gender issues and victim-perpetrator dynamics conducted during the past decade, Fergusson and Mullen (1999) found that for *female victims* of child sexual abuse between 92 percent and 99 percent of the perpetrators were men, while for *male victims* between 63 percent and 86 percent of the perpetrators were male. In their research on documented child abuse in day-care settings, Finkelhor and Williams (1988) found that female perpetrators were much more common in child-care settings than elsewhere: approximately 20 percent of the abuse of both boys and girls was by a female perpetrator acting alone or with other females, and approximately 33 percent of the abuse involved female perpetrators acting in concert with male perpetrators. Greenfield's (1996) survey of incarcerated criminals reveals that males were the perpetrator in 97 percent of cases. In Groth's (1979) study of con-

victed male sex offenders, of the 60 percent who claimed to have been victimized in childhood, 20 percent of the victimization was committed by females. In the Burgess et al. (1987) study of serial rapists, *of the 56* percent who claimed to have been sexually abused, 40 percent reported female perpetrators. For detailed discussion about female perpetrators, see Elliott (1994).

CHAPTER 3

1. In actual clinical work with dissociative patients, understanding the exaggeration of external reality as a defense against intrapsychic conflict (Inderbitzin and Levy, 1994) must be balanced against the dissociation of painful reality, the use of intrapsychic conflict as a defense against historical reality, and the disturbing intrapsychic fantasies that arise from traumatic experiences. Neither the use of fantasy as a defense against reality nor the use of reality as a defense against fantasy should come to dominate the field or our clinical formulations about trauma and dissociation.

2. Revulsion and disbelief sometimes prevent clinicians from asking questions and listening effectively (Ganzarain and Buchele, 1989). In the psychoanalytic community, the intergenerational transmission of blind spots regarding sexual abuse (Kramer, 1994) and severe dissociative disorders has produced contemptuous, marginalizing references to this patient population— "bad borderlines," "bad" hysterics, litigious feminist zealots, easily suggestible patients with identity diffusion, fantasy-prone confabulators, disability and welfare chiselers, manipulators, attention-seekers, liars, members of "a cult of victimization" exercising "the abuse excuse."

3. The iatrogenic hypothesis has never been empirically validated (Kluft, 1989; Kluft and Foote, 1999; Ross, 1997), and there is not one documented case of iatrogenic MPD in the clinical literature; still, it is repeatedly invoked in the ongoing debates about DID, recovered memory, and trauma therapy. Although some critics have argued that DID is a North American culture-bound condition (for example, Fahy, 1988), Kluft and Foote (1999) describe how numerous studies including cohorts from the United States, Canada, the Netherlands, Norway, and Turkey consistently demonstrate comparable findings that previously undiagnosed DID occurs in 3 to 6 percent of psychiatric inpatients and 5 to 18 percent of patients in substance-abuse treatment settings. According to these authors, if DID were a culture-bound syndrome, predominantly iatrogenic and primarily determined by social psychological factors, then one would expect variations across cultures with more DID patients being found in those nations in which the disorder had become part of the professional cultural idioms and in which professionals would presumably have become more "adept" at inducing (or implanting) the features of DID. Research has consistently documented the role of trauma-related events in precipitating dissociative features and dissociative disorders, however. Ross (1997) claims that "the quality of argument used by DID skeptics is evidence of the failure of liberal arts education in the English-speaking world. None of the published critiques of DID have any base in research or data" (p. 226). Kluft (1996a) deconstructs their circularity: "Since DID cannot be legitimate, it must be artifactual, and then it is merely a matter of assigning blame for the initiation and perpetuation of the clinical picture" (p. 354). While recognizing the possibility that extremely bad therapy could conceivably create an iatrogenic pathway to some of the patterns of DID, and while questioning the creation of analogs of alter personalities among college students as proof of the iatrogenic hypothesis, both Ross and Kluft continue to caution therapists to be aware of the potential for secondary gains for some patients from displaying DID symptoms and, accordingly, to avoid amplifying them unnecessarily.

4. McHugh (1997), a particularly vituperative critic, contends that the "twisted logic" of the DID literature has "deranged the discourse of psychiatry and cultivated a Sherlock Holmes fantasy among many psychotherapists" (p. ix). Piper (1997) likens support for the MPD/DID paradigm to psychiatry's embrace of lobotomy and he warns that it may drain the lifeblood of, and permanently damage the public trust in, the wisdom of the mental health professions.

5. A document issued by the U.S. Advisory Board on Child Abuse and Neglect Worldwide (cited in Cavaliere, 1995), and presented to Congress and the Clinton administration, concluded that "at least 2000 children a year—five each day—die at the hands of their parents or caretakers; more pre-school children are killed by their parents than die from falls, choking, suffocation, drowning or fires" (p. 34). Moreover, as the U.S. Advisory Report indicates, some 18,000 children annually are permanently disabled and another 142,000 are seriously injured from severe abuse.

6. Recent breakthroughs in brain research reveal alarming dimensions to trauma's effect on mind and body, particularly in young children. Developmental traumatologist DeBellis and colleagues (1999) recently documented that the overwhelming stress of maltreatment experiences in childhood is associated with adverse brain development: specifically, PTSD subjects had smaller intracranial and cerebral volumes than matched controls; the total midsagittal area of the corpus collosum and middle and posterior regions remained smaller, while right, left, and total lateral ventricles were proportionately larger than controls after adjustment for intracranial volume. Brain volume robustly and positively correlated with age of onset of PTSD trauma and negatively correlated with duration of abuse. Results of a prospective longitudinal study of 166 abused girls age six to fifteen conducted by Putnam (1999) found that compared to matched controls, the abused girls demonstrated permanent biological system abnormalities (hypothalamic-pituitary-adrenal axis, sympathetic nervous system, physical growth and development, immune system function, hypothalamic-pituitary-gonadal axis). These biological changes relate to the psychopathologies of affect regulation, attentional problems, and possibly disturbances in sense of self or identity. Directly experiencing and/or witnessing violence can alter the brain's anatomy and chemistry in ways that inhibit learning, concentration, attachment, empathy; consequences include impairment of the immune system and shortening of the life span. Accordingly the results of a study by Felitti and colleagues (1998) investigating the relationship between childhood abuse (and household dysfunction) and adult medical problems found a strong graded relationship between breadth of exposure to abuse and multiple risk factors for several of the leading causes of death in adulthood (including ischemic heart disease, cancer, chronic lung disease, skeletal fractures, liver disease, and HIV). In essence, experience can become biology, so the traumatization of children is a public health and human rights issue, not just a law-enforcement problem.

7. Discussing the painful irony in the dissociative disorders field when in the past decade the mental health professions have at their disposal an unprecedented amount of knowledge about how to diagnose and treat patients with severe dissociative disorders, Kluft and Foote (1999) note that profound impediments continue to exist limiting optimal utilization of this information in the service of patient care (for example, lack of widespread knowledge about dissociative disorders in the professional community, ongoing skepticism about the legitimacy of the disorder, the recent backlash against trauma treatment and traumatic memories, the rise of managed care with its devaluation of intensive forms of psychotherapy, the lack of mental health research funds available to study severe dissociative disorders, and the ongoing dominance within the mental health professions of paradigms that do not accord a place of value and importance—including in training curricula of the mental health professions' educational endeavors—to traumatic stress and the spectrum of disorders resulting from interpersonal violence). According to these authors, these forces have a detrimental effect on the well-being and treatment of patients with DID and other severe dissociative disorders and compromise their access to appropriate care, thereby revictimizing a victim population.

8. According to Ross (1995b) the name of the disorder was changed (in discussions of the American Psychiatric Association committee revising the *Diagnostic and Statistical Manual (DSM IV)* "in an effort to neutralize the pervasive fixed negative cathexis in psychiatry of the term multiple personality disorder. . . . Whether this will prove to be a successful political strategy or not, time will tell" (p. 66). In his discussion comparing *DSM IV* with *ICD–10*, Ross articulates the highly political nature of attitudes, inclusion criteria, and classification of certain disorders,

which he views as ideologically—not scientifically—based; he suggests that *DSM IV* still suffers from "the vestigial effects of Freudian theory" (p. 66).

9. Discussing the debates over the legitimacy of ritual abuse, Noblitt and Perskin (1995) explain the many arguments supporting the existence of ritual abuse. Among the most important are ample historical and anthropological evidence that ritual abuse has occurred in a variety of cultures throughout history; confessions by some perpetrators of ritual abuse and other cult-based criminal activity; convictions in criminal cases and guilty verdicts in civil cases against individuals accused of ritual abuse; cases of ritual murder (e.g., Matamoros) are a matter of public record, as are cult abuses by for example, the People's Temple, the Branch Davidians; survivors from all over report similar ritual, torture, and mind-control experiences, and respond to exactly the same trigger words, programmed cues, and invocations.

10. Bowart (1994) identifies problems with FBI Special Agent Ken Lanning's (1992) public conclusions, often cited (by backlash writers), that there is no evidence of any truth to reports of ritual abuse: Lanning's story and conclusions have changed; the FBI cannot find abuse because they won't come to a crime scene to see it when called (sometimes they arrest the complainant); Lanning admits (in a *Vanity Fair* dialogue with Leslie Bennets, 1993, p. 42) to having never interviewed one survivor, to confining his search for evidence to conversations with other law enforcement officers and a few therapists. Bowart further reports that Lanning rushed out to interview "several dozen" victims as soon as his "oversight" was pointed out, only to conclude that there was still no evidence of any truth to their reports of ritual abuse. Given the numerous testimonies of survivors suggesting that a large, well-organized cryptocracy is using mind control to guard its secrets (Bowart, 1994; Noblitt and Perskin, 1995; Ryder, 1994) and that law enforcement agencies such as the FBI are part of that cryptocracy, Lanning's arguments—citing the difficulties of successfully committing large-scale conspiracy crimes and the limitations of human nature in terms of maintaining cult secrets—hardly hold water.

11. The phenomena of collusion and collaboration are so central to the social facilitation of child abuse and to the maintenance of the internal world of severely dissociative patients—who internalize and identify as much with collaboration and collusion as with "the aggressor"—that we must be as interested in elucidating forms of collaboration as we are in understanding forms of perpetration. In fact, among the most recalcitrant, self-defeating aspects of DID patients' personality systems are those part-selves or alters insistent on denying negative realities. Much of their "psychotic blindness" is rooted in their internalization of the disavowal, dismissiveness, and incredulity projected by their nonabusing or colluding caretakers and by family members and the society at large; it is bolstered by their adamant desire to be normal, regardless of the intrapsychic cost in self-betrayal. The tenacity of these internalized collaborator parts of severely dissociative trauma survivors is greater, although subtler, than that of acting-out parts associated with identification with the aggressor. *Collaboration* is defined as "a cooperation with an enemy invader," *collusion* as "a secret agreement for fraudulent or illegal purposes," and *complicity* as "the fact or state of being an accomplice; a partnership in wrongdoing" (Webster, 1989).

12. For others, the abuse of a daughter or son may break open years of denial; realization and action may save both parent and child, ending collaboration.

13. A few studies (Brosig and Kalichman, 1992; Kim, 1986) of mental health professionals' compliance with mandatory reporting of child-abuse laws show that more than 30 percent of clinicians sometimes suspect that one of their cases involves child maltreatment but fail to report it. Nationally, child protective services are under siege (explosive increases in cases, poor staff morale, public blame for the failure of the system as a whole), and constrained by limited resources despite the legal requirement that all reports be investigated (Melton et al., 1995).

14. Literature reviews (e.g., Everson and Boat, 1989) cite documented prevalence rates of false allegations ranging from 2 to 50 percent, and these wide discrepancies have been attributed to biased and small samples in prior studies.

15. Peterson and Briggs (1997) studied problems related to asking of "specific" questions when interviewing children about trauma. They found that preschool children are much less

likely to be veridical when they say "no," as they may do to influence the interviewer's evaluation of them, because they cannot remember, because they do not understand the referent being queried, because young children like the word no, because rapport is not well established, because the child wants to agree with an adult, or because the child wants the questioning terminated. Hence when young children deny a queried proposition they are often seriously misrepresenting the truth of what actually occurred, or their answers could potentially be manipulated because of their syntactic, intellectual, or social confusion. Peterson and Briggs conclude that, since yes/no questions are often used by law enforcement personnel and others asking about forensically relevant events, the risks that children will deny that child abuse has taken place must be taken into account.

16. Sorenson and Snow (1991) investigated 116 confirmed cases of child sexual-abuse disclosures. They found that in 22 percent of the cases, children recanted their allegations, but that 92 percent of those who recanted eventually reaffirmed their abuse allegations.

CHAPTER 4

1. Normal and pathological multiplicity define a continuum that extends from fluid movement, healthy dynamic interplay, and simultaneous awareness of multiple self-states in varying relationships to one another, to the fragmentation-disturbances of severe dissociative disorders, which always involve a collapse of flexibility, paradoxical experiencing (Bromberg, 1994; Schwartz, 1994; Pizer, 1992; 1996a; Davies, 1996a; 1996b), and a "scotomatous narrowing of consciousness"(Davies, 1996a, p. 566). By extension, unconscious life is conceptualized as dissociatively based, rather than as primarily repression-based.

2. Bromberg (1994, p. 520) eloquently describes the dissociative dialectic between knowing and not knowing: "Where drastically incompatible emotions or perceptions are required to be cognitively processed within the same relationship and such processing is adaptationally beyond the capacity of the individual to contain . . . within a unitary self-experience, one of the competing algorithms is hypnoidally denied access to consciousness to preserve sanity and survival. When ordinary adaptational adjustment to the task at hand is not possible, dissociation comes into play. The experience that is causing the incompatible perception and emotion is unhooked from the cognitive processing system and remains raw data . . . cognitively unsymbolized within that particular self-other representation except as a survival reaction."

3. One important corollary is the relationship between childhood violence and adolescent or adult entrance into prostitution: from 60 percent to 90 percent of those in prostitution were sexually assaulted in childhood (Harlan, Rodgers, and Slattery, 1981; Murphy, 1993; Silbert and Pines, 1983; Giobbe, 1991). From 62 percent to 90 percent of women in prostitution have been physically battered in childhood (Bagley and Young, 1987; Silbert and Pines, 1981; Giobbe, 1991). Hunter (1994) reports on a study of more than a hundred survivors of prostitution at the Council for Prostitution Alternatives in Portland: 85 percent reported a history of incest, 90 percent a history of physical abuse, and 98 percent a history of emotional abuse. Sixty-seven percent of prostitutes interviewed in five countries (South Africa, Thailand, Turkey, Zambia, and the United States) met diagnostic criteria for PTSD (Farley et al., 1998).

4. Bromberg's emphasis, from the relational perspective, on staying the same while changing is paralleled by Briere's (1996) pragmatic trauma-theory emphasis on balancing safety and engagement in the treatment of sexual abuse survivors: "good therapy must acknowledge and honor the survivor's competing needs to maintain safety and inner stability, while at the same time, being open to information and experiences so that he or she may heal and grow" (p. 112).

5. Caruth (1995) describes one of several moral dilemmas at the heart of the difficult task of recognition and reparation of trauma. "How do we help relieve the suffering of victims, and learn to understand the nature of suffering, without eliminating the force and truth of the reality that trauma survivors face and quite often try to transmit to us? . . . The difficulty of listening and responding to traumatic stories in a way that does not lose their impact, that does not

reduce them to clichés or turn them all into versions of the same story, is a problem that remains central to the task of therapists, literary critics, neurobiologists, and filmmakers alike" (1995, p. vii).

6. I felt this to be a vivid illustration of what Bromberg (1995a) calls the patient's need to "stay the same while changing."

CHAPTER 5

1. "One simply never talks to an alter" (McHugh, 1995, p. 114); "When you want a particular behavior to stop, you stop reinforcing it" (Loftus, 1995, p.208); "Paying attention to the alters does not always make them disappear" (ibid.)—as if such disappearing per se were the goal of therapy.

2. See Boon (1997), Van der Hart and Boon (1997), and Kluft (1999a) for discussions of supportive versus uncovering therapy for DID patients, and for a review of the prognostic criteria for making decisions over whether (and when) to proceed with trauma work.

3. The dichotomy between those who use hypnosis and those who do not is better bridged when therapy is defined as facilitating a more fluid and creative relationship for the patient with self and others. Most DID patients are so gifted at self-hypnosis—even to the extent of self-inducing impermeable trance states bordering on the autistic—that orchestrated hypnotic interventions may not be necessary.

4. These formulations are products of a relational revisioning of the notion of neutrality where the effects of the therapist's influences are regarded as inevitable and working with the dynamics of reciprocal influence is regarded as essential to moderate the intrusiveness of the therapist's values and beliefs and to temper the therapist's use of power over the patient in any way.

5. This view corresponds to Ogden's (1989) description of how a more primitive mode of experiencing (the paranoid-schizoid mode, for example) may be useful in certain situations and may inform and help articulate other modes (e.g., the depressive).

6. Within each of these essential aspects of the traumatized self there are solid and immovable structures of aggression organized around attachments and identifications with perpetrators (as well as islands of insight, self-soothing, and self-protection that appear both mystical and transcendent in their wisdom and serenity).

7. Many theorists (Herman, 1992; Ross, 1989; 1997; Putnam, 1989; Harvey, 1996; Kluft, 1998; 1999b) posit systematic stage models of treatment to guide both clinicians and patients through the complexities of the treatment process. Most of the systems break treatment down into early, middle, and late phases (for example, Herman's "safety stage," "remembrance and mourning stage," and "reconnection stage"). One of the most inclusive and articulated in terms of guiding the treatment of complex posttraumatic and dissociative disorders is the model proposed by Chu (1992b; 1998): early stage—focusing on self-care and symptom control, acknowledgment of trauma and its effects, maintaining functioning, verbal expressivity, development of capacity for healthy relatedness; middle stage—defined by exploration and abreactive work, breakdown of denial and dissociative defenses, and development of new perspectives about the past, the self, and relationships, and often including mourning and grieving, which extend into the final treatment phase; late stage—reflecting consolidating gains and increasing skills in creating healthy interactions with the world, self-empowerment and self-confidence, and an ability to move forward in the world relatively unencumbered by the past.

8. Discussing the confusion in the field over the catch-all word *abreaction* and ultimately recommending its abandonment in favor of more appropriate and specific terminology, Van der Hart and Steele (2000) summarize the most frequent usages: reactivated traumatic memories are called *spontaneous abreactions*; the treating or processing of traumatic memories refers to *planned abreactions*; the products of gradual, carefully paced work on trauma are called *fractionated abreaction*; therapy patients are helped to *abreact* their traumatic experiences. Van der Hart and Steele note that the dissociative disorder field prefers *spontaneous abreactions* while the post-

traumatic stress disorders field speaks of *flashbacks* and more recently also of intrusions, intrusive recall, or intrusive traumatic memories (e.g., Van der Kolk, McFarlane, and Weisaeth, 1996); however, when the term *flashback* is used, it is often unclear whether the author is referring to its visual, sensorimotor, or intrusive dimensions or just how encompassing the phenomena might be. Van der Hart and Steele favor *traumatic memories,* which they view as "representations of experiences that are either not integrated or insufficiently integrated in consciousness, memory, and identity, and thus are clearly dissociative in nature" (p. 4).

9. To represent all work with regressive states, memory material, or any posttraumatic affect as dangerous and ill-advised is to *mis*represent it, even though excessive abreactions (those "conducted" or "directed" by well-intended, overzealous, naïve, or incompetent clinicians) can indeed lead to losses, temporary or long term. It is important to note here that *failure* to access and rework past traumas can also lead to losses in functioning.

10. A flashback is defined by Sonnenberg (1985, p. 5) as "an altered state of consciousness in which the individual believes he or she is again experiencing the traumatic event." Sonnenberg notes that in spite of its dramatic manifestations, a full-blown flashback is only one point on a spectrum of more or less subtle alterations in consciousness experienced by individuals suffering from various forms of posttraumatic stress disorder.

11. Van der Hart and his colleagues (1993) describe a three-stage process (synthesis, realization, and integration) for moderating abreactions: in the *synthesis* phase, the therapist guides the patient to associate elementary and fragmented psychological phenomena (e.g., sensations, affects, behaviors, thoughts, images, etc.) into more complex and coherent mental structures; in the *realization* phase, the patient develops increased ability to give autobiographical accounts (rather than sensorimotor and behavioral reenactments) of his/her past trauma, becomes aware that the trauma is indeed over, and is able to assign meaning to the past experience in such a way that s/he has some understanding of the implications of the event(s) for his/her past, present, and future existence; *integration* phase of abreaction refers to the ongoing process of returning to various aspects of the trauma and its consequences to redefine its meanings within the patient's autobiographical self.

12. The healing effects of fantasies of retaliation or fantasies of forgiveness or notions about healing the perpetrators are more powerful if they arise spontaneously after frozen trauma has been unfrozen, relived, and then worked through in one way or another. If such fantasies are prompted before the painful memories are revisited, they may bolster dissociation rather than help restore unity in the traumatized, dissociative self.

13. In the dissociative disorders, some alternative, independent, mutually exclusive ego- or self-states are associatively unavailable and/or antagonistic to each other. Which one predominates depends on the patient's emotional condition, on whether traumatic memories have been stimulated, on current life circumstances, and on the specific transference/countertransference patterns operating at the time (Davies and Frawley, 1991).

14. Among the most useful of these models with clear application to most severely dissociative trauma survivors is Harvey's (1996) "ecological" view of trauma therapy. According to Harvey, the primary elements of the recovery and integration process include: establishing authority over the remembering process; integrating memory and affect; developing affect tolerance; mastering symptoms and distressing stimuli; developing self-esteem and self-cohesion; developing and repairing relational capacities, including the ability to negotiate realistic attachments; and developing the capacity for meaning-making, including mourning the traumatic past and imbuing it somehow with life-affirming and self-affirming meanings.

CHAPTER 6

1. Such respect for the patient's subjectivity is of course inconsistent with the insistent avoidance and suppression of alter personalities and dissociative symptoms enjoined by Loftus (1995) and other supporters of the false memory syndrome movement, who fear reification of the disorder. They define a willingness to work with DID on its own terms, including talking

with alter personalities, as representative of the negative influence of therapists (Loftus, 1995; McHugh, 1993a; 1993b; Brenneis, 1997; Ofshe and Watters, 1994); they do not address the influence and domination involved in denying the legitimacy of the patient's memories or his/her subjectively compelling experience of alter personalities. The suggestion (Loftus, 1993; Loftus and Ketcham, 1994) that avoiding a patient's dissociative aspects will result in that patient's suppressing posttraumatic behavior can be viewed as countertransferential acting out and as concretizing traumatic relational paradigms of subjugation; moreover, it may lead to retraumatization. ("Therapists who are skeptical about MPD but partially accept its reality often talk about strengthening the patient and eliminating the need for the alter personalities, when what they are actually doing is reinforcing the degree of separation between the host and other alter[s]" [Ross, 1995b, p. 133].) Finally, dissociation is not in any case something to be eradicated or conditioned out of existence. In the transitional zone of the therapy relationship, the realness or falseness of the part-selves is not a central issue; it is only central for the skeptics and the legalists who require a world organized into absolute truths and absolute lies.

2. Clinicians disagree about the similarities between DID and borderline personality disorder (Fink and Golinkoff, 1990; Kemp, Gilvertson, and Torem, 1988; Ross, 1989; Young, 1988). Many DID patients meet BPD diagnostic criteria—with the regrettable result that DID critics accuse DID specialists of creating a disorder that is merely an epiphenomenon of BPD. The position that DID patients are essentially borderlines-run-amok often hinges on dismissing the veracity of the trauma-based etiology of DID. Chu (1996), discussing the fact that many BPD patients report extensive histories of childhood abuse (emotional, physical, and sexual) and profound neglect as well as the witnessing of violence, concludes that it is not trauma that produces borderline disorder but the accompanying gross disruptions of familial attachments and the massive failures in appropriate caregiving and protection. This book shares Ross's (1997) view that BPD should be regarded as a trauma disorder that entails the use of many of the forms of dissociation used by DID patients (not, however, excessive dissociation of knowledge), but to a lesser extent. In order to articulate the intrinsic overlap between the two more precisely, Ross (1997) recommends that future research identify three subgroups: DID with BPD, DID without BPD, and BPD without DID. According to Ross, neither DID patients nor borderlines have anything particularly wrong with their personalities: they both have dissociative disorders involving numerous psychic functions, and both DID and borderline personality are features of chronic trauma disorders in the majority of patients treated by mental health professionals. If and when the dissociative anxieties and depressive symptoms of the alleged borderline patient are successfully treated the "borderline" personality will melt away. Likewise, if and when the DID patient's addictions, underlying needs for dissociation, and traumatic attachments are addressed, the borderline features will dissipate, and the "management" of the patient can turn into effective treatment. Ross (1997) describes how DID patients typically fall into one of three Axis II groups: (1) those with no serious character pathology or management problems where only occasional or no inpatient care is required; (2) an intermediate group with more severe Axis I and II pathology early in treatment but a favorable prognosis; and (3) a poor-prognosis group where character pathology and treatment-resistant Axis I symptoms predominate, and where mental health resource utilization is high. See Kluft (1994a; 1994b) for discussion of treatment trajectories in DID patients, which essentially parallels Ross's (1997) findings; Kluft has developed the Dimensions of Therapeutic Movement Instrument (DTMI)—to assess (and track) DID patients' prognosis and progress. In examining Axis II and prognosis issues in the treatment of DID, Ross finds that "An important consequence of the DID diagnosis is that many people regarded as high-character pathology/poor prognosis cases by other psychiatrists prove to have a good prognosis when the DID and the childhood trauma are addressed systematically by a skilled treatment team" (p. 134).

3. Personal clinical experience reveals that the developmental trajectory from domination, disavowal, and dissociation toward recognition either between alters (or self-states) and in the individual's relationship with his/her self as a whole passes through (or becomes fixed at one

of) four basic developmental stages: *Noticing* (limited self-observation, inconsistent memory, minimal pattern recognition or insight); *Acknowledging* (intellectual insight, more continuous memory, curiosity with minimal affective engagement); *Embracing* (affective resonance, internal empathy, self-forgiveness, consolidated memories, capacity for intrapsychic conflict); and *Integrating* (psychological communion, an integration of wisdom and compassion, dissolution of all dissociative barriers).

CHAPTER 7

1. Winnicott's (1951, p. 2) seminal paper on "Transitional Objects and Transitional Phenomena" identifies "an intermediate area of experiencing, to which inner reality and external life both contribute, . . . [that] shall exist as a resting-place for the individual engaged in the perpetual human task of keeping inner and outer reality separate yet interrelated." Many psychoanalytic theorists believe that the potential for creative play, intersubjectivity, and the use of fantasy and imagination for creative problem solving and other important developmental achievements are the result of the individual's capacity for transitional experiencing.

2. The presence or absence of a stuffed animal in the room may not be the only observation to be made about it—independent of such iatrogenic situations as when a therapist refuses to allow it into the office and a stuffed animal becomes the basis of a power struggle, or when a therapist inadvertently reinforces the patient's narcissistic investment in separateness by instigating excessive play therapy with child-alters.

3. Evidence reviewed by Whalen and Nash (1996) reveals that fantasy-proneness is only moderately correlated with DID, and recent research by Leavitt (1997) reveals that patients who recover memories of abuse in psychotherapy are less suggestible than other psychiatric patients.

4. Brenneis (1997) and Haaken (1998) propose in contrast that many of the transference manifestations, including aggressive ones, of alleged trauma survivors and DID patients are actually the result of invasive, controlling, and inappropriate therapeutic techniques visited by a zealous practitioner on a malleable patient. Brenneis insists that many of the posttraumatic symptoms are the patient's way of saying that s/he feels mistreated and abused by the therapist's interventions—which is entirely possible (and not only in DID- or trauma-oriented therapies), especially when the therapist dominates with his/her point of view and leaves little room for other ones or for protest or for multiple narratives. The bulk of disturbed aggressive responses of DID patients, however, are based on profound rage, suppressed protest responses, lack of integration and maturation of the aggressive drive, enactments of the original traumatic relational paradigms within the transference, and therapists' errors other than indoctrination (e.g., empathic failures, poor timing and pacing, and unbalanced treatment alliances that do not take all of the patient's alter personalities into account, etc.). It is important that all therapists discriminate between unconscious communications and reenactments that reveal the patient's camouflaged feelings toward the therapist and those that reveal as yet unsymbolized, or unformulated, dissociated aspects of prior relational or traumatic experience. Sometimes both are going on at once, and the therapy dyad must enter a long period of mutual reflection and collaboration to untie all the knots.

5. Howell (1997) points out how an unconscious need for resonance can lead masochistic aspects of the dissociative self to form bonds with antisocial others.

6. Grand (2000) describes the result of situations in which trauma victims are welcomed back into the perpetrator's or perpetrators' "approving embrace" following moral transgression. Under conditions where the victim's own torture ceases following the moral transgression (Grand refers to this coerced perpetration as "the bestial gesture," p. 113), and if the victim had no cohorts with whom to make a reparative gesture, and particularly if this annihilation occurred in early childhood, the capacity for healthy guilt may be permanently eradicated. According to Grand, this developmental deficit is not merely the result of identification with the aggressor

with its attending states of terror, pain, and confusion. Rather, it is due to the victim's inventing of an empathic other in the perpetrator who becomes the victim's only mirroring object, the only human link; the only outlet for the victim's need to make a reparative gesture is the perpetrator.

CHAPTER 8

1. Based on my own clinical experience and observations, and contrary to the allegations of critics who fail to understand the power of trauma-bonding, the abuse survivor is more likely to become a protector and caretaker of the perpetrator and family system (or pimp) than s/he is to initiate confrontations or lawsuits or even to leave home and break connections—(*viz.*, cases cited by Cheit [1999] and Gartner [1999], in which abused children as adults could not override the trauma bond [or did so and then, in the face of a guilty verdict, attempted to recant] when asked to testify against their perpetrator-fathers in accusations brought by others). I have never met or consulted on a severely traumatized dissociative patient who did not have at least one powerful alter identified with, or at the very least with a profoundly protective attitude toward, his/her perpetrators.

2. Many dissociative trauma survivors of organized perpetrator groups report that medical professionals were often actively involved in the groups' activities and were utilized by group leaders to perform emergency surgeries and other medical interventions on traumatized children. These interventions were designed to disguise evidence of the abuse or to save the life of a child whose death might have brought suspicion onto the cult or perpetrator group. Finally, many survivors report that medical professionals were used in mind-control training sessions since they had the skills and means of measuring alterations in brain waves, breathing, heart rates, and so on. important in evaluating optimal conditions for various aspects of coercive thought reform and brainwashing.

3. Examples of the truths tacitly agreed on include the abuse was the child's fault because of his/her behavior, personality, or gender ("Girls and women drive men wild"), or because the child's body responded physically to the perpetrator's manipulations, proving that s/he obviously wanted to have sex and thus was responsible for it in the first place, or because the child responded by "freezing" rather than by fighting or running away; the offender could not control his/her behavior or was under stress, sick, drunk, and so on, and so not responsible; the abuse was the fault of the perpetrator's wife for not having more frequent or better sex with him; the offender never intended to hurt the victim; it was up to the child to stop the offender, or to take care of the adult's sexual needs; the victim overreacted to the abuse; the victim should feel bad if s/he is unable to forgive the offender (Salter, 1995, pp. 213–214).

4. One of the most sophisticated instances of mind-control programming, often associated with the now-renowned MKUltra projects of the CIA, documented the engineering of *Manchurian Candidate*–like "marionette operatives" (Marks, 1979; Bowart, 1994; Thomas, 1989). Bowart (1994), cautioning us to remember that only failures of mind control survived to tell the stories—because when mind control is successful, there is no memory left at all—hints at the sinister extent of just this one operation when he notes that virtually every government agency became involved eventually, wittingly or unwittingly.

5. "Patricia Hearst was rebaptized Tania, the revolutionary; Linda Boreman was renamed Linda Lovelace, the whore" (Herman, 1992, p. 93).

6. The therapist and patient should maintain a focus on self-reflection, the patient's (and therapist's) automatic state changes, extreme shifts between feeling and deadness or between terror and blankness, and the patient's rapid changes in feelings toward the therapist. Specifically, a patient's sudden, intense, and unexpected or intrusive homicidal and suicidal feelings, or uncanny flight reactions may, if reflected and not acted upon, reveal perpetrator-implanted thought patterning. (This is not, however, to suggest that patient and therapist avoid intense rage and hate emerging in the transference by labeling these emotions "programming.")

CHAPTER 9

1. See Noblitt and Perskin (2000) for documentation of Dr. Noblitt's disturbing experiences with the media.

2. Analyzing the various meanings of John's use of FMS ideologies, while important, would have been insufficient to produce some of his longer-lasting changes. Playing with the originally concretized material on the other hand, turned it into a version of Winnicott's (1971) *squiggle game*, whereby partners take turns drawing and modifying each other's scribbles.

3. Systematic summaries of research on memory consistently indicate that basic memory processes in adults, and to a lesser degree in children, can and should be considered generally accurate but subject to distortion under pressure. Hence it is possible for memories of abuse that have been forgotten for a long time to be remembered and it is also possible to construct convincing pseudomemories for events that have never occurred (Alpert et al., 1996). Research on the accuracy of recovered memories of abuse by Dalenberg (1996) found that recovered and continuous memories of abuse are equally likely to be supported by objective evidence and that the therapy setting does not tend to foster the recovery of inaccurate memories. Results of her study also indicated that recovered or delayed memories tended to involve shame or terror whereas continuous memories tended to include sadness or loss.

4. Laura Brown (1996) points out that a good deal of the public thrashing of therapists and their influence—by Ofshe and Watters (1994), and Loftus and Ketcham (1994), for example—is rooted in references to self-help books and to reports made by third parties who were never present at the therapy in question, or to so-called scholarly material based primarily on analysis of popular press sources or on the accounts of third parties who almost always are accused parents with clear investments in how therapy is portrayed. Anything can be made to look good or bad by being redescribed (Rorty, 1989)—and as Spezzano (1993a) writes, even "truth resides not in the observations or measurements but in the discussion" (p. 204).

5. Safran (1999) describes how in order to be able to tolerate the depths of the patient's despair, therapists must be able to tolerate whatever personal feelings of despair are evoked. Safran understands the therapist's despair as: (1) despair experienced in relation to, or based on empathic resonance with, the patient's despair; and (2) despair related to the therapist's feelings of impotence vis-à-vis the patient. Emphasizing an essential element of what is involved in surviving destruction, Safran explains that therapists need to be familiar with the experience of working with helplessness, hopelessness, and despair in their own lives, and they need to have developed a significant degree of compassion for themselves in their own despair. Without this developmental achievement, Safran warns, the therapist might be prone to avoid real contact with the patient's despair, retreating to the safety of formulations, or engaging in futile efforts to take away the patient's despair through "interpretation, consolation, hollow empathy, or reassurance" (p. 7). Similarly, without tolerance for his/her own impotence as helper/healer and his/her inability to take away the patient's pain or solve problems for the patient, the therapist may retreat to magical rituals of completion, restitution, or transformation, never fully confronting his/her limitations or the limitations of psychotherapy.

CHAPTER 10

1. Ogden (1990) suggests that deliberate remembering can be a form of mourning where the patient can acknowledge that past events no longer exist in their original forms. He believes the analysis of the transference can transform repetition into a memory that shifts experience from more paranoid-schizoid modes of relating—and hence rigid and impermeable—to depressive position modes, thus expanding historicity and the capacity for affect tolerance. Clinicians from diverse theoretical orientations underscore similar requirements for transforming trauma, such as using language that subjectively validates connections to previously dissociated experience,

and reworking traumatic experience in the here-and-now of the therapy interaction where old and new object relational experience collide and are eventually disentangled.

2. Subtle or overt shaming of a trauma survivor for his/her "failure" to forgive the abuser(s) is unfortunately a far too common, culturally sanctioned form of revictimization. Grand's (2000) important contributions to the psychology of trauma and redemption of both victims and perpetrators emphasize that for many victims of unspeakable acts, forgiveness violates rather than restores. For many victims and perpetrators alike, forgiveness—especially forgiveness that transpires without a dialogue with the perpetrator's repentance—is tantamount to an abandonment of memory and an invitation to redissociation and renewed violations. For Grand, forgiveness of the unrepentant facilitates malignant dissociative contagion and fosters the reproduction of evil. Not only can the victim be retraumatized by pressures to (prematurely) forgive his/her perpetrator, but any hope for the healing of the perpetrator may also be lost, especially if the culpability of the perpetrator remains occluded and he/she is never "required to meet the real other, or to know himself as real. To embrace the unrepentent perpetrator in the soft envelope of forgiveness is to abandon the perpetrator to the loneliness of his own depravity" (p. 157).

3. In a group of normal undergraduate males, Briere and Runtz (1989) found 21 percent who reported sexual attraction to children. Seven percent of the subjects revealed that they might engage in sex with a child if they could do so without being discovered or punished. Factors associated with sexual interest or intent toward children aside from the ability to evade detection included having a traditional view of women and children as objects or property without feelings to be taken into account, or with feelings to be manipulated or invented for convenience.

4. Our culture's ambivalence about recognizing and making reparations for childhood trauma is no different from our denial and confusion over making reparations for so many historical violations—the annihilation of Native American populations; slavery; our refusal to rescue victims of the Nazi holocaust before and during World War II and our granting of citizenship (and government, military, and intelligence positions) to Nazi perpetrators and Nazi scientists (Hunt, 1991); war atrocities (Dresden, Hiroshima and Nagasaki, Vietnam); the betrayals of the McCarthy era; and government/CIA-sponsored military mind control, LSD, sterilization, and radiation research on human subjects.

5. Although I have not found any data documenting the frequency of occurrence of perpetrator-identified states in DID patients (which measurement would surely be confounded by the intense cover-up and camouflage these alters enjoy within DID systems), Ross's (1997) report on 236 DID cases reveals the presence of the related phenomenon of persecutory alters in 84 percent of them.

6. Similarly, the therapist treating the survivor of severe childhood trauma will inevitably end up feeling that s/he is victim, collaborator, and perpetrator within the therapeutic relationship. Even the most well-intentioned therapist "will be experienced as abusing his/her power at some point, and will certainly feel like, and possibly even be, the patient's victim at others" (Hegeman, 1995, p. 409). In concrete and symbolic ways the therapist will feel guilt, shame, and confusion about these roles—many times before the journey of therapy is concluded. The shrapnel of the patient's trauma may land squarely in the heart of the therapist's most vulnerable psychological territory.

7. For whatever combination of reasons, in my clinical experience, severely dissociative male patients use the false memory syndrome ideology much more frequently than their female counterparts do (and for more prolonged periods of time) in their struggles to decide what to believe and to engage their therapists in enactments around betrayal, boundary violation, mind control, and domination/submission.

References

Abel, G.G., Becker, J.V., Mittelman, M., Cunningham-Rathner, J., Rouleau, J.L., and Murphy, W.D. (1987). Self-reported sex crimes of nonincarcerated paraphiliacs. *Journal of Interpersonal Violence*, 2(1), 3–25.

Adams, M.A. (1989). Internal self-helpers of persons with multiple personality disorder. *Dissociation*, 2(3), 138–143.

Alexander, F., and French, T.M. (1946). *Psychoanalytic Therapy: Principles and applications*. New York: Ronald Press.

Alexander, P., and Friedrich, W.N. (Eds.) (1991). *The Role of the Extended Family in the Evaluation and Treatment of Incest*. New York. W.W. Norton.

Allen, J.G. (1995). Dissociative processes: Theoretical underpinnings of a working model for clinicians and patients. In J.G. Allen and W.H. Smith (Eds.). *Diagnosis and Treatment of Dissociative Disorders* (pp. 1–24). Northvale, NJ: Jason Aronson, Inc.

Allison, R.B. (1980). *Minds in Many Pieces*. New York: Rawson, Wade.

Alpert, J.L. (1995). Criteria: Signposts toward the sexual abuse hypothesis. In J.L. Alpert (Ed.), *Sexual Abuse Recalled: Treating trauma in the era of the recovered memory debate* (pp. 63–96). Northvale, NJ: Jason Aronson, Inc.

Alpert, J.L. (1996). Informed clinical practice and the recovered memory debate. In K. Pezdek and W.P. Banks (Eds.), *The Recovered Memory/False Memory Debate* (pp. 325–340). San Diego, CA: Academic Press.

Alpert, J.L., Brown, L.S., Ceci, S.J., Courtois, C.A. Loftus, E.F., and Ornstein, P.A. (Eds.) (1996). *American Psychological Association Working Group on Investigation of Memories of Childhood Abuse: Final report*. Washington, DC. American Psychological Association.

Althof, S.E. (1994). A therapist's perspective on the false memory controversy. *Journal of Sex Education*, 20(4), 246–254.

Altman, N. (1995). *The Psychoanalyst in the Inner City*. Hillsdale, NJ: Analytic Press.

Alvarez, L. (1996). After death of six-year old girl: Report shows system collapse. *New York Times*, April 9, p. 1.

Amnesty International (1973). *Report on Torture*. London: Gerald Duckworth.

Araji, S., and Finkelhor, D. (1986). Abusers: A review of the research. In D. Finkelhor (Ed.), *A Sourcebook on Child Sexual Abuse* (pp. 89–118). Beverly Hills, CA: Sage.

Armstrong, J.G. (1999). False memories and true lies: The psychology of a recanter. *Journal of Psychiatry and Law*, 27, 519–548.

Aron, L. (1992). Interpretation as the expression of the analyst's subjectivity. *Psychoanalytic Dialogues*, 2, 475–508.

Aron, L. (1996). *A Meeting of Minds: Mutuality in psychoanalysis*. Hillsdale, NJ: Analytic Press.

Aron, L. (1999). Clinical choices and the relational matrix. *Psychoanalytic Dialogues*, 9(1), 1–30.

Atwood, G., and Stolorow, R. (1984). *Structures of Subjectivity: Explorations in psychoanalytic phenomenology*. Hillsdale, NJ: Analytic Press.

Auerhahn, N.C., and Laub, D. (1987). Play and playfulness in holocaust survivors. *Psychoanalytic Study of the Child*, 42, 45–58.

Bagley, C., and King, K. (1990). *Child Sexual Abuse*. New York: Tavistock/Routledge.

Bagley, C., and Young, L. (1987). Juvenile prostitution and child sexual abuse: A controlled study. *Canadian Journal of Community Mental Health*, 6(1), 5–26.

Bak, R. (1974). Distortions of the concept of fetishism. *Psychoanalytic Study of the Child*, 24, 191–214.

Barach, P.M. (1991). Multiple personality disorder as an attachment disorder. *Dissociation*, 4(3), 117–124.

Barach, P.M. (1999a). President's message. *The International Society for the Study of Dissociation News*, 17(3), 1.

Barach, P.M. (1999b). President's message. *The International Society for the Study of Dissociation News*, 17(4), 1.

Barach, P.M. (1999c). President's message. *The International Society for the Study of Dissociation News*, 17(5), 1.

Barach, P.M. (1999d). President's message. *The International Society for the Study of Dissociation News*, 17(6), 1.

Barach, P.M., and Comstock, C.M. (1996). Psychodynamic psychotherapy of dissociative identity disorder. In L.K. Michelson and W.J. Ray (Eds.), *Handbook of Dissociation: Theoretical, empirical, and clinical perspectives* (pp. 413–429). New York: Plenum Press.

Bargh, J.A., and Chartrand, T.L. (1999). The unbearable automaticity of being. *American Psychologist*, 54(7), 462–479.

Basch, M.F. (1983). The perception of reality and the disavowal of meaning. *Annual of Psychoanalysis*, 11, 125–153.

Bateson, G. (1972). *Steps Towards an Ecology of Mind: Collected Essays in Anthropology, Psychiatry, Evolution, and Epistemology*. New York: Ballantine.

Beahrs, J.O. (1994). Dissociative identity disorder: Adaptive deception of self and others. *Bulletin of the American Academy of Psychiatry and the Law*, 22(2), 22–237.

Becker, D. (1996). The deficiency of the concept of posttraumatic stress disorder when dealing with victims of human rights violations. In R.J. Kleber, C.R. Figley, and B.P.R. Gersons (Eds.), *Beyond Trauma: Cultural and societal dynamics* (pp. 99–109). New York: Plenum Press.

Becker, J.V., and Quinsey, V.L. (1993). Assessing suspected child molesters. *Child Abuse and Neglect*, 17(1), 169–194.

Beebe, B., Jeffrey, J., and Lachmann, F.M. (1992). A dyadic systems view of communication. In N. Skolnick and S. Warshaw (Eds.), *Relational Perspectives in Psychoanalysis* (pp. 61–81). Hillsdale, NJ: Analytic Press.

Beere, D. (1995). Loss of background: A perceptual theory of dissociative disorders. *Dissociation*, 8(3), 165–174.

Benedek, E.P., and Schetky, D.H. (1987a). Problems in validating allegations of sexual abuse. Part 1: Factors affecting perception and recall of events. *Journal of the American Academy of Child and Adolescent Psychiatry*, 26, 912–915.

Benedek, E.P., and Schetky, D.H. (1987b). Problems in validating allegations of sexual abuse. Part 2: Clinical evaluation. *Journal of the American Academy of Child and Adolescent Psychiatry*, 26, 916–921.

Benjamin, J. (1988). *The Bonds of Love: Psychoanalysis, feminism, and the problem of domination*. New York: Pantheon.

Benjamin, J. (1990). An outline of intersubjectivity: The development of recognition. *Psychoanalytic Psychology*, 7, 33–46.

Benjamin, J. (1995). Comment. *Psychoanalytic Psychology*, 12(4), 595–598.

Bennets, L. (1993). Nightmares on Main Street. *Vanity Fair*, June, p. 42.

Bentovim, A., and Tranter, M. (1994). A systematic approach. In V. Sinason (Ed.), *Treating Survivors of Satanic Abuse*. New York: Routledge.

Berger, L.S. (1996). Cultural psychopathology and the "false memory syndrome" debate: A view from psychoanalysis. *American Journal of Psychotherapy*, 50(2), 167–177.

Biderman, A.D. (1957). Communist attempts to elicit false confessions from Air Force prisoners of war. *Bulletin of the New York Academy of Medicine*, 33, 616–625.

Bigras, J. (1990). Psychoanalysis as incestuous repetition: Some technical considerations. In H.B. Levine (Ed.), *Adult Analysis and Childhood Sexual Abuse* (pp. 173–196). Hillsdale, NJ: Analytic Press.

Bion, W.R. (1959). Attacks on linking. *International Journal of Psychoanalysis*, 40, 308–315.

Bion, W.R. (1993). *Second Thoughts: Selected papers on psycho-analysis*. Northvale, NJ: Jason Aronson, Inc.

Bishop, S.J., Murphy, J.M., Jellinek, M.S., Quinn, D., and Poltrast, F. (1992). Protecting seriously maltreated children: Time delays in a court sample. *Child Abuse and Neglect*, 16, 465–474.

Bliss, E.L. (1980). Multiple personalities. *Archives of General Psychiatry*, 37, 1388–1397.

Bliss, E.L. (1984). A symptom profile of patients with multiple personalities, including MMPI results. *Journal of Nervous and Mental Disease*, 174, 727–735.

Bliss, E.L. (1986). *Multiple Personality, Allied Disorders, and Hypnosis*. New York: Oxford University Press.

Blizard, R.A., and Bluhn, A.M. (1994). Attachment to the abuse: Integrating object relations and trauma theories in treatment of abuse survivors. *Psychotherapy*, 31(3), 383–390.

Bloom, S.L. (1994). Hearing the survivor's voice: Sundering the wall of denial. *Journal of Psychohistory*, 21(4), 461–468.

Bloom, S. (1997). *Creating Sanctuary: Toward the evolution of sane societies*. New York: Routledge.

Bluhm, H.O. (1999/1948). How did they survive? Mechanisms of defense in Nazi concentration camp survivors. *American Journal of Psychotherapy*, 53(1), 96–122.

Blume, E.S. (1995). The ownership of truth. *Journal of Psychohistory*, 23(2), 131–140.

Bollas, C. (1987). *The Shadow of the Object*. New York: Columbia University Press.

Bollas, C. (1989). *Forces of Destiny: Psychoanalysis and human idiom*. Northvale, NJ: Jason Aronson, Inc.

Bollas, C. (1992). *Being a Character: Psychoanalysis and self experience*. New York: Hill and Wang.

Bollas, C. (1995). The structure of evil. In C.Bollas, *Cracking Up* (pp. 180–220). New York: Hill and Wang.

Boon, S. (1997). The treatment of traumatic memories in DID: Indications and contraindications. *Dissociation*, 10, 65–80.

Boonpala, P. (1996). The role of the International Labor Organization. *The Prostitution of Children* (pp. 53–62). Symposium Proceedings, U.S. Department of Labor, Bureau of International Affairs, 1996.

Bowart, W.H. (1994/1978). *Operation Mind Control: Researcher's Edition*. Fort Bragg, CA: Flatland Editions. (Previously published, 1978: New York: Dell Publishing Company.)

Bowlby, J. (1969). *Attachment and Loss. Vol. 1 Attachment*. New York: Basic Books.

Bowlby, J. (1982). *Attachment*. New York: Basic Books.

Boyer, L.B. (1979). Countertransference with the severely regressed. In L. Epstein and A.H. Feiner (Eds.), *Countertransference: The therapist's contribution to the therapeutic situation* (pp. 347–374). Northvale, NJ: Jason Aronson, Inc.

Brandchaft, B. (1994). To free the spirit from its cell. In R.D. Stolorow, G.E. Atwood, and B. Brandchaft (Eds.) *The Intersubjective Perspective* (pp. 57–76). Northvale, NJ: Jason Aronson, Inc.

Brandchaft, B., and Stolorow, R. (1990). Varieties of therapeutic alliance. *The Annual of Psychoanalysis*, 18, 99–114. Hillsdale, NJ: Analytic Press.

Braude, S.E. (1995) *First Person Plural: Multiple personality and the philosophy of mind*. (Rev. Ed.) London: Rowman and Littlefield.

Braun, B.G. (1984). Towards a theory of multiple personality and other dissociative phenomena. *Psychiatric Clinics of North America*, 7, 171–193.

Braun, B.G. (1989). Letter to the editor. *International Society for the Study of Multiple Personality and Dissociation Newsletter* (p. 11). Chicago, IL: ISSMPD.

Braun, B.G., and Grey, G. (1987). Report on the 1986 questionnaire on multiple personality disorder and cult involvement. Paper presented at the 4th International Conference on Multiple Personality Disorder and Dissociation, Fall, 1987, Chicago.

Bremner, J.D., and Brett, E. (1997). Trauma-related dissociative states and long-term psychopathology in posttraumatic stress disorder. *Journal of Traumatic Stress*, 10(1), 37–49.

Bremner, J.D., Randall, P., Scott, T.M., Bronen, R.A., Delaney, R.C., Seibyl, J.P., Southwick, S.M., McCarthy, G., Charney, D.S., and Innis, R.B. (1995). MRI based measurement of hippocampal volume in posttraumatic stress disorder. *American Journal of Psychiatry*, 152, 973–981.

Bremner, J.D., Randall, P., Vermetten, E., Staib, L., Bronen, R.A., Mazure, C., Capelli, S., McCarthy, G., Innis, R.B., and Charney, D.S. (1997). MRI based measurements of hippocampal volume in post-traumatic stress disorder related and childhood physical and sexual abuse. *Biological Psychiatry*, 41, 23–32.

Brenneis, C.B. (1994). Belief and suggestion in the recovery of memories of childhood sexual abuse. *Journal of the American Psychoanalytic Association*, 42, 1027–1053.

Brenneis, C.B. (1997). *Recovered Memories of Trauma: Transferring the present to the past*. Madison, CT: International Universities Press.

Brenner, I. (1994). A twentieth century demonological neurosis. *Journal of Psychohistory*, 21(4), 501–504.

Brenner, I. (1996). The characterological basis of multiple personality. *American Journal of Psychotherapy*, 50(2), 154–166.

Breslau, N., and Davis, G.C. (1992). Posttraumatic stress disorder in an urban population of young adults: Risk factors for chronicity. *American Journal of Psychiatry*, 149, 671–675.

Brett, E.A. (1993). Classification of posttraumatic stress disorder in DSM IV: Anxiety disorder, dissociative disorder, or stress disorder. In J.R.T. Davidson and E.B. Foa (Eds.), *Posttraumatic Stress Disorder: DSM IV and Beyond* (pp. 191–206). Washington, DC: American Psychiatric Press.

Briere, J.N. (1989). *Therapy for Adults Molested as Children*. New York: Springer.

Briere, J.N. (1992a). Methodological issues in the study of sexual abuse effects. *Journal of Consulting and Clinical Psychology*, 60(2), 196–203.

Briere, J.N. (1992b). *Child Abuse Trauma: Theory and treatment of the lasting effects*. Newbury Park, CA: Sage.

Briere, J.N. (1995). Child abuse, memory, and recall: A commentary. *Consciousness and Cognition*, 4, 83–87.

Briere, J.N. (1996). *Treatment of Adults Sexually Molested as Children: Beyond survival*. New York: Springer.

Briere, J., Henschel, D., and Smiljanich, K. (1992). Attitudes towards sexual abuse: Sex differences and construct validity. *Journal of Research on Personality*, 26, 398–406.

Briere, J.N., and Runtz, M. (1987). Post sexual abuse trauma: Data and implications for clinical practice. *Journal of Interpersonal Violence*, 2, 367–379.

Briere, J.N., and Runtz, M. (1989). University males' sexual interest in children: Predicting potential indices of "pedophilia" in a non-forensic sample. *Child Abuse and Neglect*, 13, 65–75.

Briere, J.N., and Smiljanich, K., and Henschel, D. (1994). Sexual fantasies, gender, and molestation history. *Child Abuse and Neglect*, 18, 131–137.

Bromberg, P.M. (1980). Empathy, anxiety, and reality: A view from the bridge. *Contemporary Psychoanalysis*, 16, 223–236.

Bromberg, P.M. (1991). On knowing one's patient inside out: The aesthetics of unconscious communication. *Psychoanalytic Dialogues*, 1, 399–422.

Bromberg, P.M. (1993). Shadow and substance: A relational perspective on clinical process. *Psychoanalytic Psychology*, 10, 147–168.

Bromberg, P.M. (1994). Speak! That I may hear you: Some reflections on dissociation, reality, and psychoanalytic listening. *Psychoanalytic Dialogues*, 4, 517–547.

Bromberg, P.M. (1995a). Dissociation and personality organization: Reflections on Peter Goldberg's essay. *Psychoanalytic Dialogues*, 5(3), 511–528.

Bromberg, P.M. (1995b). Resistance, object usage, and human relatedness. *Contemporary Psychoanalysis*, 31, 173–192.

Bromberg, P.M. (1996a). Hysteria, dissociation and cure: Emmy von N revisited. *Psychoanalytic Dialogues*, 6(1), 55–72.

Bromberg, P.M. (1996b). Standing in the spaces: The multiplicity of self and the psychoanalytic relationship. *Contemporary Psychoanalysis*, 32(4), 509–536.

Bromberg, P.M. (1998). Introduction. In P.M. Bromberg, *Standing in the Spaces: Essays on clinical process, trauma, and dissociation* (pp. 1–16). Hillsdale, NJ: Analytic Press.

Brosig, C.L., and Kalichman, S.C. (1992). Clinicians' reporting of suspected child abuse. A review of the empirical literature. *Clinical Psychology Review*, 12, 155–168.

Brown, D. (1995). Sources of suggestion and their applicability to psychotherapy. In J.L. Alpert (Ed.), *Sexual Abuse Recalled: Treating trauma in the era of the recovered memory debate* (pp. 61–100). Northvale, NJ: Jason Aronson, Inc.

Brown, D., Frishholz, E.J., and Scheflin, A.W. (1999). Dissociative identity disorder—An evaluation of the scientific evidence. *Journal of Psychiatry and Law*, 27, 549–637.

Brown, D., and Scheflin, A.W. (1999). Factitious disorders and trauma related diagnoses. *Journal of Psychiatry and Law*, 27, 373–422.

Brown, L.S. (1994). *Subversive Dialogues*. New York: Bass Books.

Brown, L.S. (1995). Not outside the range: One feminist perspective on psychic trauma. In C. Caruth (Ed.), *Trauma: Explorations in memory* (pp. 100–112). Baltimore, MD: Johns Hopkins University Press.

Brown, L.S. (1996). Your therapy client as plaintiff: Clinical and legal issues for the treating therapist. *Sexual Abuse Recalled: Treating trauma in the era of the recovered memory debate* (pp. 337–362). Northvale, NJ: Jason Aronson, Inc.

Burgess, A.W., and Grant, R.N. (1988). *Children Traumatized in Sex Rings*. Washington, DC: National Center for Missing and Exploited Children.

Burgess, A.W., Groth, A.N., Holmstrom, E.L., and Sgroi, S.M. (1987). *Sexual Assault of Children and Adolescents*. Lexington, MA: Lexington Books.

Burgess, A.W., Groth, A.N., and McCausland, M.P. (1981). Child sex initiation rings. *American Journal of Orthopsychiatry*, 51, 110–119.

Burgess, A.W., Hazelwood, R.R., Rokous, F.E., Hartman, C.R., and Burgess, A.G. (1988). Serial rapists and their victims: reenactment and repetition. In R.A. Prentky and V.L. Quinsey (Eds.). *Human Sexual Aggression: Current perspectives*. Annals of the New York Academy of Science (pp. 277–295), Vol. 528, August 12. New York: New York Academy of Science.

Bybee, D., and Mowbray, C. (1993). An analysis of allegations of sexual abuse in a multi-victim day-care case. *Child Abuse and Neglect*, 17, 767–783.

Cameron, M. (1995). *Broken Child*. New York: Kensington Publishing Corp.

Carlson, E.B., and Putnam, F.W. (1989). Integrating research in dissociation and hypnotic susceptibility. Are there two pathways to hypnotizability? *Dissociation*, 2(1), 32–38.

Carlson, E.B., Putnam, F.W., Ross, C.A., Torem, M., Coons, P., Bowman, E.S., Chu, J., Dill, D.L., Loewenstein, R.J., and Braun, B.G. (1993). Predictive validity of Dissociative Experiences Scale. *American Journal of Psychiatry*, 150, 1030–1036.

Caruth, C. (1995). Preface. In C. Caruth (Ed.), *Trauma: Explorations in memory* (pp. vii–ix). Baltimore, MD: Johns Hopkins University Press.

Caruth, C. (1995a). Introduction. In C. Caruth (Ed.), *Trauma: Explorations in memory* (pp, 3–12). Baltimore, MD: Johns Hopkins University Press.

Caruth, C. (1995b). Recapturing the past. In C. Caruth (Ed.), *Trauma: Explorations in Memory* (pp. 151–157). Baltimore, MD: Johns Hopkins University Press.

Cavaliere, F. (1995). Parents killing kids: A nation's shame. *APA Monitor*, August, 1995, 34.

Ceci, S.J., and Bruck, M. (1993). Suggestibility of the child witness: A historical review and synthesis. *Psychological Bulletin*, 113(3), 403–439.

Ceci, S.J., Huffman, M.L.C., Smith, E., and Loftus, E.F. (1994). Repeatedly thinking about a non-event: Source misattribution among preschoolers. *Consciousness and Cognition*, 3, 388–407.

Charles, G. (1995). The assessment and investigation of ritual abuse. In Ney, C.T. (Ed.), *True and False Allegations of Child Abuse*. New York: Bruner/Mazel.

Charney, D.S., Deutch, A.Y., Krystal, J.H., Southwick, S.M., and Davis, M. (1993). Psychobiological mechanisms of post-traumatic stress disorder. *Archives of General Psychiatry*, 50, 294–305.

Chassay, S. (1996). Trauma as initiation: A shamanic perspective on sexual abuse. *Shamanic Applications Review*, 2, 3–12.

Chefetz, R.A. (1997). Special case transferences and counter-transferences in the treatment of dissociative disorders. *Dissociation*, 10(4), 255–265.

Cheit, R. (1999). Junk skepticism and recovered memory. Plenary Paper presented at the 16th annual Fall Conference of the International Society for the Study of Dissociation (ISSD). Miami, FL, November 1999.

Chodron, P. (1994). *Start Where You Are: A guide to compassionate living*. Boston, MA: Shambala.

Chu, J.A. (1988). Ten traps for therapists in the treatment of trauma survivors. *Dissociation*, 1(4), 24–32.

Chu, J.A. (1992a). Empathic confrontation in the treatment of childhood abuse survivors, including a tribute to the legacy of Dr. David Caul. *Dissociation*, 5(2), 98–103.

Chu, J.A. (1992b). The therapeutic roller-coaster: Dilemmas in the treatment of childhood abuse survivors. *Journal of Psychotherapy Practice and Research*, 1, 351–370.

Chu, J.A. (1996). Posttraumatic responses to childhood abuse and implications for treatment. In L.K. Michelson, and W.J. Ray (Eds.), *Handbook of Dissociation: Theoretical, empirical, and clinical perspectives* (pp. 381–400). New York: Plenum Press.

Chu, J.A. (1998). *Rebuilding Shattered Lives: The responsible treatment of complex post-traumatic and dissociative disorders*. New York: John Wiley and Sons, Inc.

Chu, J.A., and Dill, D.L. (1990). Dissociative symptoms in relation to childhood physical and sexual abuse. *American Journal of Psychiatry*, 147, 887–892.

Chu, J.A., Frey, L.M., Ganzel, B.L., and Matthews, J.A. (1999). Memories of childhood abuse: dissociation, amnesia, and corroboration. *American Journal of Psychiatry*, 156(5), 749–755.

Chu, J.A., Matthews, J.A., Frey, L. M., and Ganzel, B. (1996). The nature of traumatic memories of childhood abuse. Dissociation, 9(1), 2–17.

Cohen, B.M. (1996). Art and the dissociative paracosm: Uncommon realities. In L.K. Michelson, and W.J. Ray (Eds.), *Handbook of Dissociation: Theoretical, Empirical, and Clinical Perspectives* (pp. 525–544). New York: Plenum Press.

Comstock, C. (1992). Response to the centrality of relationship: What's not being said. *Dissociation*, 5, 171–172.

Conway, A. (1994). Trance formations of abuse. In Sinason, V. (Ed.), *Treating Survivors of Satanist Abuse* (pp. 254–264). New York, NY: Routledge.

Coons, P.M. (1986). Treatment progress in 20 patients with multiple personality disorder. *Journal of Nervous and Mental Diseases*, 174, 715–721.

Coons, P.M. (1994). Confirmation of childhood abuse in child and adolescent cases of multiple personality disorder and dissociative disorder not otherwise specified. *Journal of Nervous and Mental Diseases*, 182, 441–464.

Coons, P.M., Bowman, E.S., and Milstein, V. (1988). Multiple personality disorder: A clinical investigation of 50 cases. *Journal of Nervous and Mental Diseases*, 176, 519–527.

Coons, P.M., and Milstein, V. (1986). Psycho-sexual disturbances in multiple personality: Characteristics, etiology, and treatment. *Journal of Clinical Psychiatry*, 47, 106–110.

Corwin, D.L., Berliner, L. Goodman, G., Goodwin, J., and White, S. (1987). Child sexual abuse and custody disputes: No easy answers. *Journal of Interpersonal Violence*, 2(1), 91–105.

Courtois, C. (1988). *Healing the Incest Wound: Adult survivors in therapy*. New York: Norton.

Courtois, C. (1992). The memory retrieval process in incest survivor therapy. *Journal of Child Sexual Abuse*, 1(1), 15–32.

Cozolino, L.J. (1989). The ritual abuse of children: Implications for clinical practice and research. *Journal of Sex Research*, 26 (1), 131–138.

Creamer, M.A. (1996). A cognitive processing formulation of posttraumatic stress reactions. In R.J. Kleber, C.R. Figley, and B.P.R. Gersons (Eds.), *Beyond Trauma: Cultural and societal dynamics* (pp. 55–73). New York: Plenum Press.

Crewdson, J. (1988). *By Silence Betrayed: Sexual abuse of children in America*. New York: Harper and Row.

Crossley, N.C. (1996). *Intersubjectivity: The fabric of social becoming*. Thousand Oaks, CA: Sage Publications.

Cushman, P. (1994). Confronting Sullivan's spider: Hermeneutics and the politics of therapy. *Contemporary Psychoanalysis*, 30, 800–844.

Cushman, P. (1994a). *Constructing the Self, Constructing America: A cultural history of psychotherapy*. New York: Addison-Wesley.

Dalenberg, C. (1996). Are memories recovered in therapy as accurate as continuous memories of abuse? *Journal of Psychiatry and Law*, 24(2), 229–275.

Danieli, Y. (1988). Confronting the unimaginable: Psychotherapists' reactions to victims of the Nazi Holocaust. In J.P. Wilson, Z. Harel, and B. Kahana, (Eds.), *Human Adaptation to Extreme Stress: From the Holocaust to Vietnam* (pp. 224–225). New York: Plenum Publishing.

Daro, D., and McCurdy, K. (1993). *Current Trends in Child Abuse Reporting and Fatalities: The results of the 1993 Annual Fifty State Survey*. Chicago: National Committee for the Prevention of Child Abuse and Neglect.

Daskovsky, D. (1998). The Abuser and the abused: Sources of resistance to resolving splits in the countertransference in the treatment of adults who were sexually abused as children. *Psychoanalytic Psychology*, 15(1), 3–13.

Davies, J.M. (1996a). Linking the "psychoanalytic" with the postclassical: Integration, dissociation, and the multiplicity of unconscious process. *Contemporary Psychoanalysis*, 32(4), 553–576.

Davies, J.M. (1996b). Maintaining complexities: A reply to Crews, Brenneis, and Stern. *Psychoanalytic Dialogues*, 6(2), 281–294.

Davies, J.M. (1997). Dissociation, repression, and reality testing in the countertransference. In R.B. Gartner (Ed.), *Memories of Sexual Betrayal: Truth, fantasy, repression and dissociation* (pp. 45–76). Northvale, NJ: Jason Aronson, Inc.

Davies, J.M., and Frawley, M.G. (1991). Dissociation processes and transference-countertransference paradigms in the psychoanalytically oriented treatment of adult survivors of sexual abuse. *Psychoanalytic Dialogues*, 2(1), 5–36.

Davies, J.M., and Frawley, M.G. (1994). *Treating Adult Survivors of Childhood Sexual Abuse*. New York: Basic Books.

DeBellis, M.D., Chrousous, G.P., Dorn, L.D., Burke, L., Helmes, K., Kling, M.A., Tirckett, P.K., and Putnam, F.W. (1994a). Hypothalamic-pituitary-adrenal axis dysregulation in sexually abused girls. *Journal of Clinical Endocrinology and Metabolism*, 78, 249–255.

DeBellis, M.D., Lefter, L., Trickett, P.K., and Putnam, F.W. (1994b). Urinary catecholamines excretion in sexually abused girls. *Journal of the American Academy of Child and Adolescent Psychiatry*, 33, 320–327.

DeBellis, M.D., Keshavan, M.S., Clark, D.B., Casey, B.J., Giedd, J.N., Boring, A.M., Frustaci, K., and Ryan, N.D. (1999). A.E. Bennett Research Award. Developmental traumatology. Part II: Brain development. *Biological Psychiatry*, 45(10), 1271–1284.

DeMause, L. (1974). The evolution of childhood. In L. DeMause (Ed.), *The History of Childhood*. New York: Psychohistory Press.

DeMause, L. (1991). The universality of incest. *Journal of Psychohistory*, 19, 123–164.

DeMause, L. (1994). Why cults terrorize children. *Journal of Psychohistory*, 21(4), 505–518.

DeMause, L. (1996). Restaging early traumas in war and social violence. *Journal of Psychohistory*, 23(4), 344–391.

DeYoung, M. (1986). A conceptual model for judging the truthfulness of a young child's allegation of sexual abuse. *American Journal of Orthopsychiatry*, 56(4), 550–559.

Dimenstein, G. (1996). The role of the media. *The prostitution of children* (72–75). Symposium Proceedings, U.S. Department of Labor, Bureau of International Affairs, 1996.

Dorpat, T.L. (1996). *Gaslighting: The double whammy, interrogation, and other methods of covert control in psychotherapy and psychoanalysis*. Northvale, NJ: Jason Aronson, Inc.

Draijer, N., and Langeland, W. (1999). Childhood trauma and perceived parental dysfunction in the etiology of dissociative symptoms in psychiatric patients. *American Journal of Psychiatry*, 156, 379–385.

Driscoll, L.N., and Wright, L. (1991). Survivors of childhood ritual abuse: Multigenerational satanic cult involvement. *Treating Abuse Today*, 1, 5–13.

Duncan, C.W. (1993). *The Fractured Mirror: Healing multiple personality disorder*. Deerfield Beach, FL: Health Communications, Inc.

Eckhardt, M.H. (1987). Discussion of "Some problems of cross-cultural therapy with refugees seeking therapy" by C-I Dahl. *American Journal of Psychoanalysis*, 49, 33–36.

Egendorf, A. (1995). Hearing people through their pain. *Journal of Traumatic Stress*, 8(1), 5–28.

Ehrenberg, D.B. (1992). *The Intimate Edge: Extending the reach of psychoanalytic interaction*. New York: Norton.

Ehrenberg, D.B. (1996). On the analyst's emotional availability and vulnerability. *Contemporary Psychoanalysis*, 32(4), 275–286.

Eigen, M. E. (1981). The area of faith in Winnicott, Lacan, and Bion. *International Journal of Psychoanalysis*, 62, 413–433.

Eigen, M.E. (1984). On demonized aspects of the self. In M.C. Nelson and M.E. Eigen (Eds.), *Evil, Self, and Culture* (pp. 91–123: Volume IV, Self-in Process Series). New York: Human Science Press, Inc.

Eigen, M.E. (1991). Winnicott's area of freedom: The uncompromisable. In N. Schwartz-Salant and M. Stein (Eds.), *Liminality and Transitional Experiencing* (pp. 67–88). Wilmette, IL: Chiron Press.

Eigen, M.E. (1992). *Coming Through the Whirlwind: Case studies in psychotherapy*. Wilmette, IL: Chiron Press.

Eigen, M.E. (1996). *Psychic Deadness*. Northvale, NJ: Jason Aronson, Inc.

Eigen, M.E. (1998). *The Psychoanalytic Mystic*. Binghamton, NY: ESF Publishers.

Eisold, B.K. (1999). Profound recognition: Where does it fit in analytic work. *Contemporary Psychoanalysis*, 35(1), 107–130.

Elin, M.R. (1995). A developmental model for trauma. In L. Cohen, J. Berzoff, and M. Elin, (Eds.), *Dissociative Identity Disorder* (pp. 223–259). Northvale, NJ: Jason Aronson, Inc.

Elliott, D. and Briere, J.N. (1995). Posttraumatic stress associated with the delayed recall of sexual abuse: a general population study. *Journal of Traumatic Stress*, 8, 629–647.

Elliott, M. (1994). *Female Sexual Abuse of Children*. New York: Guilford.

Enns, C.Z., McNeilly, C.L., Corkery, J.M., and Gilbert, M.S. (1995). The debate about delayed memories of child sexual abuse: A feminist perspective. *The Counseling Psychologist*, 23(2), 181–279.

Everson, M.D., and Boat, B.W. (1989). False allegations of sexual abuse by children and adolescents. *Journal of the American Academy of Child and Adolescent Psychiatry*, 28(2), 230–235.

Fahy, T.A. (1988). The diagnosis of multiple personality disorder: A critical review. *British Journal of Psychiatry*, 153, 597–606.

Fairbairn, W.R.D. (1952). *Psychoanalytic Studies of the Personality*. London: Tavistock.

Faller, K.C. (1984). Is the child victim of sexual abuse telling the truth? *Child Abuse and Neglect*, 8, 473–481.

Faller, K.C. (1994). Ritual abuse: A review of research. *APSAC Advisor*, 1, 19–27.

Farley, M., Baral, I., Kiremire, M., and Sezgin, U. (1998). Prostitution in five countries: Violence and posttraumatic stress disorder. *Feminism and Psychology*, 8(4), 415–426.

Fast, I. (1998). *Selving: A relational theory of self*. Hillsdale, NJ: Analytic Press.

Federoff, J.P., and Pinkus, S. (1996). The genesis of pedophilia: Testing the abuse-to-abuser hypothesis in sex offender treatment. In E. Coleman, S.M. Dwyer, and N.J. Pollone (Eds.), *Sex Offender Treatment: Biological dysfunction, intrapsychic conflict, interpersonal violence* (pp. 85–101). New York: Haworth Press.

Feiner, A.H. (1996). Bewitched, bothered and bewildered: Some core issues in interpersonal analysis. *Contemporary Psychoanalysis*, 32(3), 411–425.

Felitti, V.J., Anda, R.F., Nordenberg, D, Williamson, D.F, Spitz, A.M., Edwards, V., Koss, M.P., and Marks, J.S. (1998). Relationship of childhood abuse and household dysfunction to many of the leading causes of death in adults. *American Journal of Preventive Medicine*, 14(4), 245–258.

Felman, S. (1995). Education and crisis or the vicissitudes of teaching. In C. Caruth (Ed.), *Trauma: Explorations in memory* (pp. 13–60). Baltimore, MD: Johns Hopkins University Press.

Ferenczi, S. (1930). Notes and fragments II. In M. Balint (Ed.), *Final Contributions to the Problems and Methods of Psychoanalysis* (pp. 219–231). New York, Bruner/Mazel, 1980.

Ferenczi, S. (1933). Confusion of tongues between adults and the child. In S. Ferenczi (1955), *Final Contributions to the Problems and Methods of Psychoanalysis* (pp. 87–101). London: Hogarth.

Ferguson, M. (1990). Mirroring processes, hypnotic processes, and multiple personality. *Psychoanalysis and Contemporary Thought*, 13, 417–450.

Fergusson, D.M. and Mullen, P.E. (1999). *Child Sexual Abuse: An Evidence Based Approach*. Thousand Oaks, CA: Sage Publishing.

Figley, C.R. (1995). *Compassion Fatigue*. New York: Bruner/Mazel.

Fine, C.G. (1994). Cognitive hypnotherapeutic intervention in the treatment of MPD. *Journal of Cognitive Psychotherapy*, 8(4), 289–298.

Fine, C.G. (1996). A cognitively based treatment model for DSM-IV dissociative identity disorder. In L.K. Michelson and W.J. Ray (Eds.), *Handbook of Dissociation: Theoretical, empirical, and clinical perspectives* (pp. 401–412). New York: Plenum Press.

Fine, C.G. (1999). The tactical-integration model for the treatment of dissociative identity disorder and allied dissociative disorders. *American Journal of Psychotherapy*, 53(3), 361–376.

Fink, D., and Golinkoff, M. (1990). Multiple personality disorder, borderline personality disorder, and schizophrenia: A comparative study of clinical features. *Dissociation*, 3(3), 127–134.

Finkelhor, D. (1994). The international epidemiology of child sexual abuse. *Child Abuse and Neglect*, 18, 409–417.

Finkelhor, D. (1998). Editorial: Improving research, policy, and practice for understanding child sexual abuse. *Journal of American Medical Association*, 280, 1865–1866.

Finkelhor, D., Hotaling, G., Lewis, I.A., and Smith, C. (1989). Sexual abuse and its relationship to later sexual satisfaction, marital status, religion, and attitudes. *Journal of Interpersonal Violence*, 4, 379–399.

Finkelhor, D., Hotaling, G., and Sedlak, A. (1990). *Missing, Abducted, Runaway, and Throwaway Children in America*. Executive Summary. Washington, DC: U.S. Department of Justice, Office of Juvenile Justice and Delinquency Prevention.

Finkelhor, D., Hotaling, G., Lewis, I.A., and Smith, C. (1990). Sexual abuse in a national survey of men and women. *Child Abuse and Neglect*, 14, 19–28.

Finkelhor, D., and Lewis, I.A. (1988). An epidemiological approach to the study of child molestation. In R.A. Prentky and V.L. Quinsey (Eds.), *Human Sexual Aggression: Current Perspectives*. Annals of the New York Academy of Science (pp. 64–78).

Finkelhor, D., Williams, L., and Burns, L. (Eds.). (1988). *Nursery Crimes: Sexual abuse in day care*. Newbury Park, CA: Sage Publications.

Finkelhor, D., and Williams, L.M. (1992). The characteristics of incestuous fathers (ERIC Document, No. 354451).

Fish-Murray, C.C., Koby, E.V., and Van der Kolk, B.A. (1987). Evolving ideas: The effect of abuse on children's thought. In B.A. Van der Kolk (Ed.), *Psychological Trauma* (pp. 89–110). Washington, DC: American Psychiatric Press.

Flax, J. (1993). *Disputed Subjects: Essays on psychoanalysis, politics, and philosophy*. New York: Routledge.

Flax, J. (1996a). Review essay. *Psychoanalytic Dialogues*, 6(6), 837–849.

Flax, J. (1996b). Taking multiplicity seriously. *Contemporary Psychoanalysis*, 32(4), 577–593.

Flores, R. (1996). Child prostitution in the U.S. In *Forced Labor: The prostitution of children* (pp. 41–52). Symposium Proceedings, U.S. Department of Labor, Bureau of International Labor Affairs, 1996.

Foa, E.B., and Hearst-Ikeda, D. (1996). Emotional dissociation in response to trauma: An information-processing approach. In L.K. Michelson and W.J. Ray, (Eds.), *Handbook of Dissociation: Theoretical, empirical, and clinical perspectives* (pp. 207–224). New York: Plenum Press.

Foa, E.B., and Kozak, M.J. (1986). Emotional processing of fear: Exposure to corrective information. *Psychological Bulletin*, 99, 20–35.

Foote, B. (1999). Dissociative identity disorder and pseudo-hysteria. *American Journal of Psychotherapy*, 53(3), 320–343.

Fosshage, J. (1992). Self psychology: The self and its vicissitudes within a relational matrix. In N. Skolnick and S. Warshaw (Eds.), *Relational Perspectives in Psychoanalysis* (pp. 21–42). Hillsdale, NJ: Analytic Press.

Fosshage, J. (1995). Interaction in psychoanalysis: A broadening horizon. *Psychoanalytic Dialogues*, 5(3), 459–478.

Fraiberg, S. (1982). Pathological defenses in infancy. *Psychoanalytic Quarterly*, 51, 612–635.

Frankel, F.H. (1994). Adult reconstruction of childhood events in the multiple personality literature. *American Journal of Psychiatry*, 150, 954–958.

Frankel, S.A., and O'Hearn, T.C. (1996). Similarities in responses to extreme and unremitting stress: Cultures of communities under siege. *Psychotherapy: Theory, research, and practice*, 33(3), 485–502.

Fraser, G.A. (1997). Visions of memories: A patient's visual representation of ritual abuse: In G.A. Fraser (Ed.), *The Dilemma of Ritual Abuse* (pp. 183–196). Washington, DC: American Psychiatric Press.

Frawley-O'Dea, M.G. (1997). Discussion: P3: Patients, politics, and psychotherapy in the true/false memory debate. In Gartner, R.B. (Ed.), *Memories of Sexual Betrayal: Truth, fantasy, repression and dissociation* (pp. 149–178). Northvale, NJ: Jason Aronson, Inc.

Frayn, D.H. (1996). Enactments: An evolving dyadic concept of acting out. *American Journal of Psychotherapy*, 50(2), 194–207.

Freud, A. (1936). *The Ego and the Mechanisms of Defense*. London: Hogarth.

Freud, S. (1912). The dynamics of the transference. *S.E.*, 12, 99–108.

Freud, S. (1930). Civilization and its discontents. *S.E.*, 21, 59–145.

Freund, K., Watson, R., and Dickey, R. (1990). Does sexual abuse in childhood cause pedophilia? An exploratory study. *Archives of Sexual Behavior*, 19, 557–568.

Freyd, J.J. (1994). Betrayal trauma: Traumatic amnesia, as an adaptive response to childhood abuse. *Ethics and Behavior*, 4(4), 307–329.

Freyd, J.J. (1996). *Betrayal Trauma: The logic of forgetting childhood abuse*. Cambridge, MA: Harvard University Press.

Fullerton, C.S., and Ursano, R.J. (1997). The other side of chaos: Understanding the pattern of posttraumatic responses. In C.S. Fullerton and R.J. Ursan (Eds.), *Posttraumatic Stress Disorder* (pp. 3–20). Washington, DC: American Psychiatric Press.

Gabbard, G.O. (1993). Countertransference and borderline patients. *The Journal of Psychotherapy Practice and Research*, 2(1), 7–18.

Gabbard, G.O. (1994). Psychotherapists who transgress sexual boundaries with patients. *Bulletin of the Menninger Clinic*, 58, 124–135.

Gadamer, H.G. (1975). *Truth and Method*. New York: Seabury Press.

Galenson, E. (1986). Some thoughts about infant psychopathology and aggressive development. *International Review of Psychoanalysis*, 13, 349–354.

Ganaway, G. (1989). Historical versus narrative truth: clarifying the role of exogenous trauma in the etiology of MPD and its variants. *Dissociation*, 2, 205–220.

Ganaway, G.K. (1994). Transference and countertransference shaping influences on dissociative syndromes. In S.J. Lynn and J.W. Rhue (Eds.), *Dissociation: Clinical and theoretical perspectives* (pp. 317–337). New York: Guilford.

Ganzarain, R.C., and Buchele, B.J. (1989). *Fugitives of Incest: A perspective from psychoanalysis and group therapy.* Madison, CT: International Universities Press.

Gardner, R. (1992). *True and False Allegations of Child Sexual Abuse.* Cresskill, NJ: Creative Therapeutics.

Gartner, R.B. (1999). *Betrayed as Boys: Psychodynamic treatment of sexually abused men.* New York: Guilford.

Gelinas, D. (1995). Dissociative identity disorder and the trauma paradigm. In L. Cohen, J. Berzoff, and M. Elin (Eds.), *Dissociative Identity Disorder: Theoretical and treatment controversies* (pp. 175–222). Northvale, NJ: Jason Aronson, Inc.

Gershuny, B.S., and Thayer, J.F. (1999). Relations among psychological trauma, dissociative phenomena, and trauma-related distress: A review and integration. *Clinical Psychology Review,* 19, 631–657.

Ghent, E. (1989). Credo: The dialectics of one-person and two-person psychologies. *Contemporary Psychoanalysis,* 25, 169–211.

Ghent, E. (1990). Masochism, submission and surrender. *Contemporary Psychoanalysis,* 26, 108–136.

Ghent, E. (1992a). Foreword. In N.J. Skolnick and S.C. Warshaw (Eds.), *Relational Perspectives in Psychoanalysis.* Hillsdale, NJ: Analytic Press.

Ghent, E. (1992b). Paradox and process. *Psychoanalytic Dialogues,* 2, 135–160.

Ghent, E. (1994). Empathy: Whence and whither? *Psychoanalytic Dialogues,* 4(3), 473–486.

Ghent, E. (1995). Interaction in the psychoanalytic situation. *Psychoanalytic Dialogues,* 5(3), 479–492.

Gilligan, C. Rogers, A, and Tolman, D. (1992). *Women, Girls, and Psychiatry.* New York: Haworth.

Giobbe, E. (1991). Prostitution: Buying the right to rape. In A.W. Burgess (Ed.), *Rape and Sexual Assault III: A research handbook.* New York: Garland Press.

Giovacchini, P.C. (1978). The impact of delusion or the delusion of impact: Ego defect and transitional phenomena. In S.A. Grolnick, L. Barkin, and W. Muensterberger (Eds.), *Between Reality and Fantasy.* Northale, NJ: Jason Aronson, Inc.

Giovacchini, P.L. (1989). *Countertransference Triumphs and Catastrophes.* Northvale, NJ: Jason Aronson, Inc.

Glenn, J. (Ed.). (1978). *Child Analysis and Therapy.* New York: Jason Aronson, Inc.

Goldberg, A. (1988). *A Fresh Look at Psychoanalysis: The view from self psychology.* Hillsdale, NJ: Analytic Press.

Goldberg, A. (1990). *The Prisonhouse of Psychoanalysis.* Hillsdale, NJ: Analytic Press.

Goldberg, P. (1995). "Successful" dissociation, pseudovitality, and inauthentic use of the senses. *Psychoanalytic Dialogues,* 5(3), 493–510.

Goldman, D. (1996). An exquisite corpse: The strain of working in and out of potential space. *Contemporary Psychoanalysis,* 32(3), 339–358.

Godwin, R. (1996). The exopsychic structure of politics. *Journal of Psychohistory,* 23(3), 252–259.

Goodwin, J.M. (1989). *Sexual Abuse: Incest victims and their families.* Chicago, IL: Yearbook Medical Publishing.

Goodwin, J.M. (1993a). Human veterans of trauma: Illustrations from the Marquis de Sade. In J.M. Goodwin (Ed.), *Rediscovering Childhood Trauma: Historical casebook and clinical applications* (pp. 95–112). Washington, DC: American Psychiatric Press.

Goodwin, J.M. (1993b). Sadistic abuse: Definition, evaluation, and treatment. *Dissociation,* 6(2/3), 181–187.

Goodwin, J.M. (1994). Credibility problems in sadistic abuse. *Journal of Psychohistory,* 21(4), 479–496.

Goodwin, J.M., and Sachs, R.G. (1996). Child abuse in the etiology of dissociative disorders. In L.K. Michelson and W.J. Ray (Eds.), *Handbook of Dissociation: Theoretical, empirical, and clinical perspectives* (pp. 91–106). New York: Plenum Press.

Gorkin, M. (1987). *Uses of Countertransference*. Northvale, NJ: Jason Aronson, Inc.

Gould, C. (1992). Diagnosis and treatment of ritually abused children. In D.K. Sakheim and S.E. Devine (Eds.), *Out of Darkness: Exploring satanism and ritual abuse* (pp. 207–248). New York: Lexington Books.

Goulding, R.A., and Schwartz, R.C. (1995). *The Mosaic Mind: Empowering the tormented selves of child abuse survivors*. New York: Norton.

Graham, D.L.R. (1994). *Loving to Survive*. New York: NYU Press.

Grand, S. (1995). Incest and the intersubjective politics of knowing history. In J.L. Alpert (Ed.), *Sexual Abuse Recalled: Treating trauma in the era of the recovered memory debate* (pp. 235–256). Northvale, NJ: Jason Aronson, Inc.

Grand, S. (1997). The paradox of innocence: Dissociative adhesive states in perpetrators of incest. *Psychoanalytic Dialogues*, 7(4), 465–490.

Grand, S. (2000). *The Reproduction of Evil: A clinical and cultural perspective*. Hillsdale, NJ: The Analytic Press.

Grand, S., and Alpert, J.L. (1993). The core trauma of incest: an object relations view. *Professional Psychology: Research and Practice*, 24(3), 330–334.

Greaves, G.B. (1992). Alternative hypotheses regarding claims of satanic cult activity. In D.K. Sakheim and S.E. Devine (Eds.). *Out of Darkness: Exploring satanism and ritual abuse* (pp. 45–72). New York: Lexington Books.

Greaves, G.B., and Faust, G.H. (1996). Legal and ethical issues in the treatment of dissociative disorders. In L.K. Michelson and W.J. Ray (Eds.), *Handbook of Dissociation: Theoretical, empirical, and clinical perspectives* (pp. 595–615). New York: Plenum Press.

Greenberg, J.R. (1986). Theoretical models and the analyst's neutrality. *Contemporary Psychoanalysis*, 22, 87–106.

Greenberg, J.R. (1991). *Oedipus and Beyond*. Cambridge, MA: Harvard University Press.

Greenberg, J.R., and Mitchell, S.A. (1983). *Object Relations in Psychoanalytic Theory*. Cambridge, MA: Harvard University Press.

Greenfield, L.A. (1996). *Child Victimizers: Violent offenders and their victims*. Justice Department Joint Publication with the Office of Juvenile Justice and Delinquency Prevention. NCJ–153258, March, 1996.

Grosch, W.N., and Olsend, D.C. (1994). *When Helping Starts to Hurt: A new look at burnout among psychotherapists*. New York: W.W. Norton.

Grossman, W.I. (1991). Pain, aggression, fantasy and concepts of sadomasochism. *Psychoanalytic Quarterly*, 40, 22–52.

Groth, A.N. (1979). *Men Who Rape*. New York: Plenum Press.

Groth, A.N., Longo, R.E., and McFadin, J.B. (1982). Undetected recidivism among rapists and child molesters. *Crime and Delinquency*, 28(3), 450–458.

Grotstein, J.S. (1984). Forgery of the soul: Psychogenesis of evil. In M.C. Nelson and M.E. Eigen (Eds.), *Evil, Self, and Culture* (pp. 203–226: volume IV, Self-in Process Series). New York: Human Science Press, Inc.

Grotstein, J.S. (1999). The fate of the unconscious in the future of psychotherapy. *American Journal of Psychotherapy*, 53(1), 52–59.

Haaken, J. (1998). *Pillar of Salt: Gender, Memory, and the Perils of Looking Back*. New Brunswick, NJ: Rutgers University Press.

Hacking, I. (1995). *Rewriting the Soul: Multiple personality and the sciences of memory*. Princeton, NJ: Princeton University Press.

Harlan, S., Rodgers, L.L., and Slattery, B. (1981). Male and female adolescent prostitution: Huckleberry House sexual minority youth services project. Department of Health and Human Services, Youth Development Bureau, Washington, DC.

Harris, A. (1996a). False memory? False memory syndrome? So-called false memory syndrome? *Psychoanalytic Dialogues*, 6(2), 155–188.

Harvey, M.R. (1996). An ecological view of psychological trauma and trauma recovery. *Journal of Traumatic Stress*, 9(1), 3–24.

Hassan, S. (1990). *Combatting Cult Mind Control. Rochester,* VT: Park Street Press.

Hedges, L.E. (1994*). Remembering, Repeating, and Working Through Childhood Trauma.* Northvale, NJ: Jason Aronson, Inc.

Hegeman, E. (1995). Resolution of traumatic transference: Two cases. *Contemporary Psychoanalysis*, 31(3), 409–422.

Hegeman, E. (1997). Reconstruction and the psychoanalytic tradition. In Gartner, R.B. (Ed.), *Memories of Sexual Betrayal: Truth, fantasy, repression and dissociation* (pp. 149–178). Northvale, NJ: Jason Aronson, Inc.

Herman, J.L. (1990). Sex offenders: A feminist perspective. In W.L. Marshall, D.R. Laws, and H.E. Barbaree (Eds.), *Handbook of Sexual Assault: Issues, theories, and treatment of the offender* (pp. 177–193). New York: Plenum Press.

Herman, J.L. (1992). *Trauma and Recovery.* Basic Books: New York.

Herman, J.L. (1992a). Complex PTSD: A syndrome of survivors of prolonged and repeated trauma. *Journal of Traumatic Stress,* 5, 377–391.

Hertzberg, J.F. (1996). Internalizing power dynamics: The wounds and the healing. *Women and Therapy,* 18(3/4), 129–148.

Hirsh, I. (1994). Dissociation and the interpersonal self. *Contemporary Psychoanalysis,* 30(4), 777–799.

Hoffman, I.Z. (1991). Discussion: Towards a social-constructivist view of the psychoanalytic situation, *Psychoanalytic Dialogues,* 1(1), 74–105.

Holmes, W.C., and Slap, G.B. (1998). Sexual abuse of male children common, under-recognized, under-treated. *Journal of American Medical Association,* 280, 1855–1862.

hooks, b. (1995). *Killing Rage: Ending racism.* New York: Henry Holt, and Co.

Horevitz, R. (1994). Dissociation and multiple personality: Conflicts and controversies. In S.J. Lynn and J.W. Rhue (Eds.), *Dissociation: Clinical and theoretical perspectives* (pp. 434–461). New York: Guilford.

Hornstein, N., and Putnam, F.W. (1992). Clinical phenomenology of child and adolescent multiple personality disorder. *Journal of the Academy of Child and Adolescent Psychiatry,* 31, 1055–1077.

Horowitz, M.J. (1986). Stress-response syndromes: A review of posttraumatic and adjustment disorder. *Hospital and Community Psychiatry,* 37, 241–249.

Howell, E.F. (1996). Dissociation in masochism and psychopathic sadism. *Contemporary Psychoanalysis,* 32(3), 427–454.

Howell, E.F. (1997). Masochism: A bridge to the other side of abuse. *Dissociation,* 10(4), 240–245.

Howitt, D. (1995). *Paedophiles and Sexual Offenses Against Children.* New York: Wiley and Sons.

Hudson, P. (1991). *Ritual Child Abuse: Discovery, diagnosis and treatment.* Sarasota, CA: R and E Publishers.

Huizenga, J. (1990). Incest as trauma: A psychoanalytic case. In H.B. Levine (Ed.), *Adult Analysis and Childhood Sexual Abuse* (pp. 117–136). Hillsdale, NJ: Analytic Press.

Hunt, L. (1991). *Secret Agenda: The United States Government, Nazi scientists, and Project Paperclip 1945 to 1990.* New York: St. Martin's Press.

Hunt, P., and Baird, M. (1990). Children of sex rings. *Child Welfare,* 419(3), 195–207.

Hunter, S.K. (1994). Prostitution is cruelty and abuse to women and children. *Michigan Journal of Gender and Law,* 1, 1–14.

Inderbitzin, L.B., and Levy, S.T. (1994). On grist for the mill: External reality as defense. *Journal of the American Psychoanalytic Association,* 42, 763–788.

International Society for the Study of Dissociation (1994). *Guidelines for Treating Dissociative Identity Disorder (multiple personality disorder) in adults (1994).* Skokie, IL: International Society for the Study of Dissociation.

Irwin, H.J. (1994). Proneness to dissociation and traumatic childhood events. *Journal of Nervous and Mental Diseases,* 182, 456–460.

Irwin, H.J. (1999). Pathological and nonpathological dissociation: The relevance of childhood trauma. *Journal of Psychology,* 133(2), 157–164.

Jacobs, T. (1986). On countertransference enactments. *Journal of the American Psychoanalytic Association*, 34, 289–302.

Janet, P. (1889). *L'automatisme Psychologique*. Paris: Felix Alcan.

Janet, P. (1986/1925). *Psychological Healing*. New York: Macmillan.

Janoff-Bulman, R. (1992). *Shattered Assumptions: Toward a new psychology of trauma*. New York: Free Press.

Jaroff, L. (1993). Lies of the mind. *Time*, November 29, 52–59.

Jellinek, M.S., Murphy, J.M., Poltrast, F., Quinn, D., Bishop, S.J., and Goshko, M. (1991). Serious child maltreatment in Massachusetts: The course of 206 children through the courts. *Child Abuse and Neglect*, 16, 179–185.

Jenkins, P. (1998). Moral Panic: *Changing Concepts of the Child Molester in Modern America*, New Haven, CT: Yale University Press.

Jones, D.P.H. (1991). Ritual child sexual abuse. *Child Abuse and Neglect*, 15, 163–170.

Jones, D.P.H. (1993). Child sexual abuse and satanism. *Newsletter of the Association of Child Psychology and Psychiatry*, 15, 207–213.

Jones, D.P.H., and McGraw, J.M. (1987). Reliable and fictitious accounts of sexual abuse of children. *Journal of Interpersonal Violence*, 2(1), 27–45.

Jonker, F., and Jonker-Bakker, I. (1997). Effects of ritual abuse: The results of three surveys in the Netherlands. *Journal of Child Abuse and Neglect*, 21, 541–556.

Jung, C.G. (1958). *The Collected Works of C.G. Jung: Vol. 3 Schizophrenia*. Princeton, NJ: Princeton University Press.

Kafka, H. (1995). Incestuous sexual abuse, memory and the organization of the self. In J.L. Alpert (Ed.), *Sexual Abuse Recalled: Treating trauma in the era of the recovered memory debate* (pp. 135–154). Northvale, NJ: Jason Aronson, Inc.

Kafka, H. (1997). Incest survival, memory disruption, and authenticity of the self. In Gartner, R. B. (Ed.), *Memories of Sexual Betrayal: Truth, fantasy, repression and dissociation* (pp. 113–128). Northvale, NJ: Jason Aronson, Inc.

Kalsched, D. (1996). *The Inner World of Trauma: Archetypal defenses of the personal spirit*. New York: Routledge.

Kardiner, A. (1941). *The Traumatic Neuroses of War*. New York: Paul Hober.

Keenan, T., and Caruth, C. (1995). The AIDS crisis is not one: A conversation with Gregg Bordowitz, Douglas Crimp, and Laura Pinsky. In C. Caruth (Ed.), *Trauma: Explorations in memory* (pp. 256–271). Baltimore, MD: Johns Hopkins University Press.

Kemp, K., Gilverston, A.D., and Torem, M. (1988). The differential diagnosis of multiple personality disorder from borderline personality disorder. *Dissociation*, 1(4), 41–46.

Kempe, C.H., Silverman, F.N., Steele, B.F., Droegemueller, W, and Silver, H.K. (1962). The battered child syndrome. *Journal of the American Medical Association*, 181, 17–24.

Kennedy, J.P. (1996). Keynote Address. Symposium Proceedings: *Forced Labor: The Prostitution of Children* (pp. 1–8), U.S. Department of Labor, Bureau of International Labor Affairs, 1996.

Kennedy, R. (1996). Aspects of consciousness: One voice or many? *Psychoanalytic Dialogues*, 4, 73–98.

Kepner, J.I. (1995). *Healing Tasks: Psychotherapy with adult survivors of childhood abuse*. San Francisco, CA: Jossey-Bass.

Kernberg, O. (1976). *Object Relations Theory and Clinical Psychoanalysis*. New York: Jason Aronson, Inc.

Kessler, R.C., Sonnega, A., Bromet, E., Hughes, M., and Nelson, L.B. (1995). Posttraumatic stress disorder in the national Comorbidity Study. *Archives of General Psychiatry*, 52, 1048–1060.

Khan, M. (1978). Secret as potential space. In S.A. Grolnick, L. Barkin, and W. Muensterberger (Eds.), *Between Reality and Fantasy* (pp. 259–270). Northvale, NJ: Jason Aronson, Inc.

Kihlstrom, J.F., Glisky, M.L., and Angiulo, M.J. (1994). Dissociative tendencies and dissociative disorders. *Journal of Abnormal Psychology*, 103, 111–124.

Kim, D.S. (1986). How physicians respond to child maltreatment cases. *Health and Social Work*, 11, 95–106.

Kincaid, J.R. (1998) *Erotic Innocence: The culture of child molesting*. Durham, NC: Duke University Press.

Kinsey, A.L., Pomerory, W.B., Martin, C.E., and Gebhard, P.H. (1948). *Sexual Behavior in the Human Male*. Philadelphia, PA: Saunders.

Kinsey, A.L., Pomerory, W.B., Martin, C.E., and Gebhard, P.H. (1953). *Sexual Behavior in the Human Female*. Philadelphia, PA: Saunders.

Kinzie, J.D., and Boehnlein, J.K. (1993). Psychotherapy with victims of massive violence: Countertransference and ethical issues. *American Journal of Psychotherapy*, 47, 90–102.

Kleber, R.J., Figley, C.R., and Gersons, B.P.R. (1996). Introduction. In R.J. Kleber, C.R. Figley, and B.P.R. Gersons (Eds.) *Beyond Trauma: Cultural and societal dynamics* (pp. 1–9). New York: Plenum Press.

Kluft, R.P. (1984). Treatment of multiple personality disorder. *Psychiatric Clinics of North America*, 7, 9–29.

Kluft, R.P. (1984a). An introduction to multiple personality disorder, *Psychiatric Annals*, 14, 19–24.

Kluft, R.P. (1985). Childhood multiple personality disorder: Predictors, clinical findings, and treatment results. In R.P. Kluft (Ed.), *Childhood Antecedents of Multiple Personality Disorder* (pp. 168–196). Washington, DC: American Psychiatric Press.

Kluft, R.P. (1985a). Childhood multiple personality disorder: Predictors, clinical findings, and treatment results. In R.P. Kluft (Ed.), *Childhood Antecedents of Multiple Personality Disorder* (pp. 167-196). Washington, DC: American Psychiatric Press.

Kluft, R.P. (1985b). Making the diagnosis of multiple personality disorder (MPD). In F.F. Flach (Ed.), *Directions in Psychiatry* (pp. 1–10). New York: Hatherleigh.

Kluft, R.P. (1987a). An update on multiple personality disorder. *Hospital and Community Psychiatry*, 38, 363–373.

Kluft, R.P. (1987b). The simulation and dissimulation of multiple personality disorder. *Journal of Clinical Hypnosis*, 30(2), 104–118.

Kluft, R.P. (1988a). Today's therapeutic pluralism. *Dissociation*, 1(2), 1–2.

Kluft, R.P. (1988b). The phenomenology and treatment of extremely complex multiple personality disorder. *Dissociation*, 1(4), 47–58.

Kluft, R.P. (1989). Iatrogenic creation of new alter personalities. *Dissociation*, 2, 83–91.

Kluft, R.P. (1990). Incest and subsequent revictimization. In R.P. Kluft (Ed.), *Incest Related Syndromes of Adult Psychopathology* (pp. 263–288). Washington, DC: American Psychiatric Press.

Kluft, R.P. (1992). Paradigm exhaustion and paradigm shift—thinking through the therapeutic impasses. *Psychiatric Annals*, 22(10), 502–508.

Kluft, R.P. (1994a). Treatment trajectories in multiple personality disorder. *Dissociation*, 7, 63–76.

Kluft, R.P. (1994b). Clinical observations on the use of the CSDS Dimensions of Therapeutic Movement Instrument (DTMI). *Dissociation*, 7, 272–283.

Kluft, R.P. (1994c). Countertransference in the treatment of multiple personality disorder. In. J.P. Wilson and J.D. Lindy (Eds.), *Countertransference and Posttraumatic Stress Disorder* (pp. 122–150). New York: Guilford.

Kluft, R.P. (1995a). The confirmation and disconfirmation of memories of abuse in dissociative identity disorder patients: A naturalistic clinical study. *Dissociation*, 8(4), 253–258.

Kluft, R.P. (1996). Dissociative identity disorder. In L.K. Michelson and W.J. Ray (Eds.), *Handbook of Dissociation: Theoretical, empirical, and clinical perspectives* (pp. 337–366). New York: Plenum Press.

Kluft, R.P. (1998). Reflections on the traumatic memories of dissociative identity disorder patients. In S. Lynn and K. McConkey (Eds.), *Truth in Memory* (pp. 304–322). New York: Guilford.

Kluft, R.P. (1999a). An overview of the psychotherapy of dissociative identity disorder. *American Journal of Psychotherapy*, 53(3), 289–319.

Kluft, R.P. (1999b). Current issues in dissociative identity disorder. *Journal of Practical Psychiatry and Behavioral Health*, 5, 3–19.

Kluft, R.P., and Fine, C.G. (1993). *Clinical Perspectives on Multiple Personality Disorder.* Washington, DC: American Psychiatric Press.

Kluft, R.P., and Foote, B. (1999). Dissociative identity disorder: Recent developments. *American Journal of Psychotherapy,* 53(3), 283–288.

Kohut, H. (1959). Introspection, empathy and psychoanalysis. *Journal of the American Psychoanalytic Association,* 7, 459–483.

Kohut, H. (1971). *The Analysis of the Self.* New York: International Universities Press.

Kohut, H. (1977). *The Restoration of the Self.* New York: International Universities Press.

Kohut, H. (1984). *How Does Analysis Cure?* Chicago, IL: University of Chicago Press.

Kornfeld, E.L. (1996). The development of a treatment approach for victims of human rights violations in Chile. In R.J. Kleber, C.R. Figley, B.P.R. Gersons (Eds.), *Beyond Trauma: Cultural and societal dynamics* (pp. 115–130). New York: Plenum Press.

Kramer, S. (1994). Further considerations on somatic and cognitive residues of incest. In A. Sugarman (Ed.), *Victims of Abuse: The emotional impact of child and adult trauma* (pp. 69–95). Madison, CT. International University Press.

Krystal, H. (1978). Trauma and affects. *The Psychoanalytic Study of the Child,* 33, 81–116.

Krystal, J.H., Bennett, A., Bremner, J.D., Southwick, A.M., and Charney, D.S. (1996). Recent developments in the neurobiology of dissociation: Implications for posttraumatic stress disorder. In L.K. Michelson and W.J. Ray (Eds.), *Handbook of Dissociation: Theoretical, empirical, and clinical perspectives* (pp. 163-190). New York, NY: Plenum Press.

Kumin, I. (1978). Developmental aspects of opposites and paradox. *International Review of Psychoanalysis,* 5, 477–483.

Lander, D. (1997). The sacrifice of the innocents. *Journal of Psychohistory,* 24(3), 214–220.

Landsberg, M. (1996). Beware of false prophets peddling false-memory hype. *Toronto Star,* February 11, p. A2.

Langer, L. (1996). *Admitting the Holocaust: Collected essays.* New York: Oxford University Press.

Langevin, R., Martentette, D., and Rosati, B. (1996). Why therapy fails with some sex offenders: Learning difficulties examined empirically. In E. Coleman, S.M. Dwyer, and N.J. Pollone (Eds.), *Sex Offender Treatment: Biological dysfunction, intrapsychic conflict, interpersonal violence* (pp. 71–84). New York: Haworth Press.

Langevin, R., and Watson, R.J. (1996). Major factors in the assessment of paraphiliacs and sex offenders. In E. Coleman, S.M. Dwyer, and N.J. Pollone (Eds.), *Sex Offender Treatment: Biological dysfunction, intrapsychic conflict, interpersonal violence* (pp. 39–70). New York: Haworth Press.

Lanning, K.V. (1984). Collectors. In A. Burgess and M. Clark (Eds.), *Child Pornography and Sex Rings* (pp. 83–92). Lexington, MA: Lexington Books, D.C. Heath and Company.

Lanning, K.V. (1992). A law enforcement perspective on allegations of religious abuse. In D.K. Sakheim and S.E. Devine (Eds.), *Out of Darkness: Exploring satanism and ritual abuse.* New York: Lexington Books.

Larson, N.R., and Maddock, J.W. (1986). Structural and functional variables in incest family systems: Implications for assessment and treatment. In T.S. Tepper and M.J. Barrett (Eds.), *Treating Incest: A multiple systems perspective.* New York: Haworth Press, Inc.

Laub, D. (1995). Truth and testimony: The process and the struggle. In C. Caruth (Ed.), *Trauma: Explorations in memory* (pp. 61–75). Baltimore, MD: Johns Hopkins University Press.

Laub, D., and Auerhahn, N. (1989). Failed empathy—A central theme in the survivor's Holocaust experiences. *Psychoanalytic Psychology,* 6, 377–400.

Laub, D., and Auerhahn, N. (1993). Knowing and not knowing massive trauma: Forms of traumatic memory. *International Journal of Psychoanalysis,* 74, 287–302.

Leavitt, F. (1997). False attribution of suggestibility to explain recovered memory of childhood sexual abuse following extended amnesia. *Child Abuse and Neglect,* 21(3), 265–272.

Leowald, H. (1988). *Sublimation.* New Haven, CT: Yale University Press.

Leowald, H.W. (1960). On the therapeutic action of psychoanalysis. *International Journal of Psychoanalysis*, 41, 16–33.

Leowald, H.W. (1972). The experience of time. *The Psychoanalytic Study of the Child*, 27, 401–410.

Leowald, H.W. (1974). Psychoanalysis as art and the fantasy nature of the psychoanalytic situation. In Leowald, H., *Papers in Psychoanalysis* (pp. 352–371). New Haven, CT: Yale University Press, 1980.

Leowald, H.W. (1980). *Papers on Psychoanalysis*. New Haven, CT: Yale University Press.

Levenson, E. (1972). *The Fallacy of Understanding*. New York: Basic Books.

Levenson, E.A. (1995/1996). A monopedal presentation of interpersonal psychoanalysis. *The Review of Interpersonal Psychoanalysis: William Alanson White Institute of Psychiatry, Psychology, and Psychoanalysis*, 1(1), 1–4.

Levenson, E.A. (1996). Aspects of self revelation and self-disclosure. *Contemporary Psychoanalysis*, 32(2), 237–248.

Levine, H.B. (1990). Introduction. In H.B. Levine (Ed.), *Adult Analysis and Childhood Sexual Abuse* (pp. 3–20). Hillsdale, NJ: Analytic Press.

Levine, H.B. (1994). Repetition, reenactment and trauma. In A. Sugarman (Ed.), *Victims of Abuse: The emotional impact of child and adult trauma* (pp. 141–164). Madison, CT: International University Press.

Lifton, R.J. (1961). *Thought Reform and the Psychology of Totalism*. New York: W.W. Norton.

Lifton, R. J. (1986). *The Nazi Doctors: Medical killing and the psychology of genocide*. New York: Basic Books.

Lindemann, E. (1944). Symptomatology and management of acute grief. *American Journal of Psychiatry*, 101, 141–148.

Lindsay, D.S., and Read, J.D. (1994). Psychotherapy and memories of childhood sexual abuse: A cognitive perspective. *Applied Cognitive Psychology*, 8, 281–338.

Lisak, D., Hopper, J., and Song, P. (1996). Factors in the cycle of violence: Gender rigidity and emotional constriction. *Journal of Traumatic Stress*, 9(4), 721–742.

Loewenstein, R.J. (1993). Anna O: Reformulation as a case of multiple personality disorder. In J.M. Goodwin (Ed.), *Rediscovering Childhood Trauma: Historical casebook and clinical applications* (pp. 139–167).

Loftus, E.F. (1993). The reality of repressed memories. *American Psychologist*, 48, 518–537.

Loftus, E.F. (1995). Remembering dangerously. *Skeptical Inquirer*, 19, 20–30.

Loftus, E.F., and Ketcham, K. (1994). *The Myth of Repressed Memory: False memories and allegations of sexual abuse*. New York: St. Martin's Press.

Loftus, E.F., Milo, E.M., and Paddock, J.R. (1995). The accidental executioner: Why psychotherapy must be influenced by science. *Counseling Psychologist*, 23(2), 300–309.

Lyon, K.A. (1992). Shattered mirror: A fragment of the treatment of a patient with multiple personality disorder. *Psychoanalytic Inquiry*, 12, 71–94.

MacKinnon, C.A. (1987). *Feminism Unmodified: Discourse on life and the law*. Cambridge, MA: Harvard University Press.

MacVicar, K. (1997). Discussion: The retrieval of repressed memories. In C. Prozan (Ed.), *Construction and reconstruction of Memory: Dilemmas of childhood sexual abuse* (pp. 189–206). Northvale, NJ: Jason Aronson, Inc.

Magid, B. (1988). The evil self. *Dynamic Psychotherapy*, 6(2), 99–113.

Main, M. (1995). Recent studies in attachment: Overview with selected implications for clinical work. In Goldberg, S., Muir, R., and Kerr, J. (Ed.), *Attachment Theory*. Hillsdale, New Jersey: Analytic Press, pp. 19–43.

Main, M., Kaplan, N., and Cassidy, J. (1985). Security in infancy, childhood, and adulthood: A move to the level of representation. In I. Bretherton and E. Waters (Eds.), *Growing Points of Attachment Theory and Research: Monography of the Society for Research in Child Development*, 50, 66–104.

Marks, J. (1979). *The Search for the "Manchurian Candidate": The CIA and Mind Control.* New York: Times Books.

Marmer, S.S. (1980). Psychoanalysis of multiple personality disorder. *International Journal of Psychoanalysis, 61,* 439–459.

Marmer, S.S. (1996). An outline for psychoanalytic treatment. In J.L. Spira (Ed.), *Treating Dissociative Identity Disorder* (pp. 183–218). San Francisco, CA: Jossey-Bass.

Marmer, S. (1999). Variations on a factitious theme. *Journal of Psychiatry and Law, 27,* 459–481.

Maroda, K.J. (1991). *The Power of Countertransference: Innovations in analytic technique.* New York: Wiley and Sons.

Maroda, K.J. (1999). *Seduction, Surrender, and Transformation: Emotional engagement in the analytic process.* Analytic Press: Hillsdale, NJ.

McCann, I.L., and Coletti, J. (1994). The dance of empathy: A hermeneutic formulation of countertransference, empathy, and understanding in the treatment of individuals who have experienced early childhood trauma. In J.P. Wilson and J.D. Lindy (Eds.), *Countertransference and Posttraumatic Stress Disorder* (pp. 87–121). New York: Guilford.

McCann, L., and Pearlman, L.A. (1990). Vicarious traumatization: A framework for understanding the psychological effects of working with victims. *Journal of Traumatic Stress, 3*(1), 131–149.

McCurdy, K., and Daro, D. (1993). *Current trends in child abuse reporting and fatalities: The results of the 1992 Fifty State Survey.* Chicago, IL: National Center on Child Abuse Prevention Research.

McFadyen, A., Hanks, H., and James, C. (1993). Ritual abuse: A definition. *Child Abuse Review, 2,* 35–41.

McHugh, P. (1997). Foreword. In A. Piper, *Hoax and Reality: The bizarre world of multiple personality* (pp. ix–x). Northvale, NJ: Jason Aronson, Inc.

McHugh, P.R. (1993a). Procedures in the diagnosis of incest in recovered memory cases. *FMS Foundation Newsletter,* May 3, p. 3.

McHugh, P.R. (1993b) To Treat. *FMS Foundation Newsletter,* October 1, p. 1.

McHugh, P.R. (1995). Witches, multiple personalities, and other psychiatric artifacts. *Nature Medicine, 1,* 110–114.

McWilliams, N. (1994) *Psychoanalytic Diagnosis: Understanding personality structure in the clinical process.* New York: Guilford.

Melamuth, N.M., Heavey, C.L., and Linz, D. (1996). The confluence model of sexual aggression: Combining hostile masculinity and impersonal sex. In E. Coleman, S.M. Dwyer, and N.J. Pollone (Eds.), *Sex Offender Treatment: Biological dysfunction, intrapsychic conflict, interpersonal violence* (pp. 13–37). New York: Haworth Press.

Meloy, R. (1988). *The Psychopathic Mind: Origins, dynamics, and treatment.* Northvale, NJ: Jason Aronson, Inc.

Melton, G.B., Goodman, G.S., Kalichman, S.C., Levine, M., Saywits, K.J., and Koocher, G.P. (1995). Empirical research on child maltreatment and the law. *Journal of Clinical Child Psychology, 24* (Suppl), 47–77.

Merskey, H. (1992). The manufacture of personalities: The production of multiple personality disorder. *British Journal of Psychiatry, 160,* 327–340.

Merskey, H. (1995). The manufacture of personalities: The production of multiple personality disorder. In L. Cohen, J. Berzoff, and M. Elin (Eds.), *Dissociative Identity Disorder: Theoretical and treatment controversies* (pp. 3–32). Northvale, NJ: Jason Aronson, Inc.

Milburn, M.A., and Conrad, S.D. (1996). The politics of denial. *Journal of Psychohistory, 23*(3), 238–251.

Miller, A. (1984). *Thou Shalt Not Be Aware.* New York: Farrar, Straus, and Giroux.

Miller, M.L. (1996). Validation, interpretation, and corrective emotional experience in psychoanalytic treatment. *Contemporary Psychoanalysis, 32*(3), 385–411.

Mitchell, S.A. (1988). *Relational Concepts in Psychoanalysis: An integration.* Cambridge, MA: Harvard University Press.

Mitchell, S.A. (1993). *Hope and Dread in Psychoanalysis*. New York: Basic.

Mitchell, S.A. (1995). Interaction in the Kleinian and Interpersonal traditions. *Contemporary Psychoanalysis*, 31(1), 65–91.

Mitchell, S.A . (1998). Letting the paradox teach us. In J.G. Teicholz and D. Kriegman (Eds.), *Trauma, Repetition, and Affect: The Work of Paul Russell*, (p.49–66). New York: The Other Press.

Mitchell, S.A. (1999). Attachment theory and the psychoanalytic tradition: Reflections on human relationality. *Psychoanalytic Dialogues*, 9(1), 85–108.

Modell, A.H. (1990). *Other Times, Other Realities*. Cambridge, MA: Harvard University Press.

Mohr, J.W., Turner, R.E., and Jerry, M.B. (1964). *Pedophilia and Exhibitionism*. Toronto: University of Toronto Press.

Moore, R. (1991). Ritual sacred space and healing: the psychoanalyst as ritual elder. In N. Schwartz-Salant and M. Stein (Eds.), *Liminality and Transitional Phenomena* (pp. 13–32). Wilmette, IL: Chiron.

Morgan, R. (1989). *The Demon Lover: On the sexuality of terrorism*. New York: Norton.

Morrison, T. (1987/1991). *Beloved*. New York: Penguin/Signet.

Muntarbhorn, V. (1996). International perspectives and child prostitution in Asia. In *Forced Labor: The Prostitution of Children* (pp. 9–31). Symposium Proceedings, U.S. Department of Labor, Bureau of International Labor Affairs, 1996.

Murphy, P. (1993). *Making the Connections: Women, work and abuse: Dramatic insight into the lives of abuse victims and practical recommendations for their successful return to work*. Orlando, FL: Paul M. Deutsch Press.

Murphy, W.D., and Smith, T.A. (1996). Sex offenders against children. In J. Briere, L. Berliner, J. Bulkley, C. Jenny, and T. Reid (Eds.), *The APSAC Handbook on Child Maltreatment*. Thousand Oaks, CA: Sage.

Myers, J.E.B., Becker, J., Belliner, L., Corwin, D.L., and Saywitz, K.J. (1989). Expert testimony in child abuse litigation. *Nebraska Law Review*, 68(1/2), 1–145.

Nachmani, G. (1995). Trauma and ignorance. *Contemporary Psychoanalysis*, 31(3), 423–450.

Nachmani, G. (1997). Discussion: Reconstructing methods of victimization. In R.B. Gartner (Ed.), *Memories of Sexual Betrayal: Truth, fantasy, repression and dissociation* (pp. 189–208). Northvale, NJ: Jason Aronson, Inc.

Nathanson, D.L. (1987). A timetable for shame. In D.L. Nathanson (Ed.), *The Many Faces of Shame* (pp. 1–62), New York: Guilford.

Nathanson, D.L. (1992). *Shame and Pride: Affect, sex, and the birth of the self*. New York: Norton.

National Center for Missing and Exploited Children. (1998). *1997 Missing Children Statistics Fact Sheet*. Arlington, VA: National Center for Missing and Exploited Children.

National Victim Center Infolink on Missing Children (1996). Vol. 1 (32). Arlington, VA: The National Center for Victims of Crime.

Natterson, J. (1991). *Beyond Countertransference: The therapist's subjectivity in the therapeutic process*. Northvale, NJ: Jason Aronson, Inc.

Nemiah, J.C. (1985). Dissociative disorders ("hysterical neurosis, dissociative type"). In H.I. Kaplan and B.J. Sadock (Eds.), *Comprehensive Textbook of Psychiatry*, 4th edition. Baltimore, MD: Williams and Wilkins.

Neumann, D.A., and Gamble, S.J. (1995). Issues in the professional development of psychotherapists: Countertransference and vicarious traumatization in the new trauma therapies. *Psychotherapy*, 32(2), 341–347.

Newton, M. (1996). Written in blood: A history of human sacrifice. *Journal of Psychohistory*, 24(2), 104–131.

Noblitt, J.R., and Perskin, P.S. (1995). *Cult and Ritual Abuse: Its anthropology and recent discovery in contemporary America*. Westport, CT: Praeger.

Noblitt, J.R., and Perskin, P.S. (2000). *Cult and Ritual Abuse: Its history, and recent discovery in contemporary America* (Rev. Ed.). Westport, CT: Praeger.

Novick, J., and Novick, K.K. (1996). Externalization as a pathological form of relating: The dynamic underpinnings of abuse. In A. Sugarman (Ed.), *Victims of Abuse: The emotional impact of child and adult trauma* (pp. 45–68). Madison, CT: International Universities Press.

Nurcombe, B., and Unutzer, J. (1991). The ritual abuse of children: Clinical features and diagnostic reasoning. *Journal of the American Academy of Child and Adolescent Psychiatry*, 30(2), 272–276.

Oates, S.R.K. (1996). *The Spectrum of Child Abuse: Assessment, treatment, prevention*. New York: Bruner/Mazel.

Ofshe, R., and Watters, E. (1994). *Making Monsters: False memory, psychotherapy, and sexual hysteria*. New York: Scribners.

Ogden, T. (1989). *The Primitive Edge of Experience*. Northvale, NJ: Jason Aronson, Inc.

Ogden, T. (1990). *The Matrix of the Mind*. Northvale, NJ: Jason Aronson, Inc.

Ogden, T. (1992). Consultation is often needed when treating severe dissociative disorders. *Psychodynamic Letter*, 1 (10), 1–4.

O'Hara, M., and Anderson, W.T. (1995). Psychotherapy's identity crisis. In W.T. Anderson (Ed.), *The Truth About Truth: De-Confusing and Re-Constructing the Postmodern World* (pp. 170–176). New York: Jeremy P. Tarcher/Putnam.

OJP (2000). Office of Justice Programs. Press Release, May 10, 2000: New Grants to Combat Internet Crimes. Justice Department's Office of Juvenile Justice and Delinquency Prevention (OJJDP), (www.ojp.usdoj.gov.).

Olafson, E., Corwin, D.L., and Summit, R.C. (1993). Modern history of child sexual abuse awareness: Cycles of discovery and suppression. *Child Abuse and Neglect*, 17, 7–24.

Olio, K.A., and Cornell, W.F. (1993). The therapeutic relationship as the foundation for treatment with adult survivors of sexual abuse. *Psychotherapy*, 30, 512–523.

Orange, D. (1995). *Emotional Understanding: Studies in psychoanalytic epistemology*. New York: Guilford.

Orange, D., Atwood, G.E., and Stolorow, R.D. (1997). *Working Intersubjectively: Contextualism in psychoanalytic practice*. Hillsdale, NJ: Analytic Press.

Orbach, S. (1999). Why is attachment in the air? *Psychoanalytic Dialogues*, 9(1), 73–84.

Orwell, G. (1949). *1984*. New York: New American Library, Signet Classic Edition, 1949.

Otero, J.F. (1996). *Forced Labor: The prostitution of children*. Symposium Proceedings, U.S. Department of Labor, Bureau of International Affairs, 1996.

Paddock, J.R. (1994). Disengaging from a blaming: Psychology in the 1990's. *Georgia Psychologist*, 47(4), 2–6.

Pearlman, L.A., and Saakvitne, K.W. (1995). *Trauma and the Therapist: Countertransference and vicarious traumatization in psychotherapy with incest survivors*. New York: Norton.

Peoples, K.M. (1992, August). Unconscious dominance and submission. In E. Cardena (Chair), *Consciousness, dissociative alterations of consciousness and trauma*. Symposium conducted at the Centennial Convention of the American Psychological Association, Washington, DC.

Perlman, S.D. (1999). *The Therapist's Emotional Survival: Dealing with the pain of exploring trauma*. Northvale, NJ: Jason Aronson, Inc.

Peters, D.S., Wyatt, G.E., and Finkelhor, D. (1986). Prevalence. In D. Finkelhor (Ed.), *A Sourcebook on Child Sexual Abuse* (pp. 15–59). Beverly Hills, CA: Sage Publishing.

Peterson, C., and Biggs, M. (1997). Interviewing children about trauma: Problems with "specific" questions. *Journal of Traumatic Stress*, 10(2), 279–290.

Phillips, A. (1994). *On Flirtation: Psychoanalytic essays on the uncommitted life*. Cambridge, MA: Harvard University Press.

Pierce, R.L. (1984). Child pornography: A hidden dimension of child abuse. *Child Abuse and Neglect*, 8, 483–493.

Piper, A. (1997). *Hoax and Reality: The bizarre world of multiple personality disorder*. Northvale, NJ: Jason Aronson, Inc.

Pithers, W.D. (1990). Relapse prevention with sexual aggressors: A method for maintaining therapeutic gain and enhancing external supervision. In W.L. Marshall, D.R. Laws, and H.E. Barbaree (Eds.), *Handbook of Sexual Assault: Issues, theories, and treatment of the offender* (pp. 343–361). New York: Plenum Press.

Pitman, R.K. (1993). Biological findings in posttraumatic stress disorder: Implications for DSM IV classification. In J.R.T. Davidson and E.B. Foa (Eds.), *Posttraumatic Stress Disorder: DSM IV and Beyond* (pp. 173–190). Washington, DC: American Psychiatric Press.

Pizer, S.A. (1992). The negotiation of paradox in the analytic patient. *Psychoanalytic Dialogues*, 2(2), 215–240.

Pizer, S.A. (1996). The distributed self: Introduction to symposium on "The multiplicity of self and analytic technique." *Contemporary Psychoanalysis*, 32(4), 499–508.

Pizer, S.A. (1996a). Negotiating potential space: illusion, play, metaphor and the subjunctive. *Psychoanalytic Dialogues*, 6(5), 689–712.

Pizer, S.A. (1998). *Building Bridges: The negotiation of paradox in psychoanalysis*. Hillsdale, NJ: Analytic Press.

Pope, K.S., and Brown, L.S. (1996). *Recovered Memories of Abuse: Assessment, therapy, forensics*. Washington, DC: American Psychological Association Press.

Price, M. (1995). Knowing and not knowing: Paradox in the construction of historical narratives. In J.L. Alpert (Ed.), *Sexual Abuse Recalled: Treating trauma in the era of the recovered memory debate* (pp. 289–309). Northvale, NJ: Jason Aronson, Inc.

Price, M. (1997). Knowing and not knowing: Paradox in the construction of historical narratives. In R.B. Gartner (Ed.), *Memories of Sexual Betrayal: Truth, fantasy, repression and dissociation* (pp. 129–144). Northvale, NJ: Jason Aronson, Inc.

Prior, S. (1996). *Object Relations in Severe Trauma: Psychotherapy of the sexually abused child*. Northvale, NJ: Jason Aronson, Inc.

Putnam, F.W. (1988). The switch process in multiple personality disorder. *Dissociation*, 1(1), 24–32.

Putnam, F.W. (1989). *The Diagnosis and Treatment of Multiple Personality Disorder*. New York: Guilford.

Putnam, F.W. (1992). Discussion: Are alter personalities fragments or fiction? *Psychoanalytic Inquiry*, 12, 95–111.

Putnam, F.W. (1994). The switch process in multiple personality disorder and other state change disorders. In R.M. Klein and B.K. Doane (Eds.), *Psychological Concepts and Dissociative Disorders* (pp. 283–304). Hillsdale, NJ: Lawrence Erlbaum and Associates.

Putnam, F. (1997). *Dissociation in Children and Adolescents: A developmental perspective*. New York: Guilford.

Putnam, F.W. (1999). Childhood maltreatment and adverse outcomes: A prospective developmental approach. Paper presented at the American Psychiatric Association Annual Meeting (Day 2, May 18, 1999).

Putnam, F.W., Guroff, J.J., Silberman, Barban, L., and Post, R.M. (1986). The clinical phenomenology of multiple personality disorder: Review of 100 recent cases. *Journal of Clinical Psychiatry*, 47, 285–293.

Putnam, F.W., and Tricket, P.K. (1997). The psychobiological effects of sexual abuse: A longitudinal study. *Annals of the New York Academy of Science*, 821, 150–159.

Pye, E. (1995). Memory and imagination: Placing imagination in the therapy of individuals with incest memories. In J.L. Alpert (Ed.), *Sexual Abuse Recalled: Treating trauma in the era of the recovered memory debate* (pp. 155–184). Northvale, NJ: Jason Aronson, Inc.

Rabin, H.M. (1995). The liberating effect on the analyst of the paradigm shift in psychoanalysis. *Psychoanalytic Psychology*, 12(4), 467–481.

Rachman, A.W. (1997). The suppression and censorship of Ferenczi's "Confusion of Tongues" paper. *Psychoanalytic Inquiry*, 17, 459–485.

Radden, J. (1996). *Divided Minds, Successive Selves: Ethical issues in disorders of identity and personality*. Cambridge, MA: MIT Press/Bradford Books.

Rascovsky, A. (1995). *Filicide: The murder, humiliation, mutilation, denigration, and abandonment of children*. New York: Jason Aronson, Inc.

Rasmussen, L.A., Burton, J.E. and Christopherson, B.J. (1992). Precursors to offending and the trauma outcome process in sexually reactive children. *Journal of Child Sexual Abuse*, 1, 33–48.

Reis, B.E. (1993). Toward a psychoanalytic understanding of multiple personality disorder. *Bulletin of the Menninger Clinic*, 57, 309–318.

Renik, O. (1995). The ideal of the anonymous analyst and the problem of self-disclosure. *Psychoanalytic Quarterly*, 64, 466–495.

Revitch, E., and Weiss, R.G. (1962). The pedophiliac offender. *Diseases of the Nervous System*, 23, 73–78.

Rhue, J.W., Lynn, S.J., and Sandberg (1995). Dissociation, fantasy, and imagination in childhood: A comparison of physically abused, sexually abused, and nonabused children. *Contemporary Hypnosis*, 12(2), 131–136.

Rieker, P.P., and Carmen, E.H. (1986). The victim to patient process: The disconfirmation and transformation of abuse. *American Journal of Orthopsychiatry*, 56(3), 360–370.

Rivera, M. (1989). Linking the psychological and the social: Feminism, poststructuralism, and multiple personality. *Dissociation*, 2(1), 24–31.

Rivera, M. (1996). *More Alike Than Different: Treating severely dissociative trauma survivors*. Toronto: University of Toronto Press.

Robbins, A.D. (1996). Sexual abuse and the epistemology of civil life. *Journal of Psychohistory*, 23(3), 307–329.

Robbins, A.D. (1997). Cults and cult abuse: Clinical realities, historical perspectives. *Journal of Psychohistory*, 24(4), 409–416.

Rogers, M.L. (1995). Factors influencing recall of childhood sexual abuse. *Journal of Traumatic Stress*, 8(4), 691–716.

Roiphe, H., and Galenson, E. (1975). Some observations on transitional object and infantile fetish. *Psychoanalytic Quarterly*, 44, 206–231.

Rorty, R. (1989). *Contingency, Irony, and Solidarity*. Cambridge: Cambridge University Press.

Rosenfeld, H. (1971). A clinical approach to the psychoanalytic theory of the life and death instincts: An investigation into the aggressive aspects of narcissism. *International Journal of Psychoanalysis*, 52(2), 174.

Rosenfeld, H. (1987). *Impasse and Interpretation: Therapeutic and anti-therapeutic factors in the psychoanalytic treatment of psychotic, borderline, and neurotic patients*. London: Tavistock.

Ross, C.A. (1989). *Multiple Personality Disorder: Diagnosis, clinical features, and treatment*. New York: Wiley.

Ross, C.A. (1991). Epidemiology of M.P.D. and dissociation. *Psychiatric Clinics of North America*, 14, 503–517.

Ross, C.A. (1992). Validity and reliability of MPD diagnoses. *California Psychologist*, September, p. 15.

Ross, C.A. (1994). *The Osiris Complex: Case studies in multiple personality disorder*. Toronto: University of Toronto Press.

Ross. C.A. (1995a). *Satanic Ritual Abuse: Principles of treatment*. Toronto: University of Toronto Press.

Ross, C.A. (1995b). The validity and reliability of dissociative identity disorder. In L. Cohen, J. Berzoff, and M. Elin (Eds.), *Dissociative Identity Disorder*. Northvale, NJ: Jason Aronson, Inc.

Ross, C.A. (1996). History, phenomenolgy, and epidemiology of dissociation. In L.K. Michelson and W.J. Ray (Eds.), *Handbook of Dissociation: Theoretical, empirical, and clinical perspectives* (pp. 3–24). New York: Plenum Press.

Ross, C.A. (1997). *Dissociative Identity Disorder: Diagnosis, clinical features, and treatment of multiple personality*. New York: John Wiley and Sons.

Van Der Kolk, B.A. (1987b). The separation cry and the trauma response: Developmental issues in the psychobiology of attachment and separation. In B.A. Van der Kolk (Ed.), *Psychological Trauma* (pp. 31–62). Washington, DC: American Psychiatric Press.

Van der Kolk, B.A. (1989). The compulsion to repeat the trauma: reenactment, revictimization, and masochism. *Psychiatric Clinics of North America*, 12(2), 389–411.

Van der Kolk, B.A. (1995). The body memory and the psychobiology of trauma. In J.L. Alpert (Ed.), *Sexual Abuse Recalled: Treating trauma in the era of the recovered memory debate* (pp. 29–60). Northvale, NJ: Jason Aronson, Inc.

Van der Kolk, B.A. (1996). The complexity of adaptation to trauma: Self-regulation, stimulus discrimination, and characterological development. In B.A. Van der Kolk, A.C. McFarlane, and L. Weisaeth (Eds.), *Traumatic Stress: The effects of overwhelming experience on mind, body, and society* (pp. 182–213). New York: Guilford.

Van der Kolk, B.A., and Fisler, R. (1995). Dissociation and the fragmentary nature of traumatic memories: Overview and exploratory study. *Journal of Traumatic Stress*, 8(4), 505–526.

Van der Kolk, B.A., McFarlane, A.C. , and Weisaeth, L. (Eds.) (1996). *Traumatic Stress: The effects of overwhelming experience on mind, body, and society*. New York: Guilford.

Van der Kolk, B.A., and Van der Hart, O. (1989). Pierre Janet and the breakdown of adaptation in psychological trauma. *American Journal of Psychiatry*, 146, 1530–1539.

Van der Kolk, B.A., and Van der Hart, O. (1991). The intrusive past: The flexibility of memory and the engraving of trauma. *American Imago*, 48, 425–454.

Van der Kolk, B.A., and Van der Hart, O. (1995). The intrusive past: The flexibility of memory and the engraving of trauma. In C. Caruth (Ed.), *Trauma: Explorations in memory* (pp. 158–182). Baltimore, MD: Johns Hopkins University Press.

Van der Kolk, B.A., Van der Hart, O., and Marmer, C. (1996). The history of trauma in psychiatry. In Van der Kolk, B.A., McFarlane, A.C., and Weisaeth, L. (Eds.) (1996), *Traumatic Stress: The effects of overwhelming experience on mind, body, and society* (pp. 47–76). New York: Guilford.

Victor, G. (1975). Grand hysteria or folie à deux? *American Journal of Psychiatry*, 132, 202.

Waites, E.A. (1993). *Trauma and Survival: Post-traumatic Stress and Dissociative Disorders in Women*. New York: W.W. Norton.

Waites, E.A. (1997). *Memory Quest: Trauma and the search for personal history*. New York: W.W. Norton.

Wakefield, H., and Underwager, R. (1993). Interview. *Paedika*, 3, pp. 2–12.

Wakefield, H., and Underwager, R. (1994). *Return of the Furies: An investigation into recovered memory therapy*. Chicago, IL: Open Court.

Waller, G., Quinton, S., and Watson, D. (1995). Dissociation and the processing of threat-related information. *Dissociation*, 8(2), 84–90.

Wang, C.T, and Daro, D. (1998). *Current Trends in Child Abuse Reporting and Fatalities: The results of the 1997 Annual Fifty State Survey*. Chicago, IL: National Center on Child Abuse Prevention Research, National Committee to Prevent Child Abuse.

Warshaw, S.C. (1992). Mutative factors in child psychoanalysis. In N.J. Skolnick and S.C. Warshaw (Eds.), *Relational Perspectives in Psychoanalysis* (pp. 147–174). Hillsdale, NJ: Analytic Press.

Waterman, J., Kelley, R., Olivieri, M.K., and McCord, J. (1993). *Beyond the Playground Walls: Sexual abuse in preschools*. New York: Guilford.

Weinberg, S.K. (1955/1976). *Incest Behavior*. New York: Citadel.

Weiner, I.B. (1962). Father-daughter incest: A clinical report. *Psychiatric Quarterly*, 36(1), 607–632.

Weiner, N., and Kurpius, S.E.R. (1995). *Shattered Innocence: A practical guide for counseling women survivors of childhood sexual abuse*. Bristol, PA: Taylor and Francis.

Weinrott, M.R., and Saylor, M. (1991). Self-report of crimes committed by sex offenders. *Journal of Interpersonal Violence*, 6(3), 286–300.

Weinstein, H.M. (1990). *Psychiatry and the CIA: Victims of Mind Control.* Washington, DC: American Psychiatric Press, Inc.

Weissman, P. (1971). The artist and his objects. *International Journal of Psychoanalysis,* 52, 401–406.

Whalen, J.E., and Nash, M.R. (1996). Hypnosis and dissociation: Theoretical, empirical and clinical perspectives. In L.K. Michelson and W.J. Ray (Eds.), *Handbook of Dissociation: Theoretical, empirical, and clinical perspectives* (pp. 191–206). New York: Plenum Press.

Whitfield, C.L. (1995). How common is traumatic forgetting? *Journal of Psychohistory,* 23(2), 119–130.

Wilber, K. (1995). *Sex, Ecology, Spirituality: The spirit of evolution.* Boston, MA: Shambhala.

Wilson, A. (1995). Mapping the mind in relational psychoanalysis: Some critiques, questions, and conjecture. *Psychoanalytic Psychology,* 12(1), 9–30.

Wilson, J.P., and Lindy, J.D. (1994). Countertransference in the treatment of posttraumatic stress disorder. In J.P. Wilson and J.D. Lindy (Eds.), *Countertransference and Posttraumatic Stress Disorder* (pp. 5–30). New York: Guilford.

Winnicott, D.W. (1953). Transitional objects and transitional phenomena. *International Journal of Psychoanalysis,* 34, 89–97.

Winnicott, D.W. (1965). *The Maturational Processes and the Facilitating Environment.* London: Hogarth.

Winnicott, D.W. (1967/1971). The location of cultural experience. In D.W. Winnicott's *Playing and Reality.* New York: Basic Books.

Winnicott, D.W. (1969). The use of an object and relating through identifications. *International Journal of Psychoanalysis,* 53, 711–716.

Winnicott, D.W. (1971). *Playing and Reality.* New York: Basic.

Wurmser, L. (1987). Shame: The veiled companion of narcissism. In D.L. Nathanson, (Ed.), *The Many Faces of Shame* (pp. 64–92). New York: Guilford.

Yochelson, S., and Samenow, S.E. (1976). *The Criminal Personality: A profile for change.* New York: Jason Aronson, Inc.

Young, W.C. (1988). Psychodynamics and dissociation: All that switches is not split. *Dissociation,* 1(1), 33–38.

Young, W.C. (1992). Treating survivors reporting ritual abuse. In D.K. Sakheim and S.E. Devine (Eds.), *Out of Darkness: Exploring satanism and ritual abuse* (pp. 249–278). New York: Lexington Books.

Young, W.C., Sachs, R.G., Braun, B.G., and Watkins, R.T. (1991). Patients reporting ritual abuse in childhood: A clinical syndrome. *International Journal of Child Abuse and Neglect,* 15, 181–189.

Youngson, S.C. (1994). Ritual abuse: The personal and professional cost for workers. In V. Sinason (Ed.), *Treating Survivors of Satanic Abuse* (pp. 292–302). New York: Routledge.

Yuille, J.C., Tymofievich, M., and Marxsen, D. (1995). The nature of allegations of child sexual abuse. In T. Ney (Ed.), *True and False Allegations of Child Abuse: Assessment and case management* (pp. 21–46). New York: Brunner/Mazel.

Zlotnick, C., Shea, M.T., Zakriski, A., Costello, E., Begin, A., Pearlstein, T., Simpsom, E. (1995). Stressors and close relationships during childhood and dissociation experiences in survivors of sexual abuse among inpatients psychiatric women. *Comparative Psychiatry,* 36, 207–212.

Index